MW00909637

Laparoscopic Hysterectomy and Pelvic Floor Reconstruction

MINIMALLY INVASIVE GYNECOLOGY SERIES

Laparoscopic Hysterectomy and Pelvic Floor Reconstruction

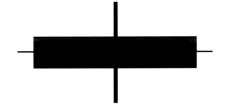

edited by

C.Y. Liu, MD
Director
Chattanooga Women's Laser Center
Chattanooga, Tennessee

b
**Blackwell
Science**

Blackwell Science

EDITORIAL OFFICES:

238 Main Street, Cambridge, Massachusetts 02142, USA

Osney Mead, Oxford OX2 0EL, England

25 John Street, London WC1N 2BL, England

23 Ainslie Place, Edinburgh EH3 6AJ, Scotland

54 University Street, Carlton, Victoria 3053, Australia

Arnette Blackwell SA, 1 rue de Lille, 75007 Paris, France

Blackwell Wissenschafts-Verlag GmbH,

   Kurfürstendamm 57, 10707 Berlin, Germany

   Feldgasse 13, A-1238 Vienna, Austria

DISTRIBUTORS:

North America

   Blackwell Science, Inc.

   238 Main Street

   Cambridge, Massachusetts 02142

   (Telephone orders: 800-215-1000 or 617-876-7000)

Australia

   Blackwell Science Pty Ltd

   54 University Street

   Carlton, Victoria 3053

   (Telephone orders: 03-347-0300)

Outside North America and Australia

   Blackwell Science, Ltd.

   c/o Marston Book Services, Ltd.

   P.O. Box 87

   Oxford OX2 0DT

   England

   (Telephone orders: 44-1865-791155)

Acquisitions: Michael Snider

Development: Debra Lance

Production: Paula Card Higginson

Manufacturing: Kathleen Grimes

Printed and bound by Walsworth Publishing Co., Marceline, MO

A catalogue record for this title is available from the Library of Congress.

I dedicate this book to my mother,
Mrs. Rei-Ru Liao,
for her loving support and selfless sacrifice
in raising her children.

Contents

Contributors

Eric J. Bieber, MD
The University of Chicago
Department of Obstetrics and
    Gynecology
The Chicago Lying-in Hospital
Chicago, Illinois

Andrew I. Brill, MD
Associate Professor
Department of Obstetrics and
    Gynecology
University of Illinois
Chicago, Illinois

Joseph R. Feste, MD
Clinical Associate Professor
Department of Obstetrics and
    Gynecology
Baylor College of Medicine
The University of Texas Health
    Science Center
Houston, Texas

Harrith M. Hasson, MD
Chairman

Department of Obstetrics and
    Gynecology
Grant Hospital
Associate Professor
Rush Medical College
Chicago, Illinois

D. Alan Johns, MD
Clinical Associate Professor
Department of Obstetrics and
    Gynecology
University of Texas Southwestern
    Medical School
Dallas, Texas
Director, GYN Laparoscopy
    Center
Harris Methodist Hospital
Forth Worth, Texas

Nicholas Kadar, MD
Director, Advanced Laparoscopic
    Surgery
Chief, Gynecologic Oncology
    and Urogynecology

The New Margaret Hague
    Women's Health Institute
Secaucus, New Jersey

Ronald L. Levine, MD,
    FACOG
Department of Obstetrics and
    Gynecology
University of Louisville School of
    Medicine
Louisville, Kentucky

C.Y. Liu, MD
Director
Chattanooga Women's Laser
    Center
Chattanooga, Tennessee

Roger C. Odell
Boulder, Colorado

David B. Redwine, MD
Director of the Endometriosis
    Institute of Oregon

St. Charles Medical Center
Bend, Oregon

Harry Reich, MD
Advanced Laparoscopic
    Consultant
Wyoming Valley Health Care
    System
Wilkes-Barre, Pennsylvania
Chief, Advanced Laparoscopic
    Surgery
New Rochelle Hospital
New Rochelle, New York

Howard C. Topel, MD
Gynecologic Endoscopist
Lutheran General Hospital
Park Ridge, Illinois

Thierry G. Vancaillie, MD
San Antonio, Texas

Foreword

Advanced laparoscopic surgery allows major intra-abdominal procedures to be performed without large abdominal incisions. Its primary benefit to the patient is a marked reduction in postoperative pain from somatic muscle and fascial disruption; this results in a rapid recovery from major surgery.

The therapeutic use of the laparoscope began in the late 1970s and early 1980s in France, Germany, and the United States as gynecologists lysed adhesions, removed ectopic pregnancies, and treated ovarian cysts and endometriosis. This laparoscopic expansion exploded in the late 1980s when first hysterectomies and then cholecystectomies were accomplished using laparoscopic techniques.

The discipline of gynecologic surgery is dynamic and continues to evolve. Modifications of standard surgical procedures done at laparotomy are usually introduced gradually into clinical practice, a process that seldom requires special training. The addition of the concept of performing these same procedures using laparoscopic visualization, usually on a video monitor, reduces the tactile abilities of the surgeon while increasing visualization by magnification. This requires additional training to integrate techniques and procedures that are new to the individual surgeon. The primary purpose of this additional surgical education is to insure safe, high-quality patient care.

As an early pioneer in advanced laparoscopic surgical procedures, it pleases me greatly to see a textbook on laparoscopic hysterectomy and repair of pelvic floor defects edited by my good friend and colleague,

C.Y. Liu. The authors of this comprehensive textbook have been very thorough, including chapters on anatomy, equipment, energy sources, hospital care, entry techniques, accepted procedures, controversial procedures, and complications. This textbook will serve as a resource to review what is available in benign gynecologic laparoscopy for removal of the uterus and repair of the pelvic floor, and the authors have admirably achieved that goal.

Harry Reich, MD

Preface

Recent advances in operative laparoscopy enable gynecologists to perform laparoscopically nearly all nonmalignant gynecological surgeries, which traditionally were performed by open laparotomy. This tremendous progress in laparoscopic surgery is due to two phenomena: 1) The increased sophistication in videography, especially the development of light-weight-chip video cameras, permits clear magnification of intraperitoneal structures. The deep pelvis and various fascial planes, which were difficult to see in traditional open laparotomy, can now be viewed in minute detail through the laparoscope. 2) Operative skills have improved. With pelvic anatomy now clear on the two-dimensional TV monitor, the gynecologist is developing increased proficiency in operating in a three-dimensional pelvis.

Many of the important operative techniques used today in laparoscopy, such as aquadissection, intraperitoneal laser and electrosurgery, and suturing with curved needles, owe their existence to our pioneers, who, despite cynicism, persevered in developing and perfecting these innovative techniques. We are indeed indebted to these individuals, for advanced laparoscopic techniques permit us to perform laparoscopically everything that heretofore required open surgery.

When I was first approached by Drs. Frank Loffer and Eric Bieber, and Mr. Michael Snider of Blackwell Science to edit a book on laparoscopic hysterectomy as part of a series on minimally invasive gynecology, I envisioned a "step-by-step how-to" text, with contributions by leading gynecologic laparoscopists on not only the various techniques of laparoscopically assisted hysterectomy but also the prevention and management of complications. In the process of our work, it became apparent that operative laparoscopy in gynecology had already entered the reparative and reconstructive fields; this holds implications for the approximately 25 to 35 percent of hysterectomies in the United States that are performed in conjunction with some type of pelvic floor defect repair. We then decided to add additional chapters to cover current practice in laparoscopic pelvic floor reconstruction. With the ever increasing aging population in our society, gynecologists will be seeing more cases of genital prolapse in their practices, which inevitably will result in an increase in pelvic floor reconstructions. It is our hope that these added chapters will serve not only as a reference but also as a stimulus for those gynecologists interested in laparoscopic pelvic floor reconstruction.

This book presents the most current techniques in laparoscopically assisted hysterectomy and pelvic floor reconstruction. In addition to detailed descriptions of the operative techniques, special emphasis is placed on anatomy critical to the surgery and on the fundamental principles of operative laparoscopy. Because the ureters are the most uncertain pelvic structures for the majority of gynecologic laparoscopists, an entire chapter is devoted to ureter identification and dissection.

My sincere appreciation is given to the contributors for sharing their insights and expertise with us. I also wish to thank my wife, Ruth, for her help in preparing the manuscript and for her endless patience and support, as well as our two delightful teenagers, Brian and Lori, for their willingness to share their dad's time with this project.

C.Y. Liu, MD

MINIMALLY INVASIVE GYNECOLOGY SERIES

Laparoscopic Hysterectomy and Pelvic Floor Reconstruction

PART ONE

Basics

1

The Role of Laparoscopic Hysterectomy in Gynecological Surgery: Present and Future

Harry Reich

W ith any new procedure, one must determine first if it can be done, then if it is safe, and, finally, if it benefits the patient. Laparoscopic hysterectomy can be done safely at great benefit to the patient. Certainly, the patient has benefited if she has less pain, spends less time in the hospital, and returns to normal daily activity sooner.

The concept of a laparoscopic approach to hysterectomy first gained national attention in 1988. Its presentation at the 1988 annual meeting of the American Association of Gynecologic Laparoscopists was reported in the January 15–31, 1989, issue of *Ob/Gyn News* (1). In that report, I noted that indications for laparoscopic hysterectomy included extensive adhesions, large fibroids, and extensive endometriosis, all of which make a vaginal approach to hysterectomy difficult. I also reported that laparoscopic hysterectomy was applicable in patients with stage 1A endometrial cancer, especially obese patients and those with risk factors for open abdominal surgery. In the discussion, Dr Steven L. Corson called my laparoscopic hysterectomy procedure "a brilliant tour de force" which he thought would have "limited appeal in the real world."

While the role of laparoscopic hysterectomy in the "present" began in 1988, I have used the laparoscope during vaginal hysterectomy since 1983 to excise endometriosis and/or ovaries and to divide adhesions and/or the upper uterine pedicles when a completely vaginal procedure was not possible (2). By 1988, I had 12 years of experience doing advanced laparoscopic surgery, including many vaginal hysterectomies during which the upper uterine blood supply was interrupted laparoscopically using bipolar desiccation (the so-called laparoscopic-assisted vaginal hysterectomy). The procedure first performed in January 1988 was significant as the uterine vessels were ligated using laparoscopic surgical techniques for the first time (3).

In 1983, I decided to use a laparoscopic approach for all benign gynecologic peritoneal cavity procedures. Since January 1988, with no selection criteria to exclude difficult cases, I have done over 300 laparoscopic hysterectomies in cases not amenable to vaginal hysterectomy. Only one case was started as a total abdominal hysterectomy, a 25-cm ovarian cystadenocarcinoma. Intraoperative conversion to laparotomy was necessary in only two instances, one because of faulty equipment in a hospital where less than 10 laparoscopic hysterectomies had been done. Complications have been published (4). Only one cuff abscess occurred, but it resulted in a laparotomy for vaginal hemorrhage at another institution.

Consumer interest in laparoscopic hysterectomy has encouraged many surgeons to attempt this procedure. As a result, initial reports indicate an alarming increase in operative complications, particularly ureteral and vascular injury. This seems to be directly related to less than adequate training, experience, equipment, and support staff. Patient safety is the surgeon's primary responsibility. Thus, "learning curve" injuries are inexcusable. Complications are an inevitable by-product of any surgical procedure, but everything possible must be done to reduce this risk.

Reduction of risk begins with a detailed patient history and comprehensive physical examination, frequently including ultrasonographic confirmation of physical findings. Medical clearance is sought on anyone with a historic or physical suggestion of possible operative compromise. Since in most cases hysterectomy is an elective procedure, the patient is extensively counseled preoperatively regarding the range of currently available options appropriate to her individual clinical situation. In 1995 it is clearly not acceptable to advocate hysterectomy without detailing the risks and benefits of other intermediary procedures.

The operative environment must be prepared for laparoscopic hysterectomy. Obviously, the surgeon requires a strong background in operative laparoscopy and sufficient training to demonstrate proficiency. Equipment must be available and functional, and a backup plan must be in place to cover any unanticipated malfunction. The competence level of the operative team is of equal importance. The anesthesiologist, nurses, and surgeon must share the same operative goals and actively cooperate to achieve them. Education of the postoperative support staff is frequently neglected.

While ureteral protection is advocated by all, how to best achieve this is hotly disputed. Isolation by ureteral dissection has been criticized as unnecessarily adding time to the procedure. We find the time well spent if ureteral risk is diminished. Our patients have not suffered adverse sequelae from this protective measure, although ureteral devascularization is a concern. As a further safeguard, a single "sentinel" stitch over the ureter placed on each side during uterine vessel ligation serves as a constant reminder of ureteral location. We have not used ureteral stents, but perform cystoscopy after indigo carmine dye injection if the ureters may be compromised. Postoperatively, early intravenous pyelogram is advised with any complaint of flank pain.

It must be emphasized that conversion to laparotomy when the surgeon becomes uncomfortable with the laparoscopic approach should never be considered a complication; rather, it is a prudent surgical decision that will profoundly decrease patient risk.

The surgical and patient advantages of laparoscopic hysterectomy are compelling and educated consumers are demanding this procedure in increasing numbers. The prudent surgeon must not place the patient at risk while mastering these techniques.

Laparoscopic hysterectomy is a substitute for abdominal hysterectomy but not for vaginal hysterectomy. Most hysterectomies currently done with an abdominal approach may be performed with laparoscopic dissection of part or all of the abdominal portion followed by vaginal removal, including fibroids weighing over 1000 gm. If the surgeon's skills are such that a vaginal hysterectomy can be done, it is always the procedure of choice. Studies comparing a laparoscopic approach to vaginal hysterectomy have never made any sense, although they are frequently cited in the literature. The indications for a laparoscopic approach to hysterectomy include a benign pathology that usually requires the selection of an abdominal approach to hysterectomy, such as extensive endometriosis, extensive adhesions, and fibroids. Stage IA endometrial cancer, stage I ovarian cancer, and stage I cervical cancer also can be done laparoscopically if the surgeon has particular expertise in the management of these cancers. If the operation is comparable, an intact abdominal wall should not compromise the end result. Laparoscopic hysterectomy is feasible in obese women, elderly women, and women with a uterus larger than 500 gm. It allows better inspection of the peritoneal cavity before and after the hysterectomy.

Presently, the concept of laparoscopic hysterectomy has resulted in a crusade by the "academic" community to discredit it, possibly to promote their academic careers. In 1994, hardly a month went by without an article discrediting laparoscopic hysterectomy. These articles suggest increased cost, increased operative time, and increased potential for complications with laparoscopic-assisted vaginal hysterectomy; they also propose that many of these operations can be done vaginally without a laparoscope. They note that the only prospective randomized clinical trial involving laparoscopic-assisted vaginal hysterectomy was their own, comparing it to standard vaginal hysterectomy; their comparison made no sense as laparoscopic hysterectomy was always meant to replace abdominal hysterectomy and should not be considered if vaginal hysterectomy is possible. Operative time for extensive pathology (adhesions and/or endometriosis) is long no matter whether open or laparoscopic surgery is done; vaginal hysterectomy for hypermenorrhea and/or prolapse takes less time.

One must realize that the concept of doing randomized control trials for laparoscopic hysterectomy is impossible. What woman would choose to have an open laparotomy incision when a laparoscopic approach is possible. To perform such a study the investigator would have to select women who have no personal regard for whether the operation results in a large incision or three puncture sites, which are often invisible.

Detractors of the laparoscopic approach to hysterectomy are quick to point out that most laparoscopic hysterectomies can be done without the laparoscope (i.e., with a vaginal approach). This is simply not true. Most hysterectomies are currently done by the abdominal approach. Even in centers with extensive experience in vaginal hysterectomy, the abdominal approach is used in over 50% of cases without prolapse (5). At the University of Vienna, from 1955 to 1985, 61% of hysterectomies were done vaginally (6078 of 9967); prolapse was present in 32% of the total number of cases.

The opponents of laparoscopic hysterectomy frequently cite increased cost when compared with a laparotomy route. Again, this is simply not true. Lawrence A. Demco, Clinical Professor at the University of Calgary (Alberta, Canada), calculated that if done by laparotomy, the cost of 682 procedures at his hospital was $1,819,280. If 90% of these operations were done laparoscopically, which was possible, the cost was $519,874. This was a savings of $1,227,475. In his calculations, Demco included the judicious use of disposable instrumentation in some cases.

Demco recently has gone further with his calculations. In both the United States and Canada, the laparoscopic approach for cholecystectomy has resulted in a 35% reduction in the hospital bill. In Canada, a laparoscopic approach to hysterectomy also resulted in a 35% savings. However, in the United States, a laparoscopic approach to hysterectomy has resulted in a 150% increase in costs. Although some of this problem is the lack of incentive hospitals have to use reusable instruments since they can charge two to three times cost for disposable instruments, many of these costs are not beyond the control of the surgeon. I suspect these costs result from inexperienced, poorly trained, and poorly educated gynecologic surgeons using a multitude of disposable instruments over a prolonged period of time. It must be emphasized that disposable trocars with retractable "safety shields" add nothing to the safety of laparoscopic procedures. In addition, laparoscopic staples for the upper uterine pedicles and the uterine vessels are never indicated; bipolar desiccation or suture ligation works better.

The most important cost expanders are disposable instruments and operative time. Expensive disposable instrument usage must be kept to a minimum as experience increases. The French word bricolage means making due with the material at hand. In the popular TV series "MacGyver," the power of bricolage is symbolized by the resourceful hero who saves the world with a minimum of raw materials and a couple of clever tricks. The gifted surgeon can take inexpensive available operating room tools and do better than others can using expensive disposable instruments. The artistic attitude that involves a healthy dose of bricolage frees the surgeon to see the possibilities of taking an ordinary instrument and making it extraordinary.

Operative time frequently is quoted at $25/min. Most operating rooms are not occupied after 3 PM; these rooms are air conditioned whether an operation takes place or not. Thus, space is not the limiting factor. Hospitals should be able to staff operating rooms around the clock with surgical technicians, licensed nurses, and nurse anesthetists working 8-hour shifts for much less than $25/min. Registered nurses cost too much for employment in the operating room; likewise, medical doctors are too expensive as surgical assistants or anesthesiologists.

Laparoscopic procedures should not deviate from the principles learned at laparotomy. Present techniques to prevent loss of pneumoperitoneum following vaginal incision while accurately delineating the junction of the cervix with the vagina will make the operation easier. Ureteral identification by dissection or illuminated stents presently serve to reduce ureteral complications.

Major questions remain to be answered in the future. Will laparoscopic surgery replace all open surgery? Will future gynecologists' experience with laparotomy be limited to cesarean sections? Should laparoscopic surgery be performed by all gynecologists? Will interdisciplinary endoscopic centers replace surgical activities in traditional specialties? Gynecologists have been replaced by general surgeons as the laparoscopic specialists in many institutions. Patient loyalty to the doctor who delivered their children has kept many women from choosing a minimally invasive procedure over laparotomy; how long will this continue? In this case I suspect that the consumer will prove to be smarter than the professor.

The indications must become better defined. The primary indication in the future for complete removal of the uterus and cervix will be extensive endometriosis, as the cervix and uterosacral ligaments are almost always involved. This will require the surgeon to have the ability to resect portions of the rectum and rectosigmoid when endometriosis has infiltrated their musculature. While hysterectomy when prolapse is present should be done with a vaginal approach, the laparoscope can be used after the uterus is out to suspend the vagina high on the uterosacral–cardinal complex and to repair paravaginal defects and the hypermobile urethra.

While the present is filled with turmoil, the future looks bright. In the future, it may be possible to selectively destroy functioning endometrium and myometrium without damaging adjacent organs. We know that the uterus can be palpated through the abdominal wall and its bottom end well visualized with a speculum. It is presently possible to image the uterus and intrauterine pathology, including fibroids and adenomyomas, but not extrauterine endometriosis. One can conceive of futuristic instrumentation that will remove this organ robotically. The key step will be a simple technique to coagulate or ligate the principal blood supply, which comes from four arteries.

The practice of laparoscopic hysterectomy is in its infancy. As younger surgeons gain more experience with this technique, the dependence on disposable stapling devices and the prolonged length of the procedure will be overcome. In addition, better training by gynecologists in urologic techniques, such as cystoscopy and insertion of ureteral stents, will serve to prevent and detect problems that may occur and possibly to help treat them. Laparoscopic and vaginal hysterectomy and endometrial ablation should make abdominal hysterectomy a rare procedure in the future.

REFERENCES

1. Reich H. Laparoscopy can be an option for some complex procedures: laparoscopic hysterectomy. Ob Gyn News 1989;24(2):1,46.
2. Reich H, McGlynn F, Sekel L. Total laparoscopic hysterectomy. Gynaecol Endoscop 1993;2:59–63.
3. Reich H, DeCaprio J, McGlynn F. Laparoscopic hysterectomy. J Gynecol Surg 1989;5:213–216.
4. Liu CY, Reich H. Complications of total laparoscopic hysterectomy in 518 cases. Gynaecol Endoscop 1994;3:203–208.
5. Gitsch G, Berger E, Tatra G. Trends in 30 years of vaginal hysterectomy. Surg Gynecol Obstet 1991;172:207–210.

2

Surgical Anatomy of the Pelvis

Nicholas Kadar

S urgical anatomy is not synonymous with topographic anatomy. Relationships between different structures are usually of interest to anatomists even if they are unimportant surgically. Moreover, topographic relationships can become altered as vital structures are dissected to expose them. A good example is provided by the relative positions of the pelvic ureter and the infundibulopelvic ligament (see below). Anatomically, the ureter lies lateral to the infundibulo-pelvic ligament on the pelvic side wall. During pelvic surgery, however, the ureter is always displaced medially from its natural position when the broad ligament is opened, and the anatomic relationship is lost.

There are also significant differences between the anatomy that can be seen through the laparoscope and that seen through an abdominal incision. The laparoscope affords a much more panoramic and anatomic view of the pelvis than is obtained at laparotomy. The uterus does not need to be displaced to the same extent to expose the pelvic structures, and a number of landmarks can be identified that are simply not visible at laparotomy (Fig 2.1).

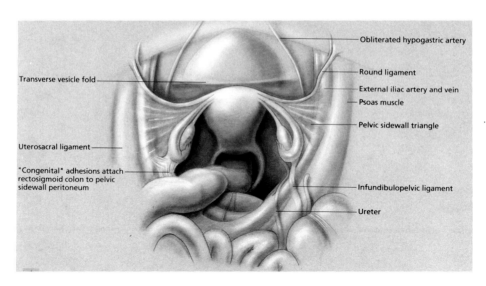

Obliterated hypogastric artery

Round ligament

External iliac artery and vein

Psoas muscle

Pelvic sidewall triangle

Transverse vesicle fold

Uterosacral ligament

"Congenital" adhesions attach rectosigmoid colon to pelvic sidewall peritoneum

Infundibulopelvic ligament

Ureter

FIGURE 2.1

Panoramic laparoscopic view of the pelvis. (Reproduced by permission from Kadar N. Atlas of laparoscopic pelvic surgery. Boston: Blackwell Science, 1995:51.)

LAPAROSCOPIC PELVIC LANDMARKS

The Anterior Pelvis

A prominent peritoneal fold is always visible in front of the uterus. It is the *transverse vesical fold*, which lies over the dome of the bladder and runs horizontally across the anterior pelvis from one superior public ramus to the other, crossing each obliterated hypogastric artery approximately an inch above where they are crossed by the round ligaments.

Prominent peritoneal folds can also be seen hanging from the anterior abdominal wall on either side of the midline. These are the *obliterated hypogastric arteries* or *lateral umbilical ligaments*. They are a continuation of the hypogastric arteries that cross the pelvic brim and run underneath the peritoneum to the umbilicus. The round ligaments cross in front of the obliterated hypogastric arteries approximately an inch medial to the internal inguinal ring. The *inferior epigastric artery*, the last

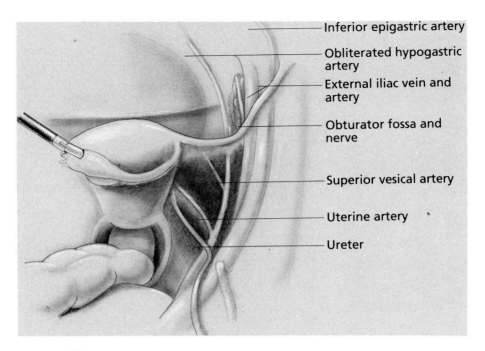

Inferior epigastric artery

Obliterated hypogastric artery

External iliac vein and artery

Obturator fossa and nerve

Superior vesical artery

Uterine artery

Ureter

FIGURE 2.2

Anatomy of the obliterated hypogastric artery and its relationships. (Reproduced by permission from Kadar N. Atlas of laparoscopic pelvic surgery. Boston: Blackwell Science, 1995:51.)

branch of the external iliac artery just proximal to the inguinal ligament, winds around the medial edge of the internal inguinal ring and also can be seen running upward and medially underneath the parietal peritoneum to enter the rectus sheath at the arcuate line. It lies lateral to the obliterated hypogastric artery on the anterior abdominal wall (Fig 2.1).

As the obliterated hypogastric arteries are traced retrogradely into the depths of the pelvis, their first important anatomic relationship is with the external iliac vessels, which lie just lateral to the obliterated hypogastric artery at the level of the pelvic inlet attached to the medial border of the psoas muscle (Fig 2.2). The external iliac vein lies directly below the external iliac artery, but the relationship becomes more inferomedial closer to the inguinal ligament. The obturator fossa is situated immediately below and somewhat lateral to the vein, a relationship that is difficult to understand if one envisages the pelvic side wall as following a vertical course below the psoas muscle. In fact, the obturator fossa is a shallow lateral recess that lies below the iliac vessels and resembles the hollow of a cupped hand. The hollow of the recess is filled out, as it were, with fatty nodal tissue through which the obturator nerve runs, and below it the obturator artery and vein, and which lies just lateral to the obliterated hypogastric artery. Slightly more proximally, the obliterated hypogastric artery meets the uterine to form the internal iliac or hypogastric artery proper (Fig 2.2). Strictly speaking, the superior vesical artery is the next branch encountered as the obliterated artery is traced proximally to the origin of the uterine artery. However, this branch of the obliterated hypogastric artery arises from its posterolateral aspect, and runs forward and upward to the bladder in the paravesical space. It cannot be seen before the paravesical space is opened medial to the obliterated hypogastric artery, the anterior surface of the uterine artery and cardinal ligament is dissected free of areolar tissue, and the obliterated hypogastric artery is deviated laterally. Throughout its pelvic course the medial border of the obliterated hypogastric artery is related to the lateral wall of the dome of the bladder, but an avascular plane can be developed between these structures (see below).

The Pelvic Side Wall

If the pelvic side wall peritoneum is put on tension by deviating the uterus to the contralateral side, the triangle of the pelvic side wall will become evident. The base of this triangle is formed by the round ligament, the lateral border by the external iliac artery, the medial border by the infundibulopelvic ligament, and the apex where the infundibulopelvic ligament crosses the common iliac artery. On the left side, so-called congenital adhesions attach the rectosigmoid to the pelvic side wall peritoneum at or just above the pelvic brim, and these usually cover the apex of the pelvic triangle (Fig 2.1). The retroperitoneum is entered laparoscopically by incising the peritoneum of the pelvic triangle, rather than by dividing the round ligament, to preserve the natural tension in the tissues and to allow blunt dissection of the retroperitoneal tissue planes (see below).

The Posterior Pelvis

If the uterus is anteverted to expose the posterior pelvis and cul-de-sac, the uterosacral ligaments will be seen easily at the base of the broad ligament on either side of the rectum running forward and slightly upward to insert into the back of the cervix (Fig 2.1). The right ureter can usually be seen through the medial leaf of the broad ligament above the uterosacral ligament and higher up, below the inferior border of the ovarian fossa, but the left ureter often is not visible. The right ureter usually can be traced along the pelvic side wall, where it lies just above the internal iliac artery, to the pelvic inlet, where it lies medial to the infundibulopelvic ligament and crosses the external iliac artery to enter the pelvis (Plate 1). The left ureter cannot be seen at the pelvic brim because it is covered by the sigmoid mesentery. If the sigmoid colon is retracted toward the left, the right common iliac artery can often be seen under the posterior parietal peritoneum, especially in thin patients, and the promontory of the sacrum can be "felt" with a probe.

PELVIC BLOOD VESSELS

The common iliac artery ends at the pelvic inlet in front of the sacroiliac joint by dividing into the external and internal iliac arteries. The *external iliac artery* runs along the pelvic brim attached to the medial border of the psoas muscle and passes under the inguinal ligament to become the femoral artery. It gives off only two branches close to the inguinal ligament: the inferior epigastric and the deep circumflex iliac arteries, both of which supply the anterior abdominal wall (Fig 2.2).

The anatomy of the *internal iliac artery* is complicated, but its surgical anatomy is straightforward because most of its branches are not encountered during pelvic surgery and dissection of the retroperitoneum. The internal iliac artery descends quite steeply into the pelvis along the pelvic side walls to where the uterine arteries are given off at the lateral attachments of the cardinal ligaments (Plate 1). They then sweep sharply upward on either side of the bladder as the obliterated hypogastric arteries (which give off the superior vesicle arteries to the bladder), cross

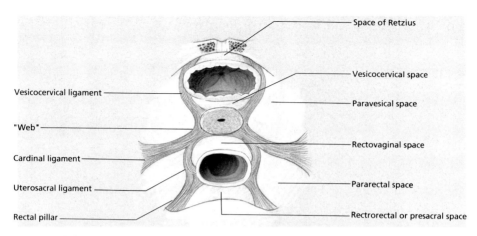

Space of Retzius

Vesicocervical space

Vesicocervical ligament

Paravesical space

"Web"

Cardinal ligament

Rectovaginal space

Uterosacral ligament

Pararectal space

Rectal pillar

Rectrorectal or presacral space

FIGURE 2.3

Tissue "spaces" and "ligaments" of the pelvic retroperitoneum. (Reproduced by permission from Kadar N. Atlas of laparoscopic pelvic surgery. Boston: Blackwell Science, 1995:54.)

the superior pubic rami, and run beneath the peritoneum of the anterior abdominal wall to the umbilicus.

RETROPERITONEAL SPACES OF THE PELVIS

The peritoneum is draped like a cape over the pelvic organs. Between the peritoneum above, the pelvic diaphragm below, and the pelvic side wall laterally, loosely packed fibrous tissue and fat surround the pelvic organs, allowing them to distend as necessary. Condensations of this retroperitoneal tissue, referred to as ligaments, divide the subperitoneal space into compartments or "spaces" (Fig 2.3). These spaces or tissue planes are only potential spaces, and a cavity or "hole" is not encountered within the tissues on opening the peritoneum. However, by blunt dissection in the correct plane, large, avascular, cavernous areas can be exposed within the retroperitoneal tissues. It is impossible to exaggerate the importance to laparoscopic surgery of knowing the anatomy of these tissue planes and how to open them correctly.

It is helpful to divide the pelvic space into two groups, the central and lateral spaces, and to think of the central spaces as those through which specific operations are carried out and of the lateral spaces as those through which vital retroperitoneal structures are identified.

The central spaces, which will be familiar to gynecologists, lie along an imaginary line connecting the symphysis pubis and the sacrum. The Retzius' space lies between the back of the pubic bone and the bladder, and must be opened to perform retropubic operations for incontinence, such as a colposuspension. The vesicovaginal space lies between the bladder and vagina and is opened during anterior colporrhaphy, whereas the rectovaginal space lies between the rectum and vagina and is opened during posterior colporrhaphy. The retrorectal or presacral space is opened during presacral neurectomy (as well as to resect the rectosigmoid colon). As these spaces are familiar to all gynecologists, they will not be discussed further.

The lateral spaces separate the pelvic viscera from the pelvic side wall; they are the paravesical and pararectal spaces. Although the paravesical space must be opened during pelvic lymphadenectomy and the pararectal space must be opened during sacrospinous ligament fixation, these spaces are usually developed to identify vital structures in the retroperitoneum, such as the ureter, uterine artery, and hypogastric artery.

THE LATERAL PELVIC SPACES

Anatomy

If an imaginary line is drawn vertically along the medial leaf of the broad ligament all the way down to the levator floor, the line will successively cross the infundibulopelvic ligament, the ureter, the uterosacral ligament and, finally, the rectal pillars. The *pararectal spaces* that are used for pelvic surgery are bounded laterally by the internal iliac arteries and medially by the ureters, and below them by the uterosacral ligaments and rectal pillars (Fig 2.4). The cardinal ligament forms the distal boundary of the pararectal space and separates it from the paravesical space, which lies in front of the pararectal space. The uterine

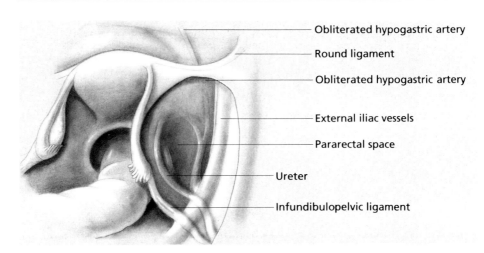

Obliterated hypogastric artery

Round ligament

Obliterated hypogastric artery

External iliac vessels

Pararectal space

Ureter

Infundibulopelvic ligament

FIGURE 2.4

Anatomy of the (lateral) pararectal space. (Reproduced by permission from Kadar N. Atlas of laparoscopic pelvic surgery. Boston: Blackwell Science, 1995:54.)

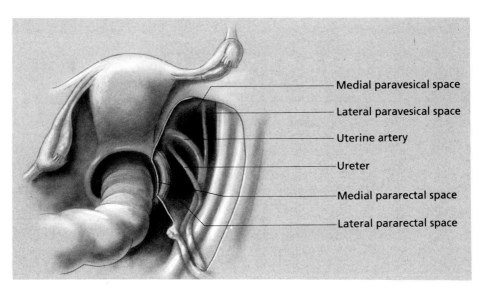

Medial paravesical space

Lateral paravesical space

Uterine artery

Ureter

Medial pararectal space

Lateral pararectal space

FIGURE 2.5

The medial and lateral pararectal and paravesical spaces. (Reproduced by permission from Kadar N. Atlas of laparoscopic pelvic surgery. Boston: Blackwell Science, 1995:55.)

artery runs on top of the cardinal ligament from the hypogastric artery to the uterus (Fig 2.5).

Prior to the development of these tissue spaces, the ureters lie just above the internal iliac arteries on the pelvic side wall (Plate 1); after the pararectal spaces are developed, the ureters mark their medial borders. Therefore, the development of the pararectal spaces always provides a reliable method of identifying the pelvic course of the ureters, as well as exposing the iliac vessels, the uterine artery, and the cardinal and uterosacral ligaments.

Another avascular tissue plane can be developed medial to each ureter and uterosacral ligament, but lateral to the peritoneum, which forms the medial portion of the broad ligament and its inferior extension into the cul-de-sac. It is this plane that the general surgeon calls the pararectal space and that he or she uses for carrying out either anterior or abdominoperineal resection of the rectum for carcinoma. In other words, our colleagues in general surgery never work laterally to the ureter when performing their pelvic operations, but leave it attached in its natural position on the lateral pelvic side wall. This medial pararectal space is also developed by pelvic surgeons during radical hysterectomy to mobilize the ureter and prepare the uterosacral ligament for division, but only after the pararectal space proper has been opened (Fig 2.6).

The *paravesical spaces* are bordered distally or caudad by the pubic bone, proximally or cephalad by the cardinal ligament, medially by the obliterated umbilical artery, laterally by the external iliac vessels and obturator fossa, and inferiorly by the levator floor. Just as a space can be developed medial to the ureter and uterosacral ligament, each being part of the same pararectal space, so a tissue plane can be developed on both sides of the obliterated hypogastric artery (Fig 2.7). The lateral portion of the space lies between the artery and pelvic side wall and is the paravesical space proper, but a plane can also be developed medially, between the obliterated hypogastric artery and the bladder. It is usually

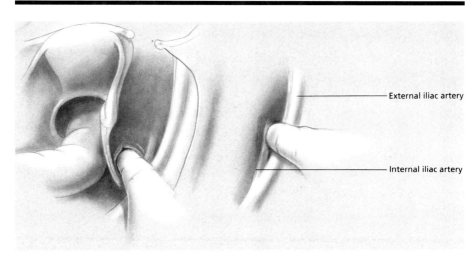

External iliac artery

Internal iliac artery

FIGURE 2.6

The pararectal space is opened at laparotomy by blunt finger dissection medial
to the internal iliac artery in the direction of the patient's contralateral femoral
head. (Reproduced by permission from Kadar N. Atlas of laparoscopic pelvic
surgery. Boston: Blackwell Science, 1995:55.)

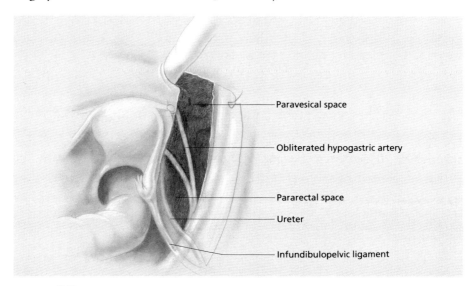

Paravesical space

Obliterated hypogastric artery

Pararectal space

Ureter

Infundibulopelvic ligament

FIGURE 2.7

The paravesical space is opened by blunt finger dissection in a medial direction
against the obliterated hypogastric artery. (Reproduced by permission from
Kadar N. Atlas of laparoscopic pelvic surgery. Boston: Blackwell Science,
1995:56.)

advantageous to open up the tissue space on both sides of the obliterated hypogastric artery to obtain good exposure of the anterior aspect of the cardinal ligament and of the uterine artery above it.

Development of the Lateral Pelvic Spaces

If the dissection is carried out in the correct plane, the lateral pelvic spaces are easily developed at laparotomy by blunt finger dissection. The round ligament is first divided and the leaves of the broad ligament separated by blunt dissection. The bifurcation of the common iliac artery is then identified by palpation, and the index finger of the dissecting hand is placed just medial to the internal iliac artery. Traction is then applied with the finger to the tissues medial to the internal iliac artery in the direction of the patient's contralateral femoral head. A bloodless space will start to develop; as it does, the plane of dissection should follow the curve of the pelvis, which, with the patient in Trendelenburg's position, is at first downward and forward, but then curves in an upward direction. The surgeon will find the ureter lying against the dissecting finger, still attached to the medial leaf of the broad ligament, for the ureter marks the medial border of the pararectal space and its lateral border is formed by the internal iliac artery.

Once the pararectal space has been opened, the index finger of the dissecting hand is placed against the medial edge of the external iliac artery and the artery is followed distally as far as the pubic ramus. On reaching the pubic bone, the direction of the dissection changes abruptly through a 90-degree angle and is again directed medially toward the patient's contralateral femoral head. A large bloodless plane (the paravesical space) will again open up and a cord-like structure will be found in the dissecting finger; this is the lateral umbilical ligament or obliterated hypogastric artery.

The pararectal spaces cannot be easily developed laparoscopically in the same way as during laparotomy. First, with each successive step of the dissection (i.e., division of the round ligament, opening of the broad ligament, separation of the areolar tissues), the tissues become progressively more slack and blunt dissection increasingly more difficult, and usually eventually impossible because the tissues cannot be maintained on tension. Second, the internal iliac artery is buried in areolar tissues and cannot be visualized at first after the broad ligament is opened, and obviously cannot be palpated. The precise level (in a cephalad–caudad sense) at which to begin dissection of the pararectal space, therefore, is not immediately apparent, and troublesome bleeding can occur if the dissection is begun over the cardinal ligament rather than proximal to it or too close to the sacrum. To overcome these difficulties, the technique of entering the retroperitoneum must be altered and a different strategy used to find the pararectal space.

LAPAROSCOPIC DISSECTION OF THE LATERAL PELVIC SPACES

Opening the Pelvic Peritoneum

To enter the retroperitoneum, the pelvic side wall triangle (see above) is first delineated by deviating the uterus to the contralateral side. The peritoneum in the middle of the triangle is then desiccated with bipolar forceps and incised with dissecting scissors; the incision is extended to the round ligament, but the round ligament is *not* divided (Fig 2.8A). The broad ligament is opened by bluntly separating the extraperitoneal areolar tissues, usually with the tip of the suction irrigator. Even tiny vessels are coagulated because the slightest amount of bleeding can stain the extraperitoneal areolar tissues and obscure view of the underlying structures (Fig 2.8B).

On the left side, so-called congenital adhesions attach the rectosigmoid to the peritoneum laterally, at or just above the pelvic brim. These usually cover the apex of the pelvic triangle. The dissection on the left side is begun by separating these adhesions from the underlying peritoneum, and the pelvic side wall triangle is opened at or near its apex (Fig 2.8C). The peritoneal incision is then carried distally to the round ligament, which is again not divided at this time.

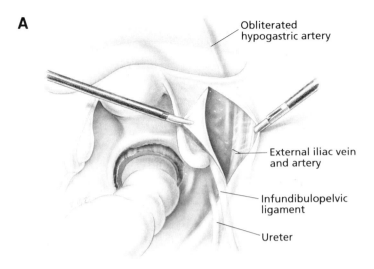

A

Obliterated
hypogastric artery

External iliac vein
and artery

Infundibulopelvic
ligament

Ureter

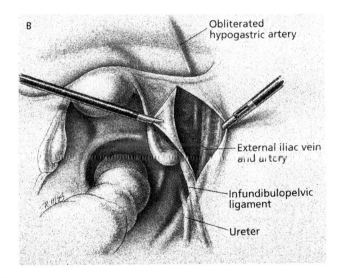

B

Obliterated
hypogastric artery

External iliac vein
and artery

Infundibulopelvic
ligament

Ureter

FIGURE 2.8

The pelvic side wall triangles are opened to gain access to the retroperitoneum.
(Reproduced by permission from Kadar N. Atlas of laparoscopic pelvic surgery.
Boston: Blackwell Science, 1995:57–58.)

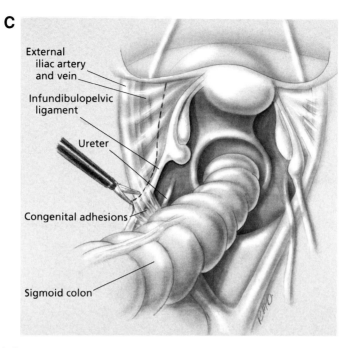

C

External iliac artery and vein

Infundibulopelvic ligament

Ureter

Congenital adhesions

Sigmoid colon

FIGURE 2.8

Continued

Dissection of the Retroperitoneum

The secret to dissecting the retroperitoneum laparoscopically is not to compartmentalize one's thinking about the dissection. The laparoscopic surgeon is already at a disadvantage by not being able to palpate retroperitoneal structures; this is compounded by the absence of reliable retroperitoneal landmarks below the peritoneum. If a technique for pelvic dissection is to be reproducible, however, reliable laparoscopic landmarks must be found, even if it means making use of structures not in the immediate vicinity of where the surgeon wants to be.

The most useful and reliable laparoscopic landmark in the pelvis is the obliterated hypogastric artery, and from its anatomy, it is easy to understand why it truly serves as a laparoscopic gateway to the retroperitoneum.

First, the obliterated hypogastric artery is nearly always identifiable, even in obese patients. In perhaps 10% of women it is not very

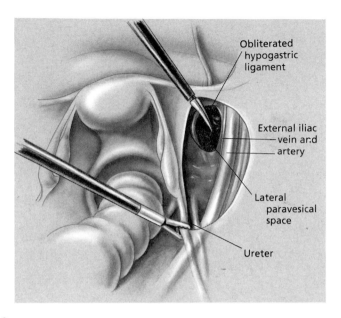

Obliterated
hypogastric
ligament

External iliac
vein and
artery

Lateral
paravesical
space

Ureter

FIGURE 2.9

The paravesical space is opened on either side of the obliterated hypogastric artery. (Reproduced by permission from Kadar N. Atlas of laparoscopic pelvic surgery. Boston: Blackwell Science, 1995:58.)

prominent, but it can still be located by making use of its anatomic relationship to the round ligament and transverse vesical fold (Figs 2.1 and 2.2).

Second, because the obliterated hypogastric artery lies within the paravesical space, it can be easily dissected free of the surrounding tissues by developing the avascular tissue planes on either side of the artery using blunt dissection (Fig 2.9).

Third, the obliterated hypogastric artery is a continuation of the hypogastric artery after it gives off the uterine artery. Therefore, once it is dissected free of the surrounding tissues in the paravesical space, the artery can be traced retrogradely to identify the uterine arteries at their origin from the internal iliac artery (Fig 2.2).

Fourth, the uterine arteries run along the cardinal ligament, which separates the paravesical and pararectal spaces. Once the uterine arteries have been identified, the paravesical spaces developed, and the anterior aspect of the cardinal ligament delineated, the dissection of the pararectal

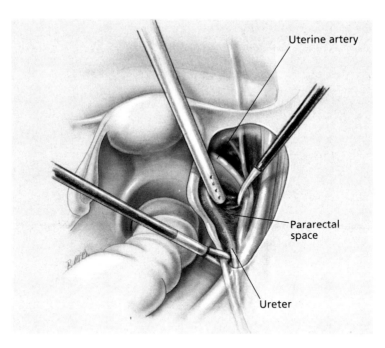

Uterine artery

Pararectal
space

Ureter

FIGURE 2.10

The obliterated hypogastric artery is traced retrogradely to the origin of the uterine artery, and the pararectal space opened by blunt dissection proximal and medial to the uterine artery. (Reproduced by permission from Kadar N. Atlas of laparoscopic pelvic surgery. Boston: Blackwell Science, 1995:59.)

space can be started accurately, proximal and medial to the cardinal ligament and uterine artery (Fig 2.10).

Thus, although at laparotomy the pararectal space can be, and usually is, opened without developing the paravesical space, at laparoscopy it is helpful to open the paravesical space first because this allows the pararectal space to be opened much more accurately with less risk of annoying, diffuse bleeding.

The pararectal space can be opened without developing the paravesical space by using the ureter, which forms the medial border of the pararectal space, as the landmark. As we shall discuss more fully in the next chapter, the key to this approach is to identify the ureter at the pelvic brim, where it lies medial to the infundibulopelvic ligament, and then trace it into the pelvis along the broad ligament, gently pushing it

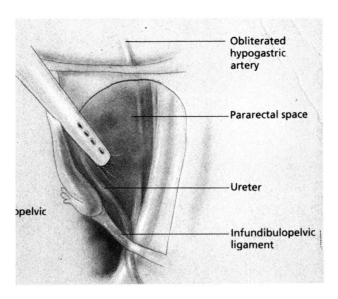

Obliterated
hypogastric
artery

Pararectal space

Ureter

ɔpelvic

Infundibulopelvic
ligament

FIGURE 2.11

The pararectal space often can be opened without developing the paravesical space, by identifying the ureter at the pelvic brim and then bluntly dissecting against the ureter in a medial direction. (Reproduced by permission from Kadar N. Atlas of laparoscopic pelvic surgery. Boston: Blackwell Science, 1995:60.)

medially with the tip of the suction irrigator or a probe, whereupon the pararectal space will open lateral to the ureter (Fig 2.11). This approach works best in thin patients who have little extraperitoneal fat, in whom the ureter and internal iliac artery are easily identified.

This is the overall strategy we use to dissect the lateral pelvic spaces laparoscopically, regardless of whether we are performing a simple laparoscopic hysterectomy or a pelvic lymphadenectomy, or are resecting a symptomatic, enlarged residual ovary (Plate 2).

The anatomy of ureter and laparoscopic identification and dissection will be discussed in detail in Chapter 8, "Identification and Dissection of the Pelvic Ureter."

SUGGESTED READING

Kadar N. Atlas of laparoscopic pelvic surgery. Boston: Blackwell Science, 1994.

3

Operating Room Setup; Instrumentation, Video, and Photographic Equipment; and Cost Analysis of Laparoscopic Hysterectomies

Ronald L. Levine

OPERATING ROOM SETUP

The operating room setup for performing a laparoscopic-assisted vaginal hysterectomy (LAVH) is no different than any other type of laparoscopic surgery, the only major difference being the type of stirrups that are used. The operating room, however, should be large enough to accommodate the equipment that is necessary. An operating room of less than 24 × 20 feet quickly becomes crowded with modern-day anesthesia equipment, a video cart, equipment carts, a back table, various electrical generators for coagulation, possibly laser equipment, and the diverse personnel needed for efficient surgery. Although Allen stirrups (Allen Medical Systems, Cleveland, OH) have been suggested for all operative laparoscopy, their use in LAVH is almost mandatory as they allow excellent surgical exposure. This type of stirrup is easily converted to different positions to facilitate the vaginal approach when needed.

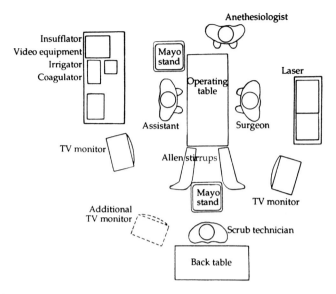

FIGURE 3.1

Suggested operating room layout. One Mayo stand is over the patient's right shoulder, opposite the surgeon, and the other is either between the patient's legs or over the left leg. The two suspended monitors are shown; however, if only one is available it may be placed near the patient's right foot.

Laparoscopic-assisted vaginal hysterectomy is best performed with the team approach. An assistant who is trained in operative laparoscopy greatly decreases the operating time and should not be regarded as a luxury, but rather an absolute necessity. Indeed, it has been shown that if the same assistant and team are used, the complication rate is reduced (1). The rest of the surgical team includes the scrub technician or nurse, who also should have training in operative laparoscopy, and at least one (but preferably two) circulating nurses, one of whom should have training in troubleshooting video problems as well as in the use of a laser in case it is needed. The recent addition of a biotechnician to the team has been found to be quite useful. This individual primarily is responsible for the care and adjustment of the technical electrical equipment, including not only the video, but also the electrical generators and irrigation and suction equipment.

The configuration of the operating room many vary according to the individual surgeon. My operating room setup is shown in Figure 3.1.

OR Setup; Instrumentation, Video, and Photographic Equipment   29

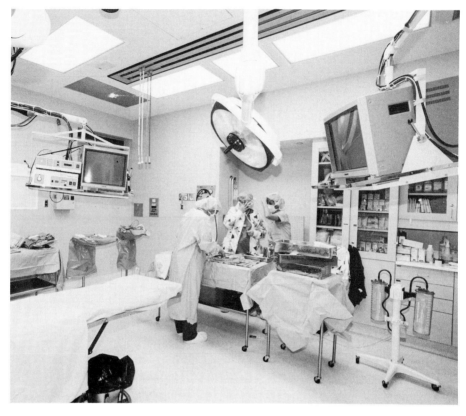

FIGURE 3.2

The monitors are on spring-loaded ceiling mounts that can be brought to a comfortable height and swung into a correct position. The left platform also holds the light source and video controls.

Two Mayo stands are used, one between the patient's legs and the other at the top of the table over the right shoulder of the patient. A large cart with the insufflator, irrigator, and various coagulating devices is placed opposite the surgeon so that he or she may view the dials with ease and so that the insufflating tubes and electrical wires have a short space to traverse. If needed, the laser may be easily swung into position from behind the surgeon. The video monitors should be effortlessly seen by the entire team without having to turn around or shift positions. Our monitors are suspended from the ceiling and

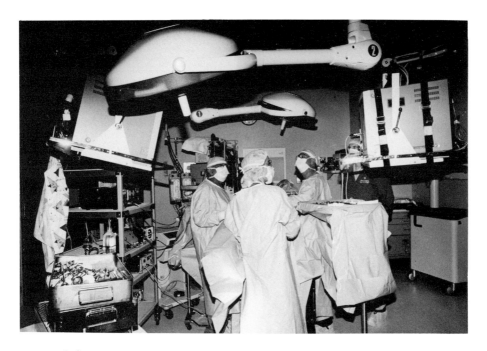

FIGURE 3.3

The surgeon and assistant are on each side of the patient and each easily sees a monitor. The scrub technician is between the patient's legs. Note that the biotechnician is also in the room.

are movable to almost any position (Fig 3.2). They are on spring-loaded mounts, allowing the monitors to be pulled down to almost any height that is comfortable for the surgeon. There are different types of ceiling mounts; they are designed to not only hold the video monitor, but to have built-in gas outlets, electrical outlets, and other adjustable platforms to hold additional equipment. One such system that can be designed to different specifications is the AMSCO Orbiter Equipment Management System (AMSCO/American Sterilizer Co, Erie, PA). If only one monitor is available it is best placed directly in front of the patient's feet. At the beginning of the procedure the scrub technician may be between the Mayo stand and the patient so that he or she may assist in moving the uterus with a manipulator if needed (Fig 3.3).

OPERATING EQUIPMENT

Trocars and Sleeves

The debate concerning reusable versus disposable trocars has produced significant controversy, with proponents of both sides equally adamant regarding advantages and disadvantages of each system. Disposable trocars have the definite superiority of a sharp tip, which many believe to offer a safety factor (2). Reusable trocars satisfy the outcry for cost containment and, because they are metal, they play a safety role in reducing the danger of capacitive coupling when using unipolar electrical energy (3). We usually begin with a 10-mm disposable port in the umbilicus for the laparoscope. Next, a midline 10-mm port is placed in the suprapubic area with step-down capability; therefore, this frequently is a disposable sleeve. The lateral ports then depend on the instruments that are anticipated to be used. If a stapler–cutter is to be used, then the lateral ports must be 12 mm; however, if the technique of desiccation and coaptation of vessels with electrosurgery is preferred, then the lateral ports should be 5-mm reusable trocars and sleeves. It is my belief that limiting the number of ports contributes nothing to the procedure and may indeed handicap the operator unnecessarily. We use a minimum of three ports, but usually four ports, including the laparoscope, are used.

Insufflator

All operative laparoscopy demands the use of a high–flow insufflator, but it is never more important than while performing an LAVH. During an LAVH there are not only frequent instrument changes, but also the likelihood of gas loss through a subsequent colpotomy incision. Loss of the pneumoperitoneum from opening into the vagina requires rates of gas flow from 6 to 10 L/min to maintain vision until the area can be resealed completely. The insufflator must operate directly from the gas cylinder supply rather than supply from an internal tank. Most current insufflators have the ability to preselect the pressure, and the machine gives some type of audible alarm if the pressure exceeds that preselection.

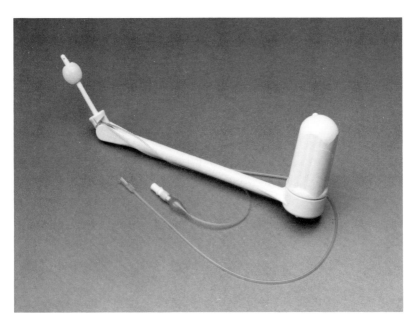

FIGURE 3.4

The Clearview Uterine Manipulator (Clinical Innovations, Murray, UT) is a completely disposable uterine manipulater. The instrument is held in place by the inflatable balloon tip. If the handle is rotated without moving the base the tip end will move in an arc, producing anteflexion. Rotating the handle will cause the uterus to rotate, with the cervix acting as the fulcrum of that rotation. A great deal of controlled motion is available with this instrument, even in a fairly large uterus.

Uterine Manipulator

A good uterine manipulator may expedite LAVH surgery. There are several types of uterine manipulators, and individual surgeons may have their personal preferences. We often use a Hodgson–type manipulator, which not only allows maximum mobilization of the uterus laterally, but also produces maximum anterior and posterior positioning. The tip is disposable and is supplied in different sizes. The Clearview Uterine Manipulator (Clinical Innovations, Murray, UT) is a completely disposable type of this instrument that is still cost effective. The second channel in the tip permits easy chromopertubation (Fig 3.4). The Valchetz instrument (Conkin Surgical Instruments, Toronto, Ontario, Canada) produces a similar result and is completely reusable.

Graspers

There are multiple types of graspers. Essentially they may be divided into traumatic and atraumatic graspers, both of which may be used in an LAVH procedure. The most commonly used instruments are 5 mm in size, however, 3-mm or as large as 10-mm graspers also may be found. Minimally, we use at least two 5-mm atraumatic graspers and two of the traumatic type. The handles vary from those that are essentially spring-loaded to the traditional box lock type of instrument. Some graspers are multipronged, such as the Hasson Bulldog-type traumatic grasper (Weck-Linvat, Chicago, IL). Traumatic-type graspers should only be used on tissue that will not bleed or that will be removed from the body.

Scissors

Sharp scissors are mandatory. We prefer those with a disposable tip and a reusable handle (Marlow Surgical Technologies, Willoughby, OH). This type of scissors is always sharp and is more cost effective than the usual disposable scissors; it also eliminates the need of having several pairs of reusable scissors of various types as the tips may be in a variety of configurations, from straight to curved Metzenbaum type (Fig 3.5).

Electrosurgical Instruments

Both unipolar and bipolar capability is important. Pedicles may be coagulated (desiccate) and vessels coapted with bipolar instrumentation, while unipolar current may be used for cutting and fulguration of small, oozing capillaries. The unipolar needle may be used to incise the cul-de-sac and may eliminate the expense of lasers. For bipolar control, Kleppinger-type forceps usually are used. The advantage of the bipolar energy system is the avoidance of a return electrode, thus increasing the margin of safety. It is important for the operating surgeon to be familiar with the appropriate energy application and to know about various complications associated with electrical energy sources. When using reusable and even disposable electrical instruments one must be aware of possible breaks in insulation. Monitoring systems, such as Electroshield (Electroscope Inc, Boulder, CO), can prevent burn injury

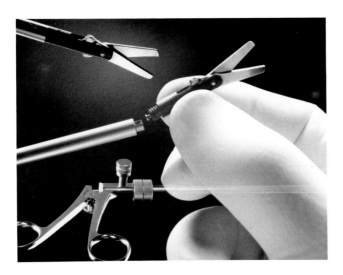

Nu-Tip (Marlow Surgical Technologies, Willoughby, OH) are laparoscopic scissors that have a reusable handle and disposable tips that are easily changed and are in different configurations, such as curved or straight. This has the advantage that sharp scissors are always available at less cost than disposable scissors.

from faulty insulation or from capacitive coupling by detecting the electrical leak.

Suction Irrigation

There are many types of suction irrigators; however, whichever system is used, it must be capable of producing enough hydraulic pressure to allow aquadissection of tissue planes. Aquadissection may be useful in dissecting the bladder from the cervix and also for dissecting the peritoneum in ureteral identification and isolation. Several varieties and lengths of instruments are helpful, so a system that can accommodate the changing of the suction–irrigation probe is desirable. We have used the Nezhat-Dorsey Hydro-Dissection System (American Hydro-Surgical Instruments, Delray Beach, FL) because multiple probes are easily put in place (Fig 3.6). The suction should be directly to wall suction, with a large reservoir to eliminate the frequent changing of the canister as large amounts of fluid may be used for irrigation. One system that may be

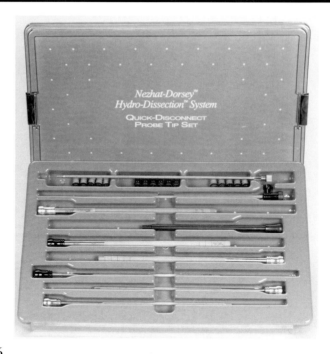

FIGURE 3.6

The multiple probes of the Nezhat-Dorsey Hydro-Dissection System (American Hydro-Surgical Instruments, Delray Beach, FL) permit easy changing of the probes to different tips and even different diameter sizes and lengths.

used, although it is difficult to clean, is the Arthroscopic Suction System (O.R. Surgical Co. Inc., Greensboro, NC), which has a suction bottle that holds 6.5 gallons and is on a special rolling stand to facilitate emptying.

Suturing

Some surgeons prefer the use of sutures to control major vessels during LAVH surgery, and certainly the ability to suture expands the operative horizon for the operative endoscopist. There are several types of needle holders; some have the traditional jaws of the regular needle holders, while others have variations of the Cook needle holder (Fig 3.7). The needle holder is usually a 5-mm instrument; it is necessary to have a needle holder and either another needle holder or a closed jaw grasper

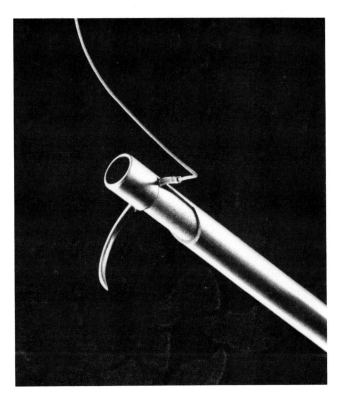

FIGURE **3.7**

The Cook Needle Holder (Cook Ob/Gyn, Bloomington, IN) has a special tip that holds the needle very firmly in position and resists twisting.

in order to suture. Although there are several methods for intracorporeal knot tying, it is very simple to use the extracorporeal technique as developed by Clarke (4) and the Clarke Knot Pusher (Marlow Surgical Technologies, Willoughby, OH) to slide a normal square knot into place (Fig 3.8).

VIDEO AND CAMERA EQUIPMENT

The use of video is no longer a separate portion of endoscopic surgery. Procedures such as LAVH are much too long and complicated to be amenable to the "one-eyed surgical approach." The surgeon must understand the basic principles of video endoscopy and be able to apply

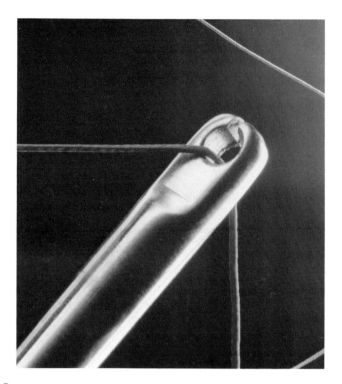

FIGURE 3.8

The Clarke Knot Pusher (Marlow Surgical Technologies), is used to push in a knot that has been tied in an extracorporeal fashion. Using this type of instrument facilitates the use of suturing if needed during LAVH.

these principles in the setup and use of the camera and video endoscopy. Today very few surgeons use a 35-mm camera in the usual laparoscopic surgical case to document their procedures. Modern chip cameras with the use of a video tape recorder and video printers have supplanted still photographic cameras. Modern video systems use the latest technology, such as digital signal processing, high-resolution cameras, and monitors coupled with light-weight camera heads and simple controls.

Basic Video Literacy

Too frequently the surgeon has little or no knowledge of the basics of modern endoscopic cameras. The following is a review of elementary

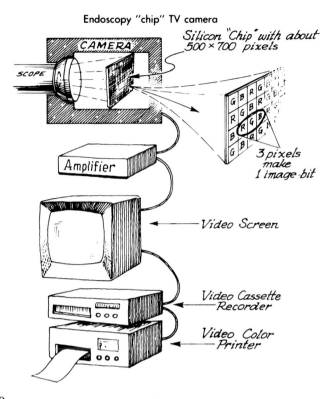

Endoscopy "chip" TV camera

FIGURE 3.9

The current video configuration consists of the scope, the camera with one or three chips, an amplifier, the video screen, and the optional video cassette recorder and video color printer. (Reproduced by permission from Hulka J. Light: Optics and television. In: Hulka J, Reich H, eds. Textbook of laparoscopy. Philadelphia; WB Saunders, 1994;21.)

terms and the mechanisms that are available in the video equipment necessary for LAVH. The most usual configuration of the modern "chip" camera system consists of the laparoscope, the camera (with one or three "chips"), the amplifier, and the monitor or screen; a video cassette recorder and a video color printer are optional (Fig 3.9). The laparoscope is attached to the camera by a coupling device that may have a beam splitter to allow the surgeon to look directly through the scope at any time without removing the coupler. This option is becoming less and less desirable as surgeons have become increasingly more adept at operating directly from the screen and as equipment allows better definition. Beam splitters supply 80% to 90% of available light to the monitor and only 10% to 20% directly to the surgeon's eye.

The camera contains the "chip," which is more accurately described as the charged coupling device or solid state sensor. The sensor has an array of light-sensitive silicon photosites known as picture elements or pixels. The charged coupling device is made up of 500 to more than 700 pixels. The camera's optics focus an image on the sensor's pixel array, and they in turn emit electrons in response to the light falling on them. The subsequent electronic emission produced is then processed by the camera controller (amplifier) to form a video signal. Each pixel can sense either red, green, or blue light in a single chip camera, and three pixels make up one image bit. In a camera with three imaging chips, each chip is responsible for picking up one of the primary colors by use of a prism or filter. The picture formed is scanned electronically, generating a signal frequency, which is transmitted to a monitor. In the monitor the signal is converted back to light.

Most surgeons have the greatest interest in resolution, as this is the index of the sharpness of the image. During endoscopic surgery it is important to be able to detect various tissue planes, and sometimes even slight nuances in sharpness and color may be important in discerning a vital structure from nonvital tissue. At times pixel numbers are used in place of the term "resolution" as the more pixels that are present, the more detail is able to be seen. The length of a diagonal line drawn between opposite corners of the photosensitive area of the sensor (chip) is referred to as the sensors's size. A sensor that measures 1/2 inch is therefore referred to as a 1/2-inch sensor. The 1/2- and 2/3-inch sensors currently are the most predominant in use.

As a rule, the larger the chip, the more pixels and the better the resolution. Usually, however, resolution is described in terms of how many separate vertical lines can be distinguished from a standard resolution chart. A modern one-chip camera may discern up to 450 lines of resolution and a three-chip camera may discern up to 600 lines. However, the limiting factor may be the ability of the monitor to discern the resolution.

Most of the good monitors available today can actually out-perform the cameras. When choosing a monitor, it should have at least a 20-inch

TABLE 3.1

Integrated systems

CAMERA		MONITOR		SYSTEM
300 lines	plus	600 lines	equal	300 lines
600 lines	plus	600 lines	equal	600 lines
300 lines	plus	600 lines	plus recorder	420 lines equal 300 lines

SOURCE: Adapted from Whelan JM, Jackson DW. Videoarthroscopy: review and state of the art. Arthroscopy 1992;8:311–319.

screen, which seems to be standard in most operating rooms, and the monitor should have a higher resolution capability than the camera. Currently monitors have resolutions of 650 to 750 lines. If the monitor has less resolution, then there will be an appreciable loss of the quality of the video image. Whelan and Jackson (5) refer to this as the "weak link theory," and have stated that no integrated system is stronger than its weakest link. If the camera has only 300 lines of resolution and the monitor has 600 lines, the system will produce only 300 lines of resolution (Table 3.1).

When choosing equipment, rather then evaluating numbers from technical data, the best method is to compare cameras and monitors in the operating room side by side and to pick the one that has the best image. Our preference is a three-chip camera and two high-resolution monitors that are suspended from the ceiling, as described above. The greatest problem with some three-chip cameras lies in the fact that the cable may be thicker and heavier than the cable for a one-chip camera.

There have been some recent technologic developments in video cameras, such as the distal chip endoscope and the three-dimensional video camera. The distal chip endoscope consists of a tube and a handle with the charged coupling device in the distal end of the tube, thus eliminating the glass rod lenses in the laparoscope. Hasson and Lynch (6) and Pelosi et al (7) have described the use of this type of camera with great success and have stated in their reports that this array allows a one-chip camera to outperform a three-chip camera. The three-dimensional camera has been adapted to laparoscopy by the American Surgical Technologies Corporation (Chelmsford, MA). The 3DSCOPE system incorporates a SteroLaparoscope which produces two images that are merged by a digital imaging process. The surgeon must wear special polarized glasses that provide the merged image to the eyes. This type of video may enhance the surgeon's ability in procedures such as laparoscopic suturing.

THE ECONOMICS OF LAPAROSCOPIC HYSTERECTOMY

The first report addressing the economics of laparoscopic surgery was published in 1985 (8) and demonstrated a 49% decrease in cost by using operative laparoscopy. The savings were possible mainly because of decreased postoperative stay, which accounted for 57% of the total savings. It is interesting that at that time there were no disposable instruments on the market; therefore, the savings that were noted in the operating room costs of an average of $53 per case meant that essentially there was no difference between the costs of the procedures. Since that time many investigators have referred to savings in hospital costs when expressing the advantages of operative laparoscopy. These savings apparently are from the decreased postoperative stay in the hospital following LAVH as opposed to abdominal hysterectomy.

However, other reports (9) have shown that despite a statistically significant decrease in postoperative hospital days after LAVH versus total abdominal hysterectomy, there was no difference in total hospital costs. Although in Howard and Sanchez's study some of the cost in the LAVH group was related to longer operative time, 60% of the additional operating room cost was attributed to equipment and supplies despite the fact that no disposable instruments or endoscopic stapler–cutters were used. In a study comparing LAVH to both vaginal and abdominal hysterectomy, Bronitsky et al (10) reported that the cost of performing an LAVH fell between the costs of the other procedures. Summitt et al (11) noted that the LAVH procedure as compared with a routine vaginal hysterectomy was almost double the cost; however, most proponents of

TABLE 3.2

Cost of TAH versus LAVH

	TAH	LAVH
LOS (days)	4.56	2.67
Total cost of OR	$3,668.75	$6,585.14
OR	$3,226.51	$4,943.80
OR drugs	141.00	330.71
OR supplies	301.24	1,310.63
Inpt room	$1,507.98	$819.33
Inpt drugs	703.26	268.94
Inpt Supplies	60.94	6.87
Laboratory	633.85	432.49
Medical imaging	331.64	0.00
Cardiology	17.10	17.10
Res therapy	50.21	0.00
Total	$6,973.73	$8,129.87

Abbreviations: TAH, total abdominal hysterectomy; LOS, length of hospital stay; OR, operating room; Inpt, inpatient, Res, respiratory therapy.

LAVH have indicated, and I agree, that LAVH is not a substitute for vaginal hysterectomy. A recent editorial criticized LAVH (12). The editorial, however, was more critical of the use of disposable instruments rather than the efficacy of LAVH.

In a comparison study in our series, the length of stay for LAVH was significantly less than that of total abdominal hysterectomy (2.67 days *v* 4.56 days) so that all charges for inpatient stay was 53.3% less for LAVH (Table 3.2). As noted in some reports, the final hospital costs were significantly higher for LAVH because the operating room charges were 55.7% higher (13). The increased cost in our study was directly related to disposable equipment and the length of the procedure. The markup charges to the patient for the disposable products vary from 1.9 to 3 times, depending on the price of the instruments (14).

OR Setup; Instrumentation, Video, and Photographic Equipment   43

The hospital charges, however, are not the only standard that one must address when evaluating the LAVH in reference to an economic advantage or an unnecessary exercise in surgical ability. One must assess the time of return to full activity to appropriately evaluate the true benefit of LAVH. Almost all authors of published data on LAVH have noted a return to the workplace at least 2 to 3 weeks earlier than patients undergoing total abdominal hysterectomy (15). To understand the overall impact on economics we must consider the return to normal activity; how that relates to economics must be carefully evaluated. Using data available from 1982 and 1988, a conservative estimate of cost savings by LAVH may be appreciated (16).

There are approximately 22 million women in the work force. The average wage for a manufacturing female employee is approximately $8/hr. For an 8-hour day, including sick time, the wage would be $64. Also consider that for each hour worked a female manufacturing employee contributes $23 of productivity to her company. In an 8-hour day the female employee produces $184 worth of product. The financial loss, therefore, of a single lost day equals $248. To put this into a national prospective, each day of return to work equals approximately $55 million in revenue per day. The return to full activity within 2 to 3 weeks therefore not only contributes multiple millions of dollars to our economy, but also positively contributes to the patient's mental well-being.

CONCLUSION

Laparoscopic-assisted vaginal hysterectomy has been shown to be advantageous both for the patient and for the economy when compared with total abdominal hysterectomy. The surgical and video equipment are essentially the same for all operative laparoscopy, and therefore should be available for all operative laparoscopists. If the patients are properly selected and the proper instruments used, the economic advantage to the third-party carriers and ultimately to the overall economy of our country will be substantial.

REFERENCES

1. See WA, Cooper CS, Fischer RJ. Predictors of laparoscopic complications after formal training in laparoscopic surgery. JAMA 1993;270:268–292.
2. Corson SL, Batzer FR, Gocial B, Maislin JF. Measurement of the force necessary for laparoscopic trocar entry. J Reprod Med 1989;34:282–284.
3. Levy BS, Soderstrom RM, Dail DH. Bowel injuries during laparoscopy. Gross anatomy and histology. J Reprod Med 1985;30:168–172.
4. Clarke HC. Laparoscopy: new instruments for suturing and ligation. Fertil Steril 1972;23:274–277.
5. Whelan JM, Jackson DW. Videoarthroscopy: review and state of the art. Arthroscopy 1992;8:311–319.
6. Hasson Hm, Lynch MA. The DistalCAM video camera. J Am Assoc Gynecol Laparosc 1993;1:58–59.
7. Pelosi MA, Kadar N, Pelosi MA III. The electronic video operative laparoscope. J Am Assoc Gynecol Laparosc 1993;1:54–57.
8. Levine RL. Economic impact of pelviscopic surgery. J Reprod Med 1985;30:655–659.
9. Howard FM, Sanchez R. A comparison of laparoscopically assisted vaginal hysterectomy and abdominal hysterectomy. J Gynecol Surg 1993;9:83–90.
10. Bronitsky C, Payne RJ, Stucky S, Wilkins D. A comparison of laparoscopically assisted vaginal hysterectomy vs traditional total abdominal hysterectomies. J Gynecol Surg 1993;9:219–225.
11. Summitt RL, Stoval TG, Lipscomb GH, et al. Randomized comparison of laparoscopy assisted vaginal hysterectomy with standard vaginal hysterectomy in an outpatient setting. Obstet Gynecol 1992;80:895–901.
12. Baggish MS. The most expensive hysterectomy. J Gynecol Surg 1992;8:57–58. Editorial.
13. Boike GM, Elfstrand EP, DelPriore G, et al. Laparoscopically assisted vaginal hysterectomy in a university hospital: report of 82 cases and comparison with abdominal and vaginal hysterectomy. Am J Obstet Gynecol 1993;168:1690–1698.
14. Levine RL. Disposable instruments for operative laparoscopy. Infertil Reprod Med Clin North Am 1993;4:221–231.

15. Carter JE, Ryoo J, Katz A. Laparoscopic-assisted vaginal hysterectomy: a case control comparative study with total abdominal hysterectomy. J Am Assoc Gynecol Laparosc 1994;1:116–121.
16. Handbook of Labor Statistics. US Department of Labor and Bureau of Labor Statistics. Bulletin 2340, August 1989.

4

Physics and Clinical Application of Electrosurgery

Roger C. Odell

E lectrosurgical energy is without question the most common form of energy used today for dissection and control of bleeding in open laparotomy and closed laparoscopy surgical procedures. Unfortunately, poor training and misconceptions about electrosurgical energy still exist, and with the latest flurry of shifting to the laparoscopy surgical technique comes quite an array of marketing and sales presentations, which further complicate a topic that was not clearly understood from the start.

The use of electrosurgical energy in laparoscopy dates back to the mid-1960s when gynecologists began operative laparoscopy through a channel within the laparoscopy (single puncture technique), which was later expanded to multiple trocar techniques. During the course of performing such procedures with electrosurgery, a number of misadventures occurred (1). The investigations of these incidents led to a number of concerns regarding the use of electrosurgery, specifically monopolar electrosurgery. For the most part monopolar electrosurgery has been discouraged in laparoscopic procedures for the past two decades. One of the objectives of this chapter is to revisit these complications so that the physics of how they occurred can be explained. Methods of minimizing these hazards as well as options available for eliminating them from being repeated in the future are also discussed.

Another key objective will be to cover the biophysics of electrosurgical energy for dissection, fulguration, and desiccation in laparoscopy to optimize efficiency in delivering this form of energy.

HISTORY

The use of high-frequency electrical energy for surgical application dates back nearly a century. Electrosurgery is the generation and delivery of radiofrequency current between an active electrode and a dispersive electrode to elevate the tissue temperature for the purpose of cutting, fulguration, and desiccation. In contrast to electrocautery, the electric current actually passes through the tissue. Harvey W. Cushing, MD, with the assistance of William T. Bovie, PhD, was the first surgeon to document the principals in depth regarding both the art as well as the biophysics pertaining to electrosurgery in 1927. These early documents detailed his appreciation of Dr Bovie's device and his encouragement regarding the versatility of this energy source. By no means did Drs Cushing and Bovie invent electrosurgery. As early as the late 1800s (D'Arsonval and Jacques, 1891), the Germans and French documented the biophysics of electrosurgical currents. A general surgeon, William L. Clark in Philadelphia in 1910, documented the removal of large benign and malignant growths of the skin, head, neck, and breast with electrosurgery. It was truly Cushing's and Bovie's documentation that changed the course of neurosurgery and other surgeons' views of the potential uses of electrosurgical energy.

TEMPERATURE AND TISSUE

Energy cannot be created or destroyed; rather, it is converted to another form of energy. In the case of electrosurgical energy, it is converted into heat at the active electrode target site for the purpose of vaporizing (cutting) and coagulation. Reviewing Table 4.1, which presents temperature increases and tissue conditions will help later with the

TABLE 4.1

The tissue effects of heating categorized by the immediate visible effect (surgeon feedback mechanism), the delayed effects, and the mechanism of injury

	TEMPERATURE (°C)					
	34–44	44–50	50–80	80–100	100–200	>200
Effect						
Visible	None	None	Blanching	Shrinkage	Steam "popcorn"	Carbonization cratering
Delayed	Edema	Necrosis	Sloughing	Sloughing	Ulceration	Larger crater
Mechanism	Vasodilatation, inflammation	Disruption of cell metabolism	Collagen denaturation	Desiccation	Vaporization	Combustion of tissue hydrocarbons

The delayed manifestation of full-thickness intestinal injury from thermal energy is the major cause of morbidity and mortality after accidental bowel burn.

discussion specific to electrosurgical modality and effect to the tissue or vessel.

HOW ELECTRICAL ENERGY AFFECTS TISSUE TEMPERATURE

The three electrical properties that cause increases in temperature are current (I), voltage (V), and resistance (impedance) (R). To help overcome the electrical energy terms and meanings, a direct analogy to water of a hydraulic energy source will be made. The water tower depicted in Figure 4.1 presents a hydraulic energy source for the purpose of performing work. Figure 4.2 shows an equivalent electrosurgical tower with the electrical terms, current, voltage, and resistance inserted. This direct relationship is important in overcoming the mystique of electrosurgical unit modalities. The reader should note that both the water tower and electrosurgical energy sources are operating with thousands of feet of head pressure and thousands of volts. This is key to recognize in performing surgery. Water towers typically are approximately 1000 feet above the ground, and all household appliances operate off 120-V, 60-cycle power sources. To be effective in all aspects of electrosurgery, the

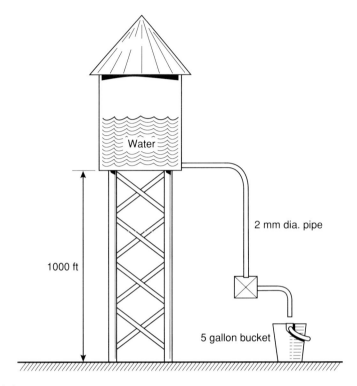

Water

2 mm dia. pipe

1000 ft

5 gallon bucket

FIGURE 4.1

Hydraulic energy source. (Electroscope, Inc, Boulder, CO.)

voltage developed in electrosurgical generators range from 1000 to 10,000 V peak to peak.

Ohms Law

The formula $I = V/R$ shows the relationship between the properties of electrosurgical energy.

Power Formula

The formula W (energy in wattage) $= V \times I$ is valuable in understanding how the three modality's waveforms (cut, fulgurate, and desiccate) are compared in performing various therapeutic effects. The voltage-current ratio of the electrosurgical waveforms is primarily responsible for the effects to tissue observed when time and electrode size are kept equal.

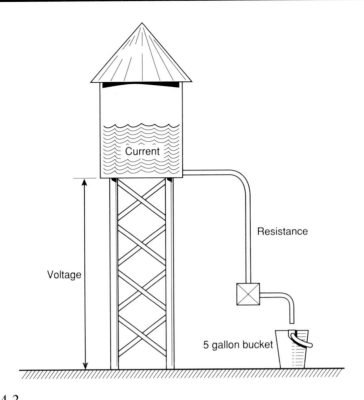

FIGURE 4.2

Electrical equivalents terms. (Electroscope, Inc, Boulder, CO.)

Power Density

Power density, which equals (current density)^2 × resistivity, is the relationship between the size of the active electrode in contact with the tissue and the effect on the tissue at a given energy setting. In noncontact modalities (i.e., cutting and fulguration), this would be equivalent to the sparking area between the active electrode and the tissue. Only when desiccating is the exact surface area of the electrode in contact with the tissue of importance when calculating power density. During fulguration and cutting, the electrode is not in contact; therefore, the power density can only be approximated. It is also worth noting that in cutting and fulguration the electrode is in motion. Therefore, the exact energy in joules is difficult to calculate at a given point.

  In general, the larger the electrode surface area, the lower the power density, and the smaller the electrode surface area, the higher the power density.

Time

The time element is the primary component for the depth and degree of tissue necrosis at a given energy setting. Many other components contribute to this discussion, but time is important, as will be demonstrated below.

CUT, FULGURATE, AND DESICCATE

Cutting, fulguration, and desiccation are the three distinct therapeutic effects to tissue for which electrosurgical energy has been used. Unfortunately, most electrosurgical units are labeled simply by two modes: "cut" and "coag." These terms do not help in the present confusion pertaining to the optimal use of this form of energy. In open procedures the optimal use often was overcome by vantage point: the surgeon has direct access to the surgical site. This is not the case in laparoscopy, which may result in far more severe complications.

Cut

Cutting is performed using a high–current, low–voltage (continuous) waveform, which rapidly elevates the tissue's temperature (100 + °C), producing vaporization or division of tissue with the least effect of lateral thermal spread (coagulation) to the walls of the incision (Fig 4.3). During optimal electrosurgical cutting, the current travels through a steam bubble between the active electrode and the tissue. Therefore, it is important to recognize that electrosurgical cutting is a *noncontact* means of dissection. The electrode floats through the tissue and there is very little tactile response transmitted to the surgeon's hand as the electrode is moved through the tissue.

The velocity of the electrode, as well as the waveform, significantly effect the depth and width of necrosis of the incision. Depths of necrosis of less than 100 μm are attainable with electrosurgical energy during dissection. The continuous waveform is analogous to the garden

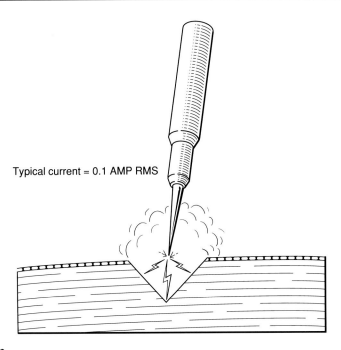

Typical current = 0.1 AMP RMS

FIGURE **4.3**

Electrosurgical cutting, with the electrode not in contact with the tissue. (Electroscope, Inc, Boulder, CO.)

valve shown in Figure 4.1, which has a constant, even flow of water delivery. Due to the constant flow of current and the lowest possible voltage to dissect, the width and depth of necrosis to the walls of the incision are minimal. Therefore, the high current–low voltage ratio within the waveform reduces the necrosis or coagulation. If the electrode is allowed to remain stationary or is slowed, the maximum temperature attained is increased, as is the depth and width of thermal damage to the walls of the incision.

Blend 1, 2, and 3: With modification of the ratio of the cutting waveform (i.e., changing the current, voltage percentage) by interrupting the current and increasing the voltage, the waveform becomes noncontinuous, with a train of packets of energy consisting of higher voltage and reduced current per time. Total energy remains the same and the voltage–current ratio is modified to increase hemostasis (coagulation) during dissection with electrosurgical current (Fig 4.4). This is

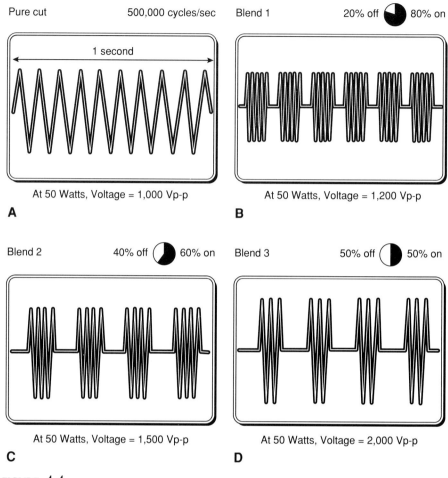

Pure cut   500,000 cycles/sec   Blend 1   20% off   80% on

1 second

At 50 Watts, Voltage = 1,000 Vp-p

A

At 50 Watts, Voltage = 1,200 Vp-p

B

Blend 2   40% off   60% on   Blend 3   50% off   50% on

At 50 Watts, Voltage = 1,500 Vp-p

C

At 50 Watts, Voltage = 2,000 Vp-p

D

FIGURE 4.4

(A) Cut waveform, (B) blend 1, (C) blend 2, and (D) blend 3. (Electroscope, Inc, Boulder, CO.)

analogous to the garden valve pulsing the water, with an increase in height of the water tower to make up for the reduction of the total water allowed to flow. Once again, total energy is not changed.

The blend waveforms will require a longer period of time to dissect the same length of incision compared with the cutting waveform. This is due to the interrupted delivery of current at the same power setting. With this increased time comes an increase in thermal spread from the voltage component of the blend waveform. This increased thermal spread improves coagulation of small vessels while dissecting. When needed, these blend modes can be a very valuable option in controlling bleeding when it is encountered while dissecting. On the other hand, if used and not needed, the increase in the width of necrosis may result in a higher risk of postoperative infection as a direct result of the increased amount of tissue necrosis. Surgical planes are destroyed; in addition, the amount of the smoke plume will be increased during laparoscopy when high-blend or coagulation modes are used to dissect. While dissecting, blend 1 has slightly increased hemostasis, blend 2 has moderate hemostasis, and blend 3 has marked increased hemostasis.

When dissecting tissue with a cut or blended mode, the electrosurgical unit should be activated first before the electrode touches the tissue. A feathering or light stroking, similar to when painting with a two-bristle paintbrush for touch-up or fine detail work, needs to be simulated. This will allow for the maximum power density as the electrode approaches the tissue just before contact, and will help initialize vaporization or dissection of tissue. In theory, and in practice with optimum technique and control setting, the force required to dissect tissue would be 0 gm of pressure between the electrode and the tissue. The key is to not let the electrode drag through the tissue.

Fulgurate

Fulguration is performed using a high-voltage, low-current, noncontinuous waveform (highly damped) designed to coagulate by means of spraying long electrical sparks outo the tissue (Fig 4.5). The most common use of fulguration is when coagulation is needed in an area that is oozing, such as in a capillary or arteriole bed, where a discrete bleeder (vessel) cannot be identified. The benefit of fulguration is its ability to arrest ooze emanating from a large area in a most efficient manner. Cardiovascular, urologic, and general surgeons have relied on fulguration for their most demanding applications (i.e., hepatic resections, bleeding from a bladder tumor resection, and surface bleeding on the heart). A very superficial eschar is produced with fulguration; therefore, the depth of necrosis is minimal as a result of the defocusing of the power density. By drawing the electrode away from the tissue, the power density goes down (defocusing the energy/current). A great deal of the energy is

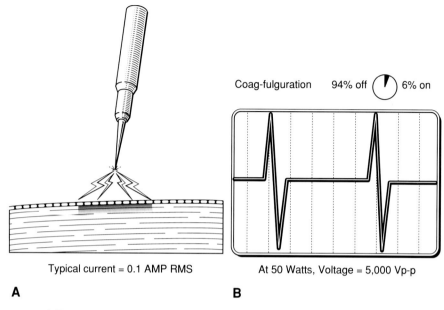

Coag-fulguration   94% off   6% on

Typical current = 0.1 AMP RMS

At 50 Watts, Voltage = 5,000 Vp-p

A   B

FIGURE 4.5

Fulguration, with the electrode not in contact with the tissue. (Electroscope, Inc, Boulder, CO.)

dissipated in heating the air between the electrode and the tissue that the current must pass through.

Fulguration and electrosurgical cutting are noncontact modalities. Fulguration can be initiated in two ways. First, by slowly approaching the tissue until a spark jumps to the tissue, whereby a raining effect of sparks will be maintained until the electrode is withdrawn or the tissue is carbonized to the point at which the sparks cease. Second, bouncing the electrode off the tissue will result in a raining effect of sparks to the tissue; this can be done without taking the pains of approaching the tissue without touching it until a spark jumps.

Electrosurgical fulguration is the most effective means of arresting the capillary/oozing type of bleeding. Time and energy are wasted by sparking to blood or saline, it is key to evacuate fluid from the target site before fulguration. Evacuation or diluting the field with nonisotonic solutions, such as glycerine or sterile distilled water, can be used to clarify the target site and optimally deliver the current to stop the bleeding most efficiently.

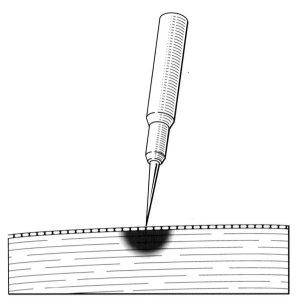

Typical current = 0.5 AMP RMS

FIGURE 4.6

Desiccation, with the electrode in contact with the tissue (no sparking between the electrode and tissue). (Electroscope, Inc, Boulder, CO.)

The depth of necrosis ranges from 0.5 mm to 1–2 mm, depending on how long the surgeon sparks to the target site. The key is to stop the sparks as soon as the bleeding stops. The energy setting on the electrosurgical unit and length of time the sparks are applied are key in controlling the depth of necrosis.

Desiccation

Any waveform will desiccate when the electrode comes in contact with the tissue (Fig 4.6). Regardless of the current-voltage ratio, with the electrode in contact with the tissue the magnitude of energy in wattage is of the greatest importance. Desiccation is another form of coagulation. Most surgeons do not make a distinction between fulguration and desiccation, but refer to both as coagulation. The application of electrosurgical current by means of direct contact with the tissue will now result in all the energy set on the electrosurgical unit being con- verted into heat within the tissue. In contrast, during both cutting and fulguration, a significant amount of the electrical energy, converted to heat, goes into the atmosphere (air/CO_2) between the electrode and the tissue. Therefore, with contact coagulation/desiccation, the increased energy delivered into the tissue results in deep necrosis (as deep as it is wide), as observed on the surface where the electrode makes contact (see Fig 4.6).

The most common application of desiccation is when a discrete bleeder is encountered; first, a hemostat is introduced to occlude the vessel by mechanical pressure, then the electrosurgical energy is applied to the body of the hemostat. This causes the current to pass through the hemostat into the tissue grasped by the jaws and back to the patient return electrode. The coaptation of vessels was documented (2) to produce a collagen chain reaction resulting in a fibrous bonding of the dehydrated denatured cells of the endothelium. Because the electrode is in good electrical contact with the tissue, the voltage-current ratio is not nearly as important as it is during cutting and fulguration, although in practical application, when desiccation is desired, the cut/blend waveforms are superior for this application to the fulguration waveform. The primary reason is that the fulguration waveform will tend to spark through the coagulated tissue, resulting in voids in the bonding to the end of the vessel. In addition, when sparks occur at the electrode in contact or near contact, the metal in the electrode will heat up rapidly, causing the tissue to adhere to the electrode when it is pulled away from the target site. Bleeding will continue each time the eschar is pulled off due to adhesion from heat within the electrode.

In bipolar desiccation, the waveform plays a far more important role. Today, for the most part, the manufacturers have incorporated a continuous low-voltage, high-current waveform in the bipolar output to maximize the effect on desiccation. In older models, the manufacturers allowed the surgeon to select either a continuous cut, blend, or fulguration waveform when bipolar desiccation was needed. The lack of understanding on the physician's part, in combination with the literature not being clear on the effect to tissue when bipolar desiccation was performed with these waveforms, led to a number of associated, documented (3) problems. Therefore, at this time the generally accepted waveform for bipolar desiccation is a continuous low-voltage, high-current waveform. I recommend that a newer-model electrosurgical unit with a dedicated, continuous bipolar waveform be used when bipolar desiccation is critical. If you must use an electrosurgical unit that allows you to select both cut/blend and fulguration bipolar currents, start with the pure cut (continuous) waveform for the best results.

When performing desiccation, patience is the key to good results. Typically the power density is much lower when desiccating. The physical size of the active electrodes is therefore larger. The larger electrode or contact area to tissue will require longer activation times to attain the desired therapeutic effect. Higher energy introduced to speed up the desiccation process will most likely be counterproductive. Higher energy levels will increase the temperature to the tissue adjacent to the electrode(s), potentially forcing the current to spark through the necrosis and resulting in fulguration rather than desiccation. Fulguration or sparking immediately stops the deep heating process and starts to carbonize the surface of the tissue only. Therefore, when sparking is observed in the process of desiccating, stop and reduce the power or pulse the current by turning the electrosurgical unit on and off to overcome this natural tendency of the electrosurgical energy. Sparking is not needed or wanted when desiccating; it causes the tissue to stick, creates uneven necrosis, and may compromise the intent to coapt the vessel. When desiccating, an ammeter (Model EPM or EM-2; Electroscope, Inc, Boulder, CO) may be used to help the surgeon determine end point coagulation/desiccation and to confirm the visual effect. The ammeter shows current flow with both visual and audible indicators, and when the electrolytic fluid within the tissue is dehydrated the meter will show no current flow. Total or complete desiccation occurs after dehydration has taken place.

INHERENT RISKS

Since the inception of monopolar electrosurgery for open surgery, there have been three potential sites for patient burns due to the presence of electrosurgical current, one intended and two unintended. The intended site is at the active electrode where the unit is used to cut, fulgurate, or desiccate the tissue during surgery. Due to its design, the active electrode has a high-power density to heat tissue rapidly. If not kept in control at all times, this electrode can burn the patient severely. Therefore, I strongly recommend that when not in use, the active electrode be stored in an insulated holster or tray.

There are two unintended sites, the first of which is a consequence of current division. Current division to alternate ground points to the patient can only occur on ground-referenced electrosurgical units. The second unintended site is due to a faulty condition at the site of the patient return electrode (i.e., partial detachment or manufacturing defect) that forces the current returning to the electrosurgical unit via a high-current density, which may cause the patient to be burned. The patient return electrode (ground plate) has a surface area of approximately 20 in^2 or larger when properly applied. Therefore, under normal conditions, very little temperature increases occur at this site. Both of these potential burn sites have been overcome by improved design within the newer electrosurgical units developed in the last two decades. These safety circuits or features are available on most units sold within the past 10 years. The two major advancements in overcoming these risks are isolated electrosurgical outputs and contact quality monitors.

Isolated Electrosurgical Outputs

Isolated electrosurgical units were introduced in the early 1970s. The primary purpose of their introduction was the prevention of alternate ground site burns due to current division. Today, because of the introduction of isolated electrosurgical units, the number of alternate site burns as a direct result of current division is essentially zero. A small percentage of hospitals use ground-referenced electrosurgical units. Therefore, it would be wise to qualify the type of electrosurgical unit in service at your hospital with regard to the type of output.

Contact Quality Monitors

Contact quality monitoring circuits were introduced in the early 1980s. The primary purpose of their introduction was to prevent burns at the patient return electrode site. The contact quality monitor incorporates a dual-section patient return electrode and circuit for the purpose of evaluating the total impedance of the patient return electrode during surgery. Therefore, during the course of surgery, if the patient return electrode becomes compromised, the contact quality circuit inhibits the electrosurgical generator's output based on the dual-section patient return electrode and circuit combination. This feature has also essentially eliminated the unintended patient burns that appear at the site of the patient return electrode.

The two technologic advancements described above have truly reduced the potential for patient burns that can occur while performing classical open electrosurgical procedures. These features are now found on electrosurgical units provided by major manufacturers, such as Aspen Labs (Englewood, CO), Birtcher Medical Systems (Irvine, CA), and Valleylab (Boulder, CO).

LAPAROSCOPIC ISSUES

As reported previously, the use of electrosurgery (4) in laparoscopic surgery has been limited to bipolar primarily for the past two decades. With the recent flurry of change in laparoscopic techniques for general, urologic, and other surgical disciplines, a major question of contention has developed: Can monopolar electrosurgical energy be used safely in laparoscopy as compared with other energy sources? The purpose of this section is to address the real issues pertaining to the safe use of electrosurgery in laparoscopy in a fashion similar to the potential hazards discussed previously regarding the general use of electrosurgery in open surgery, and to discuss the options available to help minimize or eliminate the potential of unintended burns within the peritoneal cavity during laparoscopic surgery. A discussion on the more common misconceptions in using electrosurgery in laparoscopy also will be presented.

There are three potential hazards in the use of electrosurgical energy during laparoscopy. These are a direct result of two factors: access to the peritoneal cavity is obtained through the trocar cannulas

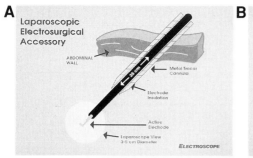

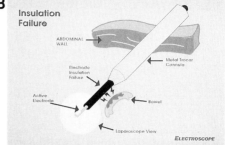

FIGURE 4.7

(A) Full view of the electrosurgical accessory passing into the peritoneal cavity. (B) Full view of the electrosurgical accessory with insulation failure. (Electroscope, Inc, Boulder, CO.)

and the laparoscope views less than 10% of the total electrosurgical device. In passing the electrosurgical active electrode through these access channels and viewed in such a fashion, the following describes the potential for unintended thermal burns as a result of energy straying out of the surgeon's control. These burn injuries are difficult to diagnose because they are delayed in presentation. In addition, the number of actual injuries reported is low as a result of medical legal implications (5,6).

Most laparoscopic accessories are approximately 35 cm long. The laparoscopic image viewed on the monitor shows a small portion, typically less than 5 cm of the distal end of the device. Therefore, the active electrode used for the delivery of the electrosurgical energy has insulation covering the majority of the electrode (Fig 4.7A). Unfortunately, 90% or more of this insulated portion of the electrode is out of the viewing image seen on the monitor. Therefore, if the insulation breakdown occurs on the shaft of the electrode, out of view from the operator, a severe burn may occur to the bowel or other organs near or touching the electrode at this site (Fig 4.7B). Insulation failures can occur for several reasons (i.e., normal wear, handling in central supply, sharp edges on trocar cannula, and corona heating as a result of the high–voltage frequency product). These burns may not be noticed during the course of surgery and may result in severe postoperative complications. It is most important to examine or have your biomedical staff set up a routine inspection of these electrodes periodically, which will minimize, but not eliminate, this hazard. Some might suggest that disposable devices will eliminate insulation failure; this cannot be relied on because the quality of the insulation typically found on disposable devices is inferior to that found on reusable instrumentation.

The second hazard that exists is one of capacitively coupled energy into other metal laparoscopic instruments or trocar cannula. The principal of how capacitance occurs requires a degree of understanding of electrical physics beyond the scope of this text. The bottom line is that 5% to 40% of the power level that the electrosurgical unit is set on to deliver can be coupled or transferred into the standard, 10-cm long trocar cannula. This energy in itself may not be dangerous, providing it is allowed to pass through a low-power density pathway, such as the all-metal (conductive) trocar cannula inserted into the abdominal wall. This will provide a conductive pathway and allow the current to return to the patient return electrode. Further tests need to be performed to assure that even with small 3- and 5-mm diameter cannula, irreversible damage does not occur.

This capacitive coupling becomes a problem when the energy is allowed or made to pass through a high-power density pathway (Fig 4.8), which can occur, for example, with the partially plastic (nonconductive) and partially metal (conductive) trocar cannulas on the market. Some trocar manufacturers supply a plastic thread to the metal cannula tube to help hold the cannula in the abdominal wall when the laparoscopic electrode is positioned in and out of the cannula port (see Fig 4.8). To avoid this hazard, I strongly recommend the use of all-metal or all-plastic trocar cannulas for the electrosurgical active laparoscopic electrode to be passed through. Capacitive coupling in conjunction with suction irrigation devices also has been addressed recently (7); up to 80% of the energy was shown on commercially available devices. Capacitive coupling to a lesser degree can occur when another laparoscopic instrument crosses the electrosurgical laparoscopic electrode within the peritoneal cavity (i.e., atraumatic grasper, etc). The energy transfer to these instruments can range from 1% to 10% of the power set on the electrosurgical unit. Some caution should be taken under this condition, especially during long activation times.

Physics and Clinical Application of Electrosurgery   63

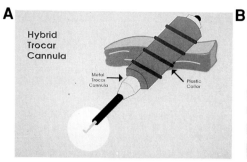 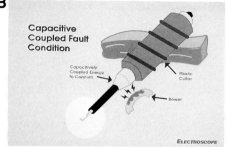

FIGURE 4.8

(A) Hybrid trocar cannula that blocks the capacitive current from the abdominal wall. (B) Capacitive coupling with a dangerous stray pathway back to the patient return electrode. (Electroscope, Inc, Boulder, CO.)

The issue of capacitive coupling was first detected during operative, single-puncture laparoscopic procedures (8,9). These laparoscopes have an operating channel (30 to 40 cm long) to pass various instruments through. It was observed that when a plastic 10- to 12-mm cannula was used to pass the operating laparoscope through, the distal end of the metal laparoscope could deliver a portion of the power (40% to 80%) set on the electrosurgical unit, and burns to adjacent tissue were documented. Therefore, during single-puncture operative laparoscopic procedures in which electrosurgery may be used, only an all-metal trocar cannula should be used to pass both the laparoscope and the electrosurgical electrode into the peritoneal cavity. The Food and Drug Administration made a strong recommendation to this effect (10).

The third potential hazard with the use of monopolar energy occurs when the active electrode is accidentally touched to the laparoscope or other conductive instruments, such as traction/countertraction devices. Where does the current/energy go if contact is made? All-metal trocar cannulas will allow the energy to pass into the abdominal wall via a low-power density pathway, which will minimize the potential for injury. If plastic cannulas are used, the current may exit to the bowel or other organs touching the laparoscope/device, out of view of the monitor. This is due to the plastic cannula blocking the directly coupled energy from being passed into the abdominal wall and back to the

64   Laparoscopic Hysterectomy and Pelvic Floor Reconstruction

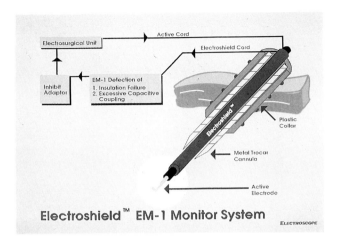

Electroshield™ EM-1 Monitor System

ELECTROSCOPE

FIGURE 4.9

The Electroshield Monitoring System features a sheath that surrounds the existing laparoscopic electrosurgical instruments. (Electroscope, Inc, Boulder, CO.)

patient return electrode. Therefore, I strongly recommend that metal cannulas always be used for the laparoscope port and for other ports that have conductive instruments inserted.

To eliminate the first two hazards in the delivery of monopolar energy, Electroscope, Inc. designed the Electroshield Monitoring System to actively monitor for insulation failure and excessive capacitive coupling out of the view of the laparoscope. The Electroshield System features either a reusable adaptive shield to the hospital's "existing" dissecting and coagulating laparoscopic electrodes or a line of totally integrated 5- and 10-mm instruments with the conductive shield built as a component of the device (Fig 4.9). These instruments are reusable or of limited use in design. The Electroshield Monitor EM-2 dynamically detects (Fig 4.10) any insulation faults and shields against the occurrence of capacitive coupling (11). If an unsafe condition exists, the Electroshield System automatically deactivates the electrosurgical unit before a burn can occur. This technologic "fail safe" advancement allows the surgeon to use monopolar electrosurgical energy in laparoscopic procedures with the same degree of confidence as in open procedures. The shielding system controls the potential hazard of stray

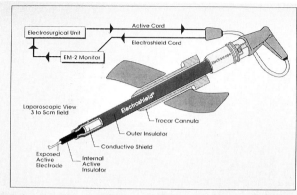

5mm Integrated Electroshield® Electrode Diagram

FIGURE 4.10

The Electroshield Monitoring System dynamically detects any insulation faults and shields against capacitive coupling. (Electroscope, Inc, Boulder, CO.)

energy out of the view of the laparoscope, which is the fundamental difference in the delivery of this energy in laparoscopy compared with open laparotomy.

MISCONCEPTIONS

There are two misconceptions that I believe need addressing with regard to the delivery of monopolar electrosurgical energy during laparoscopy. First, for some strange reason, when delivered at the target site, the electrosurgical current behaves differently in laparoscopy versus open surgical procedures, prompting statements to the effect that "The current is delivered to one origin and mysteriously exits into an adjacent origin and burns at the exit/entry point during laparoscopic procedures." The biophysics are identical with regard to the path the current takes in route to the patient return electrode in open versus laparoscopic application. Again, the key point is from the target site (i.e., the point at which the active electrode delivers the current and the path the current takes are the same; this is commonly referred to as the path of least resistance). If this fact is true, it should have surfaced in open classic procedures decades ago.

On the other hand, there are reported complications in the application of monopolar energy in both open and laparoscopic procedures in which a pedicle of tissue is created by stretching or other actions; the current is reconcentrated through this narrowing cross-section of tissue, resulting in increased temperatures applied to the tissue at that point. After thorough examination of such incidents, an interesting finding is that the complications could have been avoided if the surgeons had a better understanding of the biophysics of the delivery of energy. One such case worth reviewing is that of female laparoscopic sterilization (9), in which the complication would have been avoided if the surgeon had a better understanding of electrosurgical energy. For some unknown reason, there is a void in medical education concerning electrosurgical principles of efficacy and safety. This holds true not only for general surgeons, but for the majority of surgical disciplines. I believe this opinion is shared by surgeons more advanced in the art of this energy source as well.

The second misconception regarding monopolar electrosurgical energy is the voltage necessary to perform monopolar (coagulation) electrosurgery, which is known to range from 3000 to 5000 V peak at maximum control settings (120 W). Therefore, normal operating settings in the range of 20 to 50 W for coagulation mode (or control settings 3 to 5) may produce voltages between 1500 to 3000 V peak, invoking statements to the effect that "In a close peritoneal cavity the humidity level and other factors suggest that uncontrollable sparks may occur compared with the delivery of monopolar energy in open procedures. Therefore, this is not suitable for laparoscopy."

Physics textbooks indicate that it takes 30,000 V to spark 1 in in air under the best of conditions (12,13) and compare these distances with those of other gases. For example, in CO_2 it takes roughly 30% more voltage to spark 1 in, or 39,000 V, when compared with normal air. Humidity levels also are discussed, and the textbooks indicate that they do not play a significant factor. Hence, sparking from the active tip of the electrode can be better controlled in laparoscopy than in open procedures.

SUMMARY

Monopolar electrosurgical energy has been the gold standard for the past 50 years (14), and it has more diverse capabilities (fulguration, precise vaporization, coaptation of large vessels) than other energy sources. Medical economics also have benefitted from the electrosurgical unit. The technologic advancements in performance and safety (15,16) have positioned this device as one of the most useful tools in a surgeon's armamentarium. The adaptation of active monitoring for stray energy as a result of insulation failure or capacitive coupling and the use of all-metal trocar cannulas will increase the confidence of the surgeon in that "what you see is what you get." The adaptation of active electrode monitoring will serve as a "loss prevention" measure against medical legal issues (17). It is my opinion that the use of monopolar electrosurgical energy will again prove itself in laparoscopy. As with any surgical tool or energy source, education and skill are required. This introduction to the principles of the biophysics of electrical energy applied to tissues and its safety considerations is a start to further the understanding and to advance the usage of this powerful surgical tool.

REFERENCES

1. Peterson HB, Ory HW, Greenspan JR, Tyler CW. Deaths associated with laparoscopic sterilization by unipolar electrocoagulating devices, 1978 and 1979. Am J Obstet Gynecol 1981;139:141–143.
2. Sigel B, Dunn MR. The mechanism of blood vessel closure by hi frequency electrocoagulation. Surg Gyn Obstet 1965;121:823–831.
3. Soderstrom RM. Refinements in laparoscopic sterilization equipment. Contemp Ob/Gyn 1980;16:121–123.
4. Rioux JE. Laparoscopic tubal sterilization: sparking and its control. La Vie Med Can Franc 1973;2:760–766.
5. Wilson PD, McAnena OJ, Peters EE. A fatal complication of diathermy (electrosurgery) in laparoscopic surgery. Minimally Inv Ther 1994;3:19–20.
6. Berry SM, Ose KJ, Bell RH, Fink AS. Thermal injury of the posterior

duodenum during laparoscopic cholecystectomy. Surg Endosc 1994;8:197–200.

7. Voyles CR, et al. Unrecognized hazards of surgical electrodes passed through metal suction-irrigation devices. Surg Endosc 1994;8:185–187.

8. Corson SL. Electrosurgical hazards in laparoscopy. JAMA 1974;227:1261.

9. Engel T. Electrosurgical dynamics of laparoscopic sterilization. J Reprod Med 1975;15:33–37.

10. Federal Registry. Feb 26, 1980;45:12701.

11. Luciano AA, Soderstrom RM, Martin DC. Essential principles of electrosurgery in operative laparoscopy. Am Assoc Gynecol Laparosc 1994;1:189–195.

12. Gallagher TJ, et al. High voltage measurements testing and design. New York: Wiley, 1983:44–56.

13. Pearce JA. Electrosurgery. New York: Wiley, 1986:60–90.

14. Voyles CR, Tucker RD. Education and engineering solutions for potential problems with laparoscopic monopolar electrosurgery. Am J Surg 1992;164:57–62.

15. Tucker RD, Voyles CR, Silvis SE. Capacitive coupled stray currents during laparoscopic and endoscopic electrosurgical procedures. Biomed Instrum Technol 1993;26:303–311.

16. Sacks E. Monopolar electrosurgical safety during laparoscopy. Health Devices 1995;24(1):3–27.

17. Lap electrosurgery targeted by malpractice attorneys. Laparoscopic Surgery Update 1995;3(8):87.

5

Physics and Clinical Application of Laser Surgery

Joseph R. Feste

Although lasers have been used in medicine for years, the technique of laser surgery has received a plethora of scrutiny, criticism, and publicity. The public and professional perception of the efficacy of the surgical laser has been shaped by physicians who have touted the instrument as a panacea. Before the technique can be properly evaluated, misconceptions must be replaced by a thorough understanding of the conceptual basis and relevant applications of the surgical laser. Even so, the surgical laser is only a tool; the value of its use depends on the skills of a competent, well-trained surgeon.

It is important to review the physics of lasers before discussing their application in laparoscopic hysterectomy (1). The word "laser" originated as an acronym for "light amplification by stimulated emission of radiation." Electrons circling the nuclei of atoms usually are in a resting, or ground, state. As energy is absorbed by these atoms, the circulating electrons are raised to a higher-energy state, one in which energy is stored. This is called an excited state. This state is very unstable, and the electrons rapidly return to their resting state, releasing a burst of energy. This energy package, or quandum, is called a photon.

A laser tube contains molecules with electrons in a resting state. These electrons are excited to a higher-energy state by an external source. As these high-energy electrons decay to their normal, lower-energy state, photons are released and collide with other excited molecules, creating a cascade effect and the release of more photons. This is known as a stimulated emission. Each laser contains a substance with a specific molecular or atomic structure, and thus the photons released by each type of laser have a unique wavelength.

Laser light has three properties that distinguish it from incandescent (heated filament) light: it is monochromatic, coherent, and collimated. Monochromatic light is light of a single wavelength. If an incandescent flashlight is aimed through a prism, the light emerging will show all the colors of the spectrum, because the prism acts to break down the light into its individual wavelengths. If a laser is aimed at the same prism, however, the light emerging would look exactly like the light approaching, because it is all of one wavelength. Coherent light is light in which all the waves are exactly in phase, with the troughs and peaks of one wave occurring exactly at the time as those of other waves. Light and other forms of energy also may be described as quanta and as oscillating wave phenomena. Collimated light is light in which all rays are parallel to each other and do not diverge over long distances. This property allows laser light to be focused by lenses into very small spots.

Laser power is measured in units of power density, which is related to both the wattage and the area (spot size) at the impact site. As the wattage is increased, the depth of penetration, and thus the speed of cutting to a fixed depth, is proportionally increased. Inversely, as the spot size is increased, the power acting on the tissue is exponentially decreased. The following formula is used to calculate power density:

$$\text{Approximate power density (W/cm}^2) \; = \; \frac{\text{watts} \times 100}{\text{spot size (mm}^2)}$$

As laser light hits the tissue surface, cells at the site of impact are rapidly heated and intracellular fluid is vaporized. The cell is vaporized, and the cell particles and cell wall are heated to an extreme temperature, becoming carbonized. Around this zone of vaporization, hemostasis in small vessels occurs followed by necrosis of tissue in the area. Peripheral to the zone of vaporization, areas of change may be seen, but this tissue remains healthy.

Laser energy can be released via four different modes. The single-pulse mode releases one burst of energy for a specific length of time set by the operator (usually 0.05 to 0.50 seconds). To fire the laser again, the operator must release and step again on the foot pedal. When the repeat-pulse mode is used, the laser continues to fire intermittently as long as the foot pedal remains depressed. The continuous-wave mode releases continuous laser energy from the tube as long as the pedal remains depressed, and the superpulse mode, used primarily with the CO_2 laser, releases CO_2 laser energy in very rapid bursts (usually 250 to 750 bursts per second). This creates less heat buildup in tissue and decreases the potential for damage to surrounding tissue.

There are four lasers currently available for gynecologic surgery (Plate 3): CO_2, neodymium:yttrium-aluminum-garnet (Nd:YAG), potassium titanyl phosphate (KTP), and argon (2). Their wavelengths, and thus their properties, vary (Table 5.1). CO_2 lasers release invisible light with a wavelength of 10.6 μm (3). This light is in the far-infrared range and is invisible to the eye. A red beam (helium-neon laser) is added to allow the operator to aim and control the beam. The CO_2 beam is reflected by steel mirrors down a rigid arm. This arm can be connected to a handpiece, a micromanipulator, an operative laparoscope, a secondary puncture probe, or a wave guide. CO_2 lasers are used especially for cutting and vaporizing. They are poor coagulators, and their beams do not travel through fluids.

KTP and argon lasers are very similar in that their emitted wavelengths (0.532 and 0.458 to 0.515 μm, respectively) are very close. Both release visible light that can travel through air or fluids and that is absorbed by dark-pigmented tissue (especially green-blue). KTP and argon light can pass through flexible fibers, making these lasers convenient to use with laparoscopes and hysteroscopes (4,5).

Nd:YAG lasers emit light at 1.064 μm in the near-infrared spectrum. Nd:YAG laser light is invisible and can travel through flexible fibers and pass through fluids. These lasers penetrate deeply into tissue. They are excellent coagulators, but poor cutters unless sapphire tips

TABLE 5.1

Comparisons of the four surgical lasers used endoscopically
in gynecology

	CO_2	ND:YAG	ARGON	KTP
Tissue effect is color dependent	No	Yes	Yes	Yes
Can be passed through flexible fibers	Rigid wave guide	Yes	Yes	Yes
Beam scatters laterally	None	Moderate	Slight	Slight
Beam passes through fluid	No	Yes	Yes	Yes
Used hysteroscopically	No	Yes	Yes	Yes
Used laparoscopically	Yes	Yes	Yes	Yes
Depth of tissue effects	0.1 mm	3.0–4.0 mm	0.3–1.0 mm	0.3–1.0 mm
Allows incisions to be made	Yes (best)	Yes	Yes	Yes
Ability to stop active bleeding	Poor	Excellent	Excellent	Excellent

(special wave guides) are used. Because they pass through fluids and
penetrate deeply into tissue, they are ideal lasers for endometrial ablation
(6).

The traditional implements of surgery have been the knife, scissors,
and microneedle. The surgeon relies on both tactile and visual stimuli
when using the knife and scissors, but tactile sensation is essential for
gauging the depth and quality of the penetration. In contrast, in micro-
surgery, the virtual absence of pressure causes the surgeon to rely more
heavily on visual stimuli. In laser surgery, tactile sensation is nonexistent.
Consequently, visual perception of tissue response determines the depth
of penetration when operating. The technical aspects of the surgical laser
and the physical adjustment that the surgeon must make to use the
instrument effectively have introduced a new "state of the art" for
surgeons (7).

However, it must be remembered that the laser is not a technique;

the laser is an instrument, and it must be controlled by the surgeon. If the surgeon does not have the technical ability to use conventional techniques, he or she will not perform any better by using the laser.

In the hands of a skilled surgeon, the laser offers several distinct advantages (8). In gynecology, there are several advantages offered in all cases:

1. The laser can reduce operating time by providing hemostasis as it cuts.
2. Blood loss will be less because of its hemostatic properties.
3. If operations can be performed in a shorter time, hospitalization time and expense may be reduced.
4. Studies have shown that less postoperative pain occurs when lasers are used. This is probably a reflection of both the reduction of sutures and the thermal effect on tissues adjacent to the treated surface.

LASER SAFETY

As with any potentially hazardous technology, safety issues must be addressed. Patients and staff must be protected from laser injury. Many hospitals have found it advisable to form a committee to supervise such aspects of laser technology as maintenance of equipment, education, purchasing, scheduling, credentialing, and safety. Such committees include physicians, nurses, biomedical engineers, and risk management and administrative personnel. Policies and procedures are established, and guidelines for the safe use of lasers are developed. Many states also require the filing of specific documents by institutions in which lasers are used. Organized guidelines will help protect both patients and staff from accidents related to laser use. Inservice instructional programs for nurses and other operating room personnel are also a key aspect of laser safety. Attending periodic lectures and courses will help remind staff of the need for careful handling of this instrument.

Eye protection is needed when any laser is being used. Clear plastic or glass lenses protect the eyes from the CO_2 beam. When a KTP, Nd:YAG, or argon laser is used, glasses with specific optical densities for these wavelengths must be used. Signs should be posted to alert all personnel that lasers are being used in the operating room, and the patient's eyes should be protected with glasses or wet pads.

Protection against fires and explosions also is important. Flammable preparation materials or anesthetics should not be used. Only nonflammable drapes or wet towels should be used to drape the patient.

The laser plume, which contains carbon, water vapor cells, and, in some cases, viral DNA, must be evacuated as completely as possible. Most of the carbon particles found in laser plume are ≤ 1 μm in diameter and, if inhaled, may be deposited in the aveoli of the lungs. Like other carbon, these carbon particles may act as a carcinogen. The contents of the laser plume also can cause laryngitis or bronchitis in surgeons performing laser surgery (9).

Plume evacuators equipped with fine filters (0.1 μm) should be used to remove as much plume as possible. Suction tubing held within 1 cm of the tissue impact site will remove approximately 98% of plume; at a distance of 2 cm, approximately 50% of the plume will escape.

Although intact viral particles have been found in laser plume, no activity of these particles has been demonstrated to date. Recently, masks with a filtering ability finer than that of standard surgical masks have been introduced. However, these masks have not been shown to significantly reduce the amount of particles inhaled by the laser surgeon. Some surgeons also find that these masks are not comfortable to breathe through. Thus, careful plume evacuation should be the mainstay of inhalation safety.

Major complications secondary to gas embolization from endometrial ablation procedures were reported recently. The elimination of fibers and sapphire tips that are gas cooled would prevent these complications.

LASER APPLICATIONS FOR LAPAROSCOPIC HYSTERECTOMY

Laser energy can be used in the form of a light scalpel to perform several tasks at the time of laparoscopic hysterectomy. These include lysis of adhesions, vaporization of endometriosis, cul-de-sac dissection, and even cutting of pedicles that have been cauterized or tied with suture. However, the laser offers advantages over scissors or a knife only if there are adhesions or endometriosis. The main advantage offered by lasers of any wavelength is their ability to cut and coagulate at the same time. During dissection of adhesions and vaporization of endometriosis, no other instrument is required. This versatility of one instrument saves time in the operating room by eliminating the need for changing instruments during the procedure. Another important issue is the safety of the patient. The literature has recently substantially validated that there have been more injuries with electrosurgery than with laser energy, especially the CO_2 laser.

Adhesiolysis

In most or all cases of laparoscopically assisted vaginal hysterectomy, adhesions are present that require lysis. In the absence of adhesions or endometriosis, the efficacy of a laparoscopic procedure is questionable. There are certainly instances in which a few adhesions can be lysed and a simple vaginal hysterectomy performed.

The ultra or super pulses are preferable to continuous wave for lysing adhesions because they cause less thermal effect and produce less laser plume than the continuous wave. With the CO_2 laser, fluid or titanium rods can be used as backstops to protect the patient from injury beyond the targeted area (10).

The fiberoptic lasers, Nd:YAG, argon, and KTP, have the same potential as the CO_2 laser for lysing adhesions. However, because of the increase in scatter of laser energy with these wavelengths, care must be taken to protect structures beyond the adhesions from the laser energy.

Since all three pass through liquids, irrigating fluid will not act as a backstop for these wavelengths. Because of the ability to focus and defocus the fiberoptic lasers over a short distance, the fiberoptic laser provides greater safety in preventing the exposure to tissue distal to the adhesion. Dissection of the cul-de-sac in patients with complete cul-de-sac obliteration associated with stage 4 endometriosis or adhesive disease requires extreme caution with any of the four lasers, especially the fiberoptics. The lack of depth control will be an important consideration in dissection of the cul-de-sac (1). I prefer to use the CO_2 laser when working in this area. To prepare the patient for a vaginal hysterectomy, the cul-de-sac is completely freed of adhesions or endometriosis. Before surgery, it is important for the patient to have a complete bowel preparation (4). Care must be taken to identify the location of the ureters when the lateral cul-de-sac is dissected. Often, I have a urologist insert ureteral catheters into both ureters prior to the procedure. This makes it possible to feel the ureters with a blunt probe and also protects against inadvertent injury.

The single most common location of colon injury is the point of attachment of the ovaries to the rectosigmoid colon. This is especially common between the left ovary and rectosigmoid. I have frequently reviewed cases in which bowel perforation has occurred when unipolar scissors have been used in this location. Undoubtedly, this is not the appropriate instrument for use in dissection. In this strategic area, the CO_2 laser is more easily controlled and is much less likely to injure the colon. If one of the fiberoptic lasers is used, caution must be taken to prevent penetration of the bowel by using lower wattage and power densities, and the ovary must be used as the backstop to prevent injury to the colon as it is dissected from the attachment of the ovary.

The only other area of real concern when adhesions are lysed with laser energy is the area between the ovaries and the pelvic side walls. In this area, there are vital structures, including the ureter and branches of the internal iliac artery and vein. One must dissect the adhesions off the ovary, using the ovary as a backstop. Following the removal of adhesions, if the ovary is to be preserved, I suggest wrapping the ovary in Interceed to prevent postoperative formation of adhesions. It is important that the hemostasis be established in the ovary and pelvic side wall if the Interceed (Johnson & Johnson, New Brunswick, NJ) is to work properly.

Endometriosis

The laparoscopic treatment of endometriosis in any type of laparoscopic hysterectomy should be as complete as when the endometriosis is treated conservatively and the tubes and ovaries are left (10). All visible implants must be vaporized before the uterus, tubes, and ovaries are removed. If endometrial implants are left in the pelvis, whether or not the uterus or ovaries are removed, the implants will continue to thrive and ultimately cause symptoms. Often, the implants are intermingled with the adhesions associated with the advanced cases of endometriosis.

After adhesions are removed, the endometriosis beneath the adhesions should always be treated. Simply removing the uterus or ovaries will not affect the activity of the disease even if estrogen replacement therapy is withheld. If the ovaries are not removed, 6 months of gonadotropin-releasing hormone analog therapy should be considered. If the implants are visible, treating them will preclude the need for gonadotropin-releasing hormone therapy. If it is believed that not all endometrial implants were visible, the elimination of estrogen for 6 months would be an efficacious treatment.

CONCLUSION

As indicated by the preceding overview of the use of lasers in laparoscopic hysterectomy, various wavelengths may be appropriate for this procedure. It is obvious that laser surgery does not constitute a panacea. However, if we accept the laser as another instrument in the surgeon's armamentarium, a proper perspective can be maintained. The surgeon must be objective when evaluating the surgical laser as a potential tool. The laser undoubtedly will play a role in the future as important as the role played by other traditional surgical instruments in the past.

REFERENCES

1. Absten G. Fundamentals of laser surgery. Cincinnati: US Medical Corp, 1985.
2. Daniell JF, Feste JR. Laser laparoscopy. In: Keye WR, ed. Laser surgery in gynecology and obstetrics. Boston: GK Hall, 1985:147–164.
3. Martin DC. Infertility surgery using the carbon dioxide laser. Clin GynBriefs 1983;4(3):1.
4. Daniell JF, Miller W, Tosh R. Initial evaluation of the use of the potassium-titanyl-phosphate (KTP/532) laser in gynecologic laparoscopy. Fertil Steril 1986;46:373.
5. Keye WR, Henson LW, Astin MT, Poulson AM. Argon laser therapy of endometriosis: review of 92 consecutive patients. Fertil Steril 1987;47:208.
6. Lomano JM. Photocoagulation of early pelvic endometriosis with Nd:YAG laser through the laparoscope. J Reprod Med 1985;30:77.
7. Feste JR. Endoscopic laser surgery in gynecology. In: Reproductive surgery. Postgraduate course syllabus. Chicago: American Fertility Society, 1985:51–69.
8. Feste JR. Laser laparoscopy: A new modality. Lasers Surg Med 1983;3:170.
9. Feste JR, Lloyd JM. A new valving system for removal of laser plume during pelvic CO_2 laser endoscopic procedures. Obstet Gynecol 1987;69:669.
10. Davis GD. Management of endometriosis and its associated adhesion with the CO_2 laser laparoscope. Obstet Gynecol 1986;68:422.

6

Preoperative and Postoperative Care

Andrew I. Brill

The categorical benefit of laparoscopic hysterectomy is the transformation of abdominal into vaginal surgery. Its purported value must be supported by an acceptable level of associated morbidity and mortality. The magnitude of intraoperative and postoperative complications will directly reflect the level of diagnostic acuity exercised during the preoperative patient evaluation process. An inclusive style of informed consent provokes patient dialogue and provides an opportunity to experience and reinforce the patient's psyche. A carefully orchestrated history and physical examination provides the logic for recommending laparoscopic hysterectomy and serves to uncover risk factors known to predict patient morbidity. These factors establish the need to alter the surgical strategy and institute prophylactic measures. Supplementary diagnostic imaging studies can be used to confirm the diagnosis and reaffirm the wisdom of the laparoscopic approach. Thoughtfully chosen preoperative testing, tailored to each patient's underlying health assessment, assists to more precisely gauge the risks of surgery and reconfirm the appropriateness of the surgical plan. Comprehensive management of the postoperative period recognizes that preoperative risk factors, the stress of surgery, and the conduct of the operative procedure remain inextricably linked. Whether patient recovery is delayed by minor difficulties or more significant complications, early recognition and proactive management ideally act to preempt the evolution of more serious sequelae.

PREOPERATIVE CARE

Informed Consent

The process of obtaining informed consent culminates the preoperative covenant established between surgeon and patient. It is here that the physician's degree of commitment to the intellectual and psychologic preparation of the patient will determine her ultimate level of trust in the wisdom and plan of the proposed procedure. Sensitivity to patient ambivalence should preside over the surgeon's wish to coerce the patient to accept the recommendation for laparoscopic hysterectomy.

All patients should be fully informed of the usual risks of undergoing general anesthesia and elective surgery. These include untoward reactions to medication, hemorrhage requiring transfusion, pulmonary complications, infection, pulmonary embolism, and death. In some circumstances, it is advisable to arrange for a preoperative consultation with the anesthesiologist so that the proposed anesthesia and its attendant risks can be more fully explained.

After reviewing the pros and cons of any potential alternatives to the proposed surgery, the therapeutic necessity and potential benefits for the hysterectomy as well as the reasons for choosing the laparoscopic route to assist or complete the procedure should be explained. This requires that the patient have some basic understanding of laparoscopy and the anatomic differences between abdominal and vaginal surgery. Comparing the relative risks of abdominal versus vaginal surgery will help clarify this process. Regardless of surgeon experience or degree of pelvic pathology, the possibility and potential reasons for conversion to the laparotomic approach should be carefully explained. When appropriate, the physician should be willing to openly reveal that she or he is in the early learning phase of using the laparoscopic approach for hysterectomy.

The sequelae of hysterectomy should be understood in the most general terms of permanent sterilization and amenorrhea. The physician can elicit and be prepared to answer questions regarding the potential for changes in sexual response after hysterectomy. If bilateral adnexectomy is contemplated, the fact of castration and the advisability of postoperative estrogen replacement should be carefully reviewed. The patient must be fully aware of the inherent risks for injury to the bowel, bladder, and ureter during hysterectomy. The use of anatomic diagrams is most helpful for effectively communicating these critical facts. The more common postoperative sequelae unique to each injury should be explained.

Although the laparoscopic approach to hysterectomy promises lessened morbidity and a speedier recovery, the morbidity of laparoscopy itself must not be overlooked. The anatomic locations of trocar sites and their cosmetic effects deserve explanation. Patients must be made fully aware of the potential for inadvertent Veress needle and trocar injury to the underlying viscera, the retroperitoneal vascular structures, and the abdominal wall blood vessels with subsequent hematoma formation. The possible need for conversion to laparotomy for reparative surgery should be reviewed.

The patient should have realistic expectations about her postoperative recovery. She should anticipate that nausea, vomiting, and a clouded sensorium commonly occur after general anesthesia. The need for analgesia to relieve generalized abdominal discomfort, pain at trocar sites, and deep pelvic pain from the hysterectomy should be explained. The potential for joint soreness after prolonged Trendelenburg's positioning in stirrups and shoulder discomfort from pneumoperitoneal irritation should be reviewed. If a urinary catheter is planned for postoperative bladder drainage, its purpose and probable duration of use should be explained. Finally, the patient needs to know the expected length of hospital stay, any anticipated dietary restrictions, physical and sexual limitations, and the need for office follow-up after discharge from the hospital.

The significance of comprehensively performed informed consent goes well beyond the minimization of postoperative medicolegal conflicts. Patients empowered with knowledge and trust are better prepared for the stress of surgery and are more highly motivated for a faster postoperative recovery.

Laparoscopy as a Risk Factor

The cardiovascular and pulmonary systems in healthy patients undergoing laparoscopy are remarkably stable. Nevertheless, potentially adverse phenomena that result from the use of carbon dioxide as the distention medium, the creation and maintenance of the pneumoperitoneum, and the use of Trendelenburg's position must be seriously considered when assessing the patient for preoperative risk factors. These physiologic changes are of greatest concern when evaluating patients with known cardiac or pulmonary disease for the appropriateness of the laparoscopic approach to hysterectomy.

Several well-designed studies have established that as insufflation progresses, there is an increase in central venous return and elevation of the mean blood pressure. This trend is reversed at higher intraperitoneal pressures (>30 mm Hg) when there is a progressive decrease in mean blood pressure and cardiac output (1–3). Carbon dioxide is readily absorbed by the large peritoneal surface lining of the pelvic and abdominal cavities, resulting in a measurable decrease in blood pH and increase in the partial pressure of carbon dioxide (4). Retention of carbon dioxide may be further increased by the decrease in lung compliance and hypoventilation that results from excessive diaphragmatic elevation due to higher pneumoperitoneal pressures and the weight of the viscera while in Trendelenburg's position. Elevated blood carbon dioxide levels are associated with the release of catechols and heightened sympathetic activity (5). These changes prime the cardiovascular system for elevations in cardiac output and blood pressure, heightened myocardial sensitivity to halogenated anesthetic agents, and arrhythmias. Acute stretching of the peritoneum during insufflation can directly stimulate the sinoatrial node, causing bradyarrythmias and asystole (4).

When measured straight out of the gas cylinder, carbon dioxide has a temperature of 21.1°C (6). The surface area of the peritoneal cavity and the highly perfused splanchnic system represent a large surface area for thermal exchange. Understandably, the continuous insufflation of large volumes of uncooled carbon dioxide can potentially result in a significant decrease in the core temperature. This loss of temperature, in addition to the other hypothermic experiences in the operating room, has been measured to be as much as 0.3°C per 40–50 liters of carbon dioxide delivered to the abdominal cavity (6). While intraoperative hypothermia is protective for the brain and myocardium, normal postoperative homeostatic mechanisms can significantly stress the cardiovascular system. During recovery from general anesthesia, a lowered core temperature causes compensatory shivering and shaking. A decrease of 0.3 to 1.2°C during the postoperative period has been shown to double oxygen consumption, while shivering increased the cardiac output three to four times normal (7,8).

Higher pneumoperitoneal pressures can augment the adverse effects of general anesthesia on ventilation mechanics by elevating the diaphragm with secondary compression of lung tissue. This decreases lung compliance and worsens ventilation–perfusion inequalities. The ventilation mismatch can be further worsened by the use of Trendelenburg's position, which causes blood to accumulate in the more dependent and dorsal portions of the lungs (9).

Patient Assessment and Preparation

The preoperative history and physical examination should affirm the patient's diagnosis and logically justify the surgical plan. The decision to proceed with laparoscopic hysterectomy should reflect the presence of anatomic factors that would logically contraindicate the vaginal approach. The identification of nongynecologic conditions that commonly masquerade as pelvic complaints will help ensure that hysterectomy is the best therapeutic option for the patient. Furthermore, as the patient comes to understand which complaints are not pelvic in origin, she will develop realistic expectations about her potential for postoperative symptom relief. This process provides an excellent opportunity for the physician to develop a sense of the patient's mental state and level of preparation for the stress of the upcoming surgery. Most importantly, significant risk factors and previously undiagnosed conditions that are known to contribute to postoperative morbidity and mortality can be identified.

Patient History

A complete review of systems will help uncover important historic factors placing the patient at potentially higher risk for surgery. Communicating with the patient's primary care physician will help complete this process. If available, any summary from prior hospitalization should be reviewed for discharge diagnoses, difficulties with intubation, adverse reactions to anesthesia and medications, transfusions and transfusion reactions, postoperative urinary retention, complications such as peritonitis, and pathology report.

Cardiac and pulmonary conditions account for most surgical morbidity and mortality. Cardiopulmonary disease often manifests itself as exercise intolerance, chronic fatigue, shortness of breath, chest pain, recurrent bouts of pulmonary infection, and wheezing. It is especially important to search for these symptoms if the patient smokes cigarettes. For patients with significant underlying cardiopulmonary disease, it is wise to arrange for additional consultation with a medical specialist and the anesthesiologist. A history of valvular heart disease heralds the need to administer the appropriate prophylactic antibiotics at the time of surgery.

Patients at higher risk for developing postoperative atelectasis should be identified during the preoperative evaluation process. Acute pulmonary congestion is adversely affected by general anesthesia. Bronchial obstruction from accumulated pulmonary secretions can lead to absorption of trapped gases and significant collapse of distal pulmonary segments. Any patient with acute respiratory infections should therefore have their surgery rescheduled. Patients with chronic pulmonary disease and cigarette smokers with productive coughs should receive preoperative pulmonary physiotherapy, training for incentive spirometry, and, when appropriate, antibiotic therapy (10).

The possibility for alcohol and other substance abuse should be explored with all patients. High-risk behaviors associated with the potential for infection with the human immunodeficiency virus, hepatitis B, syphilis, and tuberculosis should be noted.

All medications taken on a regular basis and prior allergic reactions should be recorded. Due to their profound effects on platelet function, particular attention should be paid to the use of aspirin and aspirin-like compounds. Oral contraceptives should ideally be discontinued several weeks prior to surgery to avoid the possible increased risk for venous thrombosis.

Any history strongly suggestive of an underlying functional bowel disorder, especially in patients presenting with chronic pelvic pain, should be carefully evaluated. These patients should be offered a trial of dietary and/or medical therapy prior to scheduling for hysterectomy.

A history of progressive lower back pain should be investigated for possible underlying disc disease. The forces created by placement of the patient's legs in stirrups and Trendelenburg's position creates extra stress on the lower back and joints of the lower extremities. Arthritis, limitation in motion, and previous surgery of the hip and knee joints should be diligently noted. In more severe cases, plans should be made to place the lower extremities in the stirrups prior to induction of anesthesia. This will help prevent exacerbation of identified restrictive or inflammatory musculoskeletal disease.

Since the bladder will be surgically manipulated and catheterized intraoperatively, symptoms of genitourinary infection should be aggressively evaluated by urine culture and, if positive, treated with the appropriate antibiotic. A history of stress urinary incontinence warrants a careful review of present medications and a targeted examination for neurologic deficit and defective pelvic support.

It is important to document that the appropriate recommended cancer screening tests, such as mammography, Pap test, stool guaiac, and prior endometrial biopsy for abnormal uterine bleeding, have been performed. The patient's prior reproductive history, contraceptive history, and last menses should be recorded. It is preferable to perform laparoscopic surgery in the proliferative phase. This will minimize the possibility of operating in the presence of an undiagnosed early intrauterine pregnancy. Furthermore, avoiding surgery in the luteal phase removes the likelihood of creating traumatic bleeding while manipulating a highly vascularized corpus luteum. Any history of pelvic inflammatory disease must be clarified. Hospitalization for parenteral antibiosis, especially for the treatment of a pelvic abscess, may place the patient at higher risk for significant intra-abdominal and pelvic adhesions.

If the hysterectomy is being performed for hypermenorrhea, the degree of social disability, duration and character of flow, severity of dysmenorrhea, any related anemia, results of endometrial sampling, associated pathology, and any attempts at hormonal and analgesic therapies should be documented. For patients undergoing hysterectomy for chronic pelvic pain, it is important to document the chronicity, location, severity, degree of social disability or sexual dysfunction, associated pathology, recapitulation of pain on examination, and degree of relief with hormonal and analgesic medications.

Any prior abdominal or pelvic surgery should be assiduously investigated prior to laparoscopic surgery. Since most patients cannot be expected to accurately remember the findings or procedures performed during their prior surgery, it is incumbent on the physician to review the prior operative notes whenever feasible. In addition to the surgical procedures performed, attention should be focused on previously documented intra-abdominal and pelvic adhesions, the presence and anatomic distribution of endometriosis, uterine or adnexal pathologies, extirpative procedures, and any intraoperative complications. These records can be used to reaffirm the preoperative diagnosis and help reconcile abnormal findings on pelvic examination and complementary diagnostic imaging studies. If cesarean section was performed, one should anticipate significant elevation and adherence of the vesicouterine fold. Of greatest importance, prior observations of intra-abdominal adhesive disease can be used to develop a modified strategy for trocar insertion to help avert accidental injury to the underlying viscera.

Physical Examination

Outside of the genital tract, the physical examination provides supplementary information for preoperative risk assessment. It may reveal stigmata of significant underlying conditions not uncovered by the history and review of systems. The chest is examined for wheezes, rales, and diminished breath sounds or diaphragmatic excursion. The heart should be examined for the presence of arrhythmia, abnormal murmurs, and extra sounds.

In obese patients, the relative distribution of fat in the abdominal pannus should be critically appraised. Large depositions of fat in the abdominal wall between the umbilicus and mons pubis can significantly restrict trocar and instrument mobility during laparoscopic maneuvers. Since obesity is associated with a downward displacement of the umbilicus, its true anatomic relationship to the iliac crests should be noted. Any scars from prior laparotomy should be reconciled with available operative reports from prior hospitalizations. It is essential to presume that each abdominal scar may harbor underlying adhesions between it and the bowel. In patients undergoing laparoscopic hysterectomy for a large pelvic mass, topographic examination of the abdomen will establish whether realistic sites exist for trocar placement.

Since varicose veins associated with venous incompetence are a significant risk factor for postoperative deep venous thrombosis (11), the lower extremities must be examined for severe varicosities and evidence of venous stasis. Any restrictions in the range of motion of the hips and knees should be assessed and documented.

The essential pelvic examination searches for pelvic pathology and defects in supporting tissues. The plan to proceed with laparoscopic hysterectomy relies on a thorough clinical appraisal of the size, mobility, and fixation of the pelvic organs. The pubic arch should be assessed for restrictive angulation. The introitus and vagina are examined for estrogen effect, flexibility, significant defects in supportive tissues, adequacy of urethral support, and posterior nodularity. The cervix is examined for size, fixed anatomic flexions, distortion from prior surgery, and relative descent on Valsalva. The uterus is examined for size, mobility, asymmetry of the lower segment, and posterior fundal fixation. The adnexa are assessed for cystic change, fixation, and mobility. In patients with known or suspected endometriosis, the rectovaginal septum, vaginal fornices, uterosacral ligaments, and cul-de-sac must be thoroughly examined for nodularity, fixation, and point tenderness.

Once the need for hysterectomy has been established by the history and examination, the chance for successfully accomplishing this procedure by vaginal removal with the help of laparoscopic techniques must be critically weighed against the traditional approach. The ultimate decision to proceed with the laparoscopic approach must reflect a naked truthfulness about the physician's basic laparoscopic skills, prior experience in performing laparoscopic hysterectomy, and degree of comfort when operating in the midst of any identified pelvic pathology.

Diagnostic Imaging

Diagnostic imaging techniques can be used to supplement the pelvic examination and aid in the final surgical decision making. The accuracy of findings on pelvic examination often differ with those of more definitive imaging studies (12). These studies can adjunctively confirm the presence of a pelvic mass, determine the pelvic organ of origin, and elucidate internal tissue architecture. They can be especially useful for defining anatomic relationships in the significantly obese patient, when pelvic examination is inadequate secondary to abdominal guarding, and in a patient with a known adnexal or eccentrically located pelvic mass.

Ultrasound remains the primary imaging modality for pelvic masses. While transabdominal imaging techniques are better for identifying ovaries in higher positions due to leiomyomata, imaging may be obscured by obesity, bowel gas, adhesions, and acoustic blinding of the cul-de-sac from uterine retroversion. Transvaginal techniques are devoid of these problems and provide better visualization and higher resolution of the pelvic organs and related organic pathologies (13,14).

Magnetic resonance imaging should be used as a complementary imaging modality when the ultrasound results are equivocal and greater definition would influence the final surgical approach. In a patient with a large leiomyomatous uterus, magnetic resonance imaging can be used to accurately map the size and locale of potentially obstructive lower segment leiomyomata. More commonly, it can be used to definitively resolve whether an eccentrically located pelvic mass is of uterine or adnexal origin, such as a degenerated lateral wall myoma initially interpreted by sonography to be a probable adherent endometrioma. Magnetic resonance imaging also is useful for determining whether a cystic adnexal mass contains blood or fat (15).

Computed tomography is rarely indicated for the preoperative evaluation of presumed benign pelvic disease. Its primary role is for evaluating pelvic and abdominal masses suspicious for malignancy (16). Inherent disadvantages of this modality include the need for contrast dye, radiation exposure to the gonads, and the unreliability for definitive visualization of the ovaries. In cases of suspected pelvic malignancy, it is a superior modality for evaluating thick adhesions, peritoneal implants, retroperitoneal nodes, and altered ureteral anatomy (16).

Preoperative assessment of the ureters and upper renal collecting systems may be considered when a large leiomyomatous uterus tightly extends to the lateral pelvic side wall or when ureteral involvement by endometriosis is suspected by history and prior operative findings. Although intravenous urography traditionally has been used for this purpose, ultrasound has been shown to be equally efficacious in evaluation of the ureters and renal calyces for anatomic indicators of stasis (17). The absence of procedure-related morbidity and the comparative cost effectiveness makes sonographic evaluation of the urinary tract the preferred diagnostic imaging modality.

Laboratory Assessment

The purpose of preoperative laboratory testing is to reduce unnecessary preoperative risk and to detect potentially harmful conditions that are asymptomatic. It has been clearly demonstrated that the routine collection of preoperative tests in the healthy patient is not scientifically justified (18,19). In the absence of particular clinical indications, these tests contribute little to patient care and reduction of surgically related morbidity (20). Furthermore, the expense of pursuing inevitable false-positive results significantly contributes to unwarranted cost. Tradition and the fear of malpractice continues to fuel this unsubstantiated practice. The present climate of cutbacks in medical services and reimbursement demands that the surgeon's decision to order particular preoperative tests be justified by contemporary cost–benefit analyses.

Oxygen delivery to tissues is dependent on hemoglobin concentration, cardiac output, and the arteriovenous saturation difference (21). Although normal blood volume and tissue perfusion are more important than the concentration of erythrocytes for oxygen delivery to tissues (22), it is recommended that all patients have a hematocrit drawn prior to surgery (23). If anemia is identified, it must be evaluated for chronicity and severity. The source must be actively pursued. Patients with long-term anemia can tolerate much lower hemoglobin levels due to the compensation in blood volume that occurs (24). Those less likely to tolerate the intraoperative effects of significant anemia are older than

50 years and have significant atherosclerotic disease, prior myocardial infarction, and resting hypoxia (22). Surgery should be delayed in these high-risk patients. A full course of oral iron supplementation can be administered to help replenish iron stores and increase erythrocyte production. Any significant dysfunctional uterine bleeding can be treated with hormonal suppression. Although there are no data to prove that mild-to-moderate anemia contributes to surgical morbidity, it is customary to require the patient to have a hematocrit of at least 30% and a hemoglobin of 10 gm prior to elective admission for surgery (22,24).

The use of homologous red blood cell transfusion is generally indicated when significant blood loss (>1000 mL) is anticipated during the operative procedure. Given that significant hemorrhage will occur during some cases of laparoscopic hysterectomy, it is reasonable to offer the patient the opportunity to bank her own blood prior to surgery. While donation will diminish the patient's iron stores, blood collection for autologous transfusion eliminates the potential risks of viral transmission and adverse immunologic reactions associated with heterologous red blood cell transfusion (21). Up to 3 U of blood can be withdrawn during the 3 to 4-week period prior to surgery.

Routine preoperative prothrombin time, partial thromboplastin time, and platelet count have no clinical usefulness unless the clinical history or physical examination suggest a bleeding disorder (25). Agents affecting platelet function, such as aspirin, should be discontinued for at least 1 week prior to surgery.

Drawing extra blood for serum electrolytes, blood urea nitrogen, and creatinine should be restricted to patients with chronic renal disease or diabetes and to those taking diuretics (26). Unless the surgery is contraindicated in a patient with diabetes, a serum glucose or postprandial testing is justified only in patients with known diabetes mellitus (18,19). Testing for abnormal liver function should be reserved for patients with chronic liver ailments or a history of hepatitis, or if potentially hepatotoxic medications (such as danacrine) have been taken for a substantial period of time.

When caring for a patient with high-risk sexual or substance abuse behavior, the surgeon must conscientiously seize the responsibility to protect himself and associated health care personnel from the potential for transmission of infectious disease. These issues should be frankly discussed with the patient. When appropriate, testing should be strongly recommended for hepatitis B, syphilis, the human immunodeficiency virus, and tuberculosis.

Routine urinalysis for the evaluation of renal function and possible urinary tract infection is justified given that the urinary tract will be surgically manipulated, a urinary drainage catheter may be placed, and multiple medications will be administered during anesthesia. A urine pregnancy test should be considered in patients without reliable menstrual histories or methods of contraception, and if the operation will be performed in the secretory phase of the menstrual cycle.

The use of a routine preoperative electrocardiogram is discouraged. The resting electrocardiogram is an insensitive and nonspecific indicator of ischemic heart disease. Its only benefit is that it reveals a previously unrecognized myocardial infarction and detects a silent arrhythmia (27,28). Its use should be selectively applied to patients with any contributory history for cardiovascular disease or cardiac abnormality revealed on history or physical examination. The discovery of a previously unrecognized infarction by electrocardiographic examination increases in women older than 55 years and in those patients with hypertension, diabetes mellitus, peripheral vascular disease, collagen vascular disease, or chronic pulmonary disease (29). Patients on medications associated with cardiac toxicity and electrocardiographic abnormalities, and with known hypokalemia also should have this test performed.

The preoperative chest x-ray cannot be justified in patients less than 60 years of age and who are without significant risk factors for pulmonary disease (30). Radiographic assessment is indicated in patients whose history, review of systems, and physical examination reveal cardiac or respiratory disease and cigarette smoking. More thorough evaluation by preoperative pulmonary function testing should be considered for patients with chronic pulmonary disease, a heavy smoking history, or significant obesity (31). If abnormal pulmonary function is identified, a set of baseline arterial blood gases should be drawn. Smokers should be urged to stop smoking as long as possible before surgery. Those with chronic pulmonary disease may benefit from the use of preoperative bronchodilators, antibiotics, and physical therapy.

Prevention of Deep Venous Thrombosis

All patients should be evaluated for the risk of developing deep venous thrombosis and subsequent thromboembolic complications. Deep venous thrombosis is a well-documented complication of abdominal and vaginal surgery, occurring in 10% to 20% of patients undergoing benign gynecologic surgery (32,33). Up to 50% of these patients will not demonstrate clinical signs or symptoms of thrombotic disease (34).

Patients undergoing surgery develop varying degrees of hypercoagulability, decreased fibrinolytic activity, and vascular stasis (35). Despite the expected improvement in venous return from elevating the patient's legs with stirrups and using Trendelenburg's position, the normal flow of blood is nevertheless altered by some degree of venostasis, creating the potential for the local accumulation of clotting factors. Deep thrombi begin in the veins of the calf and are well established during or immediately after surgery (32). While most of these clots will spontaneously resolve, some will inevitably spread to the popliteal, femoral, and iliac veins and go on to cause pulmonary embolism (33). As many as 40% of deaths after gynecologic surgery have been attributed to pulmonary emboli (32).

Certain patients are at higher risk of developing deep vein thrombosis. Significant historic factors include age over 40 years, obesity, extensive varicosities with demonstrable venous incompetence, longer operative procedures, and higher-dose oral contraceptives (11,36). Those at greatest risk have a history of prior pulmonary embolism, deep vein thrombosis, and malignancy (11). Ideally, all obese patients older than 40 years should be considered at significant risk for developing thromboembolic complications.

It is well established that the incidence of deep vein thrombosis after surgery in high-risk patient groups can be lowered by using several different prophylactic regimens. The preoperative use of low-dose heparin has been shown to successfully decrease the incidence of small calf vein thrombi, the frequency of proximal thrombi, and major pulmonary emboli (37,38). Heparin usually is administered subcutaneously in 5000-U aliquots 2 hours preoperatively and then every 12 hours until the patient has returned to normal levels of ambulation. When choosing this medication for prophylaxis, one must balance its prophylactic effects with its known association with increased intraoperative bleeding and postoperative hematoma formation (39). The protective effects of heparin may be increased by using it in combination with graduated compression stockings (40). Stockings should ideally be placed over the legs as the extremities are lowered out of the stirrups at the completion of surgery to increase the velocity of venous flow.

The use of intermittent external pneumatic compression has been shown to be as effective as prophylactic doses of heparin in reducing venous thrombosis (41,42). While the compression sleeves require extra time for setup in the operating roon and may make it more difficult to position larger legs into stirrups, this method is devoid of the hemorrhagic side effects associated with the use of heparin. The prevention of venous thrombosis by external pneumatic compression is not improved by the addition of prophylactic heparin (43).

Prophylactic Antibiotics

The incision of the superior vaginal tissues during laparoscopic hysterectomy introduces the endogenous bacterial flora from the lower genital tract into the peritoneal cavity. Although aggressive irrigation with hydrolavage and precise hemostasis can be accomplished laparoscopically, microbial invasion of the normally sterile intraperitoneal environment in the presence of blood, serum, suture material, and ischemic pedicles can result in infection. It is appropriate to manage a patient undergoing laparoscopic hysterectomy with the same well-established principles of prophylactic antibiotics that are applied during the performance of vaginal hysterectomy (44). The rate of infectious morbidity due to cuff infections, pelvic cellulitis, and adnexal abscess is significantly decreased by the administration of preoperative antibiotics to premenopausal women undergoing vaginal hysterectomy (45,46).

Successful antimicrobial prophylaxis is dependent on the properly timed preoperative administration of an agent that has broad antimicrobial activity against the gram-negative pathogenic flora of the lower genital tract, such as a first-generation cephalosporin. Presumably due to inadequate blood and tissue levels at the time of surgical incision, the rates of infection increase if the antibiotic is given more than 2 hours preoperatively (47). It is advisable to administer an additional dose of antibiotic if the operation lasts more than 3 hours or the blood loss exceeds 1000 mL.

Bowel Preparation

While inadvertent injury to the underlying viscera is an irreducible complication of laparoscopic surgery, it is more likely to occur in patients with a history of prior abdominal surgery, inflammatory bowel disease, extensive pelvic inflammatory disease, previously documented intra–abdominal adhesions to the viscera, or a fixed pelvic mass, or when severe endometriosis involves the cul-de-sac and paravaginal tissues. In these patients, mechanical preparation and chemoprophylaxis should be considered to minimize the consequences of luminal entry and subsequent peritoneal soiling.

Preparation of the bowel prior to laparoscopic surgery is multiphasic. The first phase is mechanical when the greater bulk of stool is removed from the colon. Diminished intestinal volume is generally desirable during laparoscopic surgery and should be considered for any patient undergoing laparoscopic hysterectomy. Colonic cleansing facilitates the mobilization of the bowel out of the pelvis, especially in obese patients, in whom large pericolic fat deposits can make repositioning of the bowel superiorly very difficult.

Until recently, the repeated use of enemas with purgatives and whole gut irrigation with saline or mannitol was routinely used for preoperative mechanical preparation of the bowel. These methods are cumbersome and may require preoperative hospitalization. They can create significant patient discomfort and have the potential for changing levels of serum electrolytes (48–50). A simplified, safe, effective, and well-tolerated method using a polyethylene glycol-electrolyte lavage solution of 4 liters of Golytely (Braintree Laboratories, Braintree, MA) has been demonstrated to be superior to other forms of mechanical preparation (51). When compared with traditional protocols using whole gut lavage, purgatives, and enemas, Golytely is better at eliminating air and fluid from the bowel without creating the intestinal fluxes of water and electrolytes. This solution also has been found to measurably reduce aerobic and anaerobic colonic bacteria (51). It is best administered the night before surgery after a clear liquid diet. The patient is instructed to drink 8 oz every 10 minutes until completed. Most patients will experience watery diarrhea within 1 hour of ingestion. Some will complain of abdominal fullness, bloating, and nausea, which may prevent complete ingestion of the entire 4 liters.

For patients at extremely high risk for luminal entry during laparoscopic dissection, preoperative administration of antibiotics should be seriously considered. This second phase of preoperative bowel preparation is either by the administration of enteric antibiotics to reduce residual luminal bacteria or by the prophylactic administration of parenteral antibiotics to inhibit the proliferation of bacteria introduced into the surrounding tissues at the time of luminal entry. Although risking the emergence of resistant bacterial flora in the bowel, chemoprophylaxis can be reliably established by orally administering both neomycin sulfate 1 gm and erythromycin base 1 gm at 1:00 PM, 2:00 PM, and 11:00 PM on the day before surgery (52). The parenteral administration of a single dose of antibiotic, given within 2 hours prior to surgery, is preferred by some physicians due to patient convenience, the reduced risk of developing resistant bacterial strains, and the assurance that a high tissue concentration of antibiotic will be present at the time of surgery. The administration of various cephalosporins, metronidazole, and doxycycline has been used for this purpose with varying levels of success (53–55).

POSTOPERATIVE CARE

When compared with abdominal hysterectomy, the laparoscopic approach should result in less postoperative morbidity and accelerated postoperative recovery. These benefits can be directly attributed to the elimination of the abdominal incision and to the technical advantages afforded by using the laparoscope to help complete the procedure vaginally. Hemostasis is more precisely achieved and intraoperative bleeding is minimized. The ureters can be clearly visualized throughout the procedure. The postoperative inflammatory cascade is truncated by the elimination of most suture materials, by efficient removal of clots and tissue debris, and by the reduction of pedicle size. After vaginal cuff closure, the laparoscope allows for direct visual inspection of each vascular pedicle, the sigmoid colon and rectum, the bladder, and the ureters. Nevertheless, these putative benefits will not prevent the negative consequences of poor judgement or misguided surgical techniques.

Despite all the practical and theoretical advantages of this approach, the potential for postoperative morbidity and mortality must not be underestimated. All patients should be considered at risk for postoperative complications associated both with hysterectomy and laparoscopy. Physician alertness must not fall prey to blinding emotions of elation and triumph after successfully converting abdominal to vaginal hysterectomy with the help of the laparoscope. As complications arise, it is extremely important to promptly initiate open communication with the patient and available family members. Frank discussion empowers the patient during this period of profound vulnerability and helps minimize future medicolegal conflict.

Postoperative morbidity is directly linked to the complex interplay between any preoperative risk factors, the patient's psychological preparation, the metabolic requirements of surgery, the course of the surgical procedure, the degree of meticulous surgical technique, and the effects of anesthesia. Ultimately, each patient's postoperative course will uniquely evolve. Most patients will successfully achieve a rapid postoperative recovery and be discharged within 24 to 36 hours after surgery. Apart from those who experience definable postoperative complications, some patients will inevitably fall behind during their early recovery process. Prolonged central effects from anesthesia, significant intolerance for pain, acute hypoestrogenism after surgical castration, and unmasked pre-existing psychological conditions may all contribute to this delay. In light of most patient's expectations for a rapid recovery, the physician must make every effort to be supportive and empathically allay feelings of guilt and personal failure.

Nausea and Gastrointestinal Problems

Postoperative nausea and vomiting commonly occur after laparoscopy (56). Patient safety may be threatened by aspiration of vomitus, and postoperative recovery is often delayed by the persistence of nausea.

The stimulation of the medullary vomiting center is multifactorial and associated with a number of diverse factors (57). Gastric distention from mask ventilation prior to endotracheal intubation and further enlargement of the gastric bubble from the use of nitrous oxide may induce vomiting. The insertion of an orogastric tube for removal of the gastric contents after intubation will effectively reduce these sequelae (58). Anesthetic agents and opioids sensitize the vestibular apparatus to motion. During the immediate postoperative period, gentle handling and slow movements while repositioning the patient will help minimize these effects. The use of adequate analgesia will help alleviate the well-recognized stimulation of the vomiting center by excessive pain. The prophylactic administration of antiemetics, such as droperidol, has been shown to effectively decrease postoperative nausea and vomiting (59). The preoperative use of transdermal scopolamine has been shown to be equally efficacious and to provide more prolonged relief (60).

Since manipulation of the bowel is usually minimal during laparoscopic hysterectomy, most patients can be expected to quickly regain normal intestinal function. Clear liquids can be offered to the patient as soon as her postoperative nausea has completely subsided. Further dietary advancement depends on the degree of intestinal manipulation during surgery, patient appetite, demonstrated comfort with initial oral intake, and normal findings on abdominal examination. Extensive laparoscopic dissection of bowel away from areas of severe endometriosis and densely adherent chronic inflammatory disease may delay this process.

Abdominal Pain

Any patient complaining of progressive abdominal pain postoperatively must be carefully evaluated for possible hemorrhage and injury to the underlying visceral structures and blood vessels. Early postoperative ileus associated with diffuse peritoneal signs, regardless of white blood cell count and temperature, may indicate peritoneal soiling from a significant luminal defect in the bowel. Postoperative ileus in the absence of significant peritoneal signs may forewarn the presence of ureteral injury, retroperitoneal hematoma, or early small bowel obstruction.

Injury to the superficial and inferior epigastric vessels often presents as localized abdominal wall pain associated with induration and swelling that grows asymmetrically. Spreading ecchymotic changes within the soft tissues and skin of the abdominal wall, mons pubis, labia majora, and flanks help reinforce the diagnosis of trauma to the inferior epigastric vessel. Similar findings may be seen after significant extraperitoneal injury to the bladder.

The constellation of increasing abdominal girth, worsening peritoneal signs, tachycardia, oliguria, and postural blood pressure changes are diagnostic for hemodynamically significant postoperative hemorrhage. On the other hand, retroperitoneal hemorrhage may evolve insidiously, first revealed by vexing complaints of progressive pressure in the rectum, lower back, and flanks.

Urinary Problems

A urinary catheter commonly is used intraoperatively to decompress the bladder and provide some reliable measure of central vascular perfusion. For uncomplicated cases, postoperative urinary drainage is elective. Aside from being a valuable indicator of postoperative intravascular volume, urinary drainage alleviates some of the physical discomfort and confusion experienced by many patients in the early phases of recovery from general anesthesia. On the other hand, early mobilization, if just having to reposition on a bedpan, can initiate a valuable cycle of physical and emotional recovery. The surgeon can use the same criteria he or she typically applies after uncomplicated vaginal hysterectomy.

Postoperative oliguria usually is indicative of hypovolemia. The patient should be evaluated for inadequate fluid replacement or signs and symptoms of postoperative hemorrhage. Anuria usually indicates a kinked or clotted urinary catheter. Rarely, absent urine can be the first telltale sign of bilateral ureteral injury or a large surgical injury to the bladder. While the laparoscopic approach to hysterectomy minimizes surgical manipulation of the bladder, postoperative bladder dysfunction will inevitably occur in some patients. This temporary arrest of detrusor and periurethral mechanics can result from anxiety, postoperative pain, trauma to the bladder and associated pelvic structures, reflex spasm of the levator ani, and hypotonia caused by analgesics and relaxants used during anesthesia. In some cases, the preoperative history will have identified the patient prone to postoperative urinary retention after laparoscopy. Urinary retention is more likely to occur with a history of voiding difficulties after prior surgeries or when the patient has preoperatively ingested medications that affect bladder contractibility and urethral closure dynamics, such as beta-adrenergic drugs, central nervous system depressants, pseudoephedrine, and parasympatholytics found in various cough remedies.

It is imperative to prevent overdistention of the urinary bladder after surgery. Inordinately high bladder volumes predispose to local infection and can result in prolonged hypotonia of the detrusor muscle. If postoperative voiding difficulties are encountered, attention should be paid to the adequacy of bladder emptying. If the measured residual volume is more than 100 mL on two separate occasions prior to discharge, the patient should be taught the technique of self-catheterization or sent home with a pediatric Foley catheter, which can be removed in several days during a follow-up office visit.

Cardiopulmonary Problems

Respiratory problems are frequently encountered during the postoperative period. While the absence of the abdominal incision virtually eliminates the adverse respiratory effects from voluntary and involuntary splinting, the combination of shallow breathing from narcotics or anesthetic agents and supine positioning predisposes any patient to develop postoperative respiratory complications. Inadequate ventilatory efforts during this period of time prevent complete filling of the alveolar spaces, resulting in various degrees of alveolar collapse. If left untreated, dependent areas of alveolar collapse will eventually shunt local circulation to better ventilated lung segments, worsening any mismatches in ventilation–perfusion (61). Furthermore, tenacious mucous secretions will be steadfastly deposited.

When clinically significant, patients developing pulmonary atelectasis present with fever, tachypnea, and tachycardia. Fever during the first 24 hours of postoperative recovery usually is due to this pulmonary complication. Examination reveals diminished breath sounds at the lung bases, and audible rales and tubular breath sounds. A chest x-ray film may demonstrate plate-like streaking and basilar densities sometimes associated with segmental or lobular collapse. Progression of this condition may lead to postoperative pneumonia (61).

The evolution of clinically significant atelectasis often can be prevented by promoting measures that encourage normal ventilatory efforts in the early postoperative period. Most patients undergoing laparoscopic hysterectomy will tolerate a rapid transition from supine to sitting position and early ambulation. The use of adequate amounts of postoperative analgesia will help ensure this process. Properly guided incentive spirometry and encouragement by the nursing staff for deep diaphragmatic breathing are extremely important for successful prophylaxis (62).

Rarely, acute changes in cardiopulmonary status will occur. The sudden onset of postoperative chest pain, hypoxia, tachycardia, and tachypnea should be treated as pulmonary embolus until proven otherwise. Early diagnosis and aggressive treatment with adequate doses of anticoagulants are crucial to reduce mortality. The occurrence of postoperative pulmonary edema reflects either iatrogenic fluid overload or left ventricular dysfunction. Evaluation by a central venous catheter, invasive cardiac monitoring, and a chest x-ray film will help identify the primary etiology. Sudden cardiovascular collapse in the recovery room may be the first and final sign of significant retroperitoneal hemorrhage from trocar injury to the large retroperitoneal vessels.

REFERENCES

1. Kelman GR, Swapp GH, Smith I, et al. Cardiac output and arterial blood-gas tension during laparoscopy. BMJ 1972;44:1155–1162.
2. Marshall RL, Jebson PJR, Davie IT, Scott DB. Circulatory effects of carbon dioxide insufflation of the peritoneal cavity for laparoscopy. Br J Anaesth 1972;44:680–684.
3. Lenz RJ, Thomas TA, Wilkins DG. Cardiovascular changes during laparoscopy. Studies of stroke volume and cardiac output using impedance cardiography. Anesthesia 1976;31:4–12.

4. Scott DB, Julian DG. Observations on cardiac arrhythmias during laparoscopy. BMJ 1972;1:411–413.

5. Price HL. Effects of carbon dioxide on the cardiovascular system. Anesthesiology 1960;21:652–663.

6. Ott DE. Laparoscopic hypothermia. J Laparoendosc Surg 1991;1:127–131.

7. Roe CF, Goldberg MJ, Blair CS, et al. The influence of body temperature on early postoperative oxygen consumption. Surgery 1966;60:85.

8. Bay J, Nunn JF, Prys-Roberts C. Factors influencing arterial PO_2 during recovery from anesthesia. Br J Anaesh 1966;40:398–401.

9. Alexander GD, Noe FE, Brown WM. Anesthesia for pelvic laparoscopy. Anesth Analg 1969;48:14–18.

10. Van DeWakes JM. Preoperative and postoperative techniques in the prevention of pulmonary complications. Surg Clin North Am 1980; 60:1339–1352.

11. Kakkar VV, Howe CT, Niicolaides AN, et al. Deep vein thrombosis of the leg. Am J Surg 1970;120:527–530.

12. Carter J, Dip RA, Fowler J, et al. How accurate is the pelvic examination as compared to transvaginal sonography? J Reprod Med 1994;39:32–34.

13. Tessler FN, Schiller VL, Perrella RR, et al. Transabdominal versus endovaginal pelvic sonography: prospective study. Radiology 1989; 170:553–556.

14. Leibman AJ, Kruse B, McSweeney MB. Transvaginal sonography: comparison with transabdominal sonography in the diagnosis of pelvic masses. Am J Roentgenol 1988;151:89–92.

15. Chang YCF, Hricak H. Current status of MR imaging of the female pelvis. Crit Rev Diagn Imaging 1989;29:337–356.

16. Gross BII, Moss AA, Mihara K, et al. Computed tomography of gynecologic diseases. Am J Roentgenol 1983;141:756–773.

17. Aslaksen A, Gothlin JH, Geitung JT, et al. Ultrasonography versus urography as preoperative investigation prior to hysterectomy. Acta Obstet Gynecol Scand 1989;68:443–445.

18. Robins JA, Mushlin AI. Preoperative evaluation of the healthy patient. Med Clin North Am 1979;63:1145–1157.

19. Kaplan EB, Sheiner LB, Boeckmann AJ, et al. The usefulness of preoperative laboratory screening. JAMA 1985;253:3576–3581.

20. Narr BJ, Hansen TR, Warner MA. Preoperative laboratory screening in healthy Mayo patients: cost-effective elimination of tests and unchanged outcomes. Mayo Clin Proc 1991;66:155–159.

21. Consensus Conference. Preoperative red blood cell transfusion. JAMA 1988;260:2700–2703.
22. Watson-Williams EJ. Hematologic and hemostatic considerations before surgery. Med Clin North Am 1979;63:1165–1188.
23. Giles JDS. Anaemia and anaesthesia. Br J Anaesth 1974;46:589–602.
24. Kowalyshyn TJ, Prager D, Young J. A review of the present status of preoperative hemoglobin requirements. Anesth Analg 1972;51:75–79.
25. Eisenberg JM, Clarke JR, Sussman SA. Prothrombin and partial thromboplastin times as preoperative screening tests. Arch Surg 1982;117: 48–51.
26. Burke GR, Gulyassy PF. Surgery in the patient with renal disease and related electrolyte disorders. Med Clin North Am 1979;63:1191–1201.
27. Goldberger AL, O'Konski M. Utility of the routine electrocardiogram before surgery and on general hospital admission. Ann Intern Med 1986;105:552–5567.
28. Moorman RJ, Hlatky MA, Eddy DM, et al. The yield of the routine admission electrocardiogram. Ann Intern Med 1985;103:590–596.
29. Rose SD, Corman LC, Mason DT. Cardiac risk factors in patients undergoing noncardiac surgery. Med Clin North Am 1979;63:1271–1287.
30. Rucker L, Frye EB, Staten MA. Usefulness of screening chest roentgenograms in preoperative patients. JAMA 1983;250:3209–3211.
31. Harman E, Lillington G. Pulmonary risk factors in surgery. Med Clin North Am 1979;63:1289–1298.
32. Bonnar J. Venous thromboembolism and gynecologic surgery. Clin Obstet Gynecol 1985;28:432–446.
33. Walsh JJ, Bonnar J, Wright FW. A study of pulmonary embolism and deep vein thrombosis after major gynecological surgery using labelled fibrinogen, phlebography and lung scanning. Br J Obstet Gynaecol 1974;81:311–316.
34. Flanc C, Kakkar W, Clarke MB. The detection of venous thrombosis of the legs using ^{125}I-labelled fibrogen. Br J Surg 1968;55:742–747.
35. Thomas DP. Venous thrombogenesis. Ann Rev Med 1985;36:39–50.
36. Clarke-Pearson DL, DeLong ER, Synan IS, et al. Variables associated with postoperative deep venous thrombosis: a prospective study of 411 gynecology patients and creation of a prognostic model. Obstet Gynecol 1987;69:146–150.

37. Kakkar VV, Corrigan T, Spindler J, et al. Efficacy of low doses of heparin in prevention of deep-vein thrombosis after major surgery: a double-blind, randomized trial. Lancet 1972;2:101–106.

38. Ballard RM, Bradley-Watson PJ, Johnstone FD, et al. Low doses of subcutaneous heparin in the prevention of deep vein thrombosis after gynecological surgery. Br J Obstet Gynaecol 1973;80:469–472.

39. Pachter HL, Riles TS. Low dose heparin: bleeding and wound complications in the surgical patient. Ann Surg 1977;186:669–673.

40. Turner GM, Brooks JH. The efficacy of graduated compression stockings in the prevention of deep vein thrombosis after major gynaecological surgery. Br J Obstet Gynaecol 1984;91:588–591.

41. Clarke-Pearson DL, Synan IS, Hinshaw WM, et al. Prevention of postoperative venous thromboembolism by external pneumatic calf compression in patients with gynecologic malignancy. Obstet Gynecol 1984;63:92–98.

42. Nicholaides AN, Fernandes E, Fernandes J, Pollock AV. Intermittent sequential pneumatic compression of the legs in the prevention of venous stasis and postoperative deep venous thrombosis. Surgery 1980;87:69–72.

43. Roberts VC, Cotton LT. Failure of low-dose heparin to improve efficacy of preoperative intermittent calf compression in preventing postoperative deep vein thrombosis. BMJ 1975;3:458–461.

44. Ledger WJ, Gee C, Lewis WP. Guidelines for antibiotic prophylaxis in gynecology. Am J Obstet Gynecol 1975;121:1038–1045.

45. Hemsell DL, Cunningham FG, Kappus S, Nobles B. Cefoxitin for prophylaxis in premenopausal women undergoing vaginal hysterectomy. Obstet Gynecol 1980;56:629–634.

46. Mendleson J, Portnoy J, DeSaint VJR, et al. Effect of single and multidose cephradine prophylaxis on infectious morbidity of vaginal hysterectomy. Obstet Gynecol 1979;53:31–35.

47. Classen DC, Evans RS, Pestotnik SL, et al. The timing of prophylactic administration of antibiotics and the risk of surgical-wound infection. N Engl J Med 1992;326:281–286.

48. Panton ONM, Atkinson KG, Crichton EP, et al. Mechanical preparation of the large bowel for elective surgery. Am J Surg 1985;149:615–619.

49. Mikal S. Metabolic effects of preoperative intestinal preparation. Am J Proctol 1965;16:437–442.

50. Minervini S, Alexander-Williams J, Donovan IA, et al. Comparison of three methods of whole bowel irrigation. Am J Surg 1980;140:400–402.

51. Fleites RA, Marshall JB, Eckhauser ML, et al. The efficacy of polyethylene glycol–electrolyte lavage solution versus traditional mechanical bowel preparation for elective colonic surgery: a randomized, prospective, blinded clinical trial. Surgery 1985;98:708–716.

52. Clarke JS, Condon RE, Bartlett JG. Preoperative oral antibiotics reduce septic complications of colon operations: results of prospective randomized double-blind clinical study. Ann Surg 1977;185:251–259.

53. Keighley MRB, Arabi Y, Alexander-Williams J, et al. Comparison between systematic and oral antimicrobial prophylaxis in colorectal surgery. Lancet 1979;2:894–897.

54. Solhaug JH, Bergman L, Kylberg F. A randomized evaluation of single dose chemoprophylaxis in elective colorectal surgery—A comparison between metronidazole and doxycycline. Ann Clin Res 1983;15:15–20.

55. Bell GA, Smith JA, Murphy J. Prophylactic antibiotics in elective colon surgery. Surgery 1983;93:204–208.

56. Metter SE, Kitz DS, Young ML, et al. Nausea and vomiting after outpatient laparoscopy: incidence, impact on recovery room stay and cost. Anesth Analg 1987;661:S116.

57. Dent SJ, Ramachandra V, Stephen CR. Postoperative vomiting: incidence, analysis and therapeutic measures in 3000 patients. Anesthesiology 1955;16:564–572.

58. McCarroll SM, Mori S, Bras PJ. The effect of gastric intubation and removal of gastric contents on the incidence of postoperative nausea and vomiting. Anesth Analg 1990;70:S262.

59. Wetchler BV, Collins IS, Jacob L. The antiemetic effect of droperidol on the ambulatory surgery patient. Anesth Rev 1982;9:23–26.

60. Bailey PL, Streisand JB, Pace NL, et al. Transdermal scopolamine reduces nausea and vomiting after outpatient laparoscopy. Anesthesiology 1990;72:977–980.

61. Bartlett RH. Pulmonary pathophysiology in surgical patients. Surg Clin North Am 1980;60:1323–1338.

62. Lewis FR. Management of atelectasis and pneumonia. Surg Clin North Am 1980;60:1391–1401.

7

Insufflation Needle and Trocar Insertion Techniques in Difficult Cases

Eric J. Bieber

G reat frustration may arise when beginning a laparoscopic procedure and difficulties are encountered with either insufflation and creation of a pneumoperitoneum or insertion of primary or ancillary trocars. A knowledge of multiple alternative techniques helps to minimize these experiences and facilitate endoscopic procedures.

This chapter will review the historic development of entry techniques and the anatomy associated with the regions of entry. Various techniques will be described, with special emphasis on the management of the difficult patient.

A HISTORIC PERSPECTIVE

Throughout the 1800s, multiple clinicians and scientists experimented with novel lens and light systems to improve the evaluation of various viscera. It was not until the beginning of the 20th century that the European physician Kelling demonstrated and reported on the use of a cystoscope to examine intraperitoneal organs in dogs (1). Kelling used a needle prior to trocar insertion, creating the pneumoperitoneum with air. While Kelling performed multiple procedures, little of this information was disseminated and no direct carryover to humans occurred.

The first documented use of an endoscope to perform "laparoscopy" in a human was reported in 1910 by Stockholm physician H.C. Jacobaeus (2). Interestingly, Jacobaeus used a direct insertion technique with no prior pneumoperitoneum.

In 1920, a radiologist from Chicago, B.H. Orndoff, was one of the first to report on peritoneoscopy in the American literature (3). He described pneumoperitoneum creation prior to trocar placement and considered this essential for safe performance of the procedure.

Similarly, from 1929 and for the next 30 years, the German-born physician H. Kalk reported novel endoscopic techniques, including use of a needle for creation of a pneumoperitoneum (4,5). Kalk also was one of the initial proponents of ancillary trocars.

One of the first textbooks on laparoscopy was published in 1959 by Frangenheim (6), who had previously discussed concerns about methodology for achieving pneumoperitoneum and difficulties encountered in achieving access in patients with previous surgery. Three decades later, similar concerns are voiced by many gynecologic endoscopists.

PREPARATION PRIOR TO NEEDLE OR TROCAR INSERTION

Prior to initiating surgery, multiple steps should be taken that may decrease potential complications and increase the ease of surgery. Prior to beginning cases, the patient should be placed in a modified dorsal lithotomy position while awake to assure that there are no abnormal pressure points and that she is comfortable. While many operating rooms continue to use "candy cane" stirrups for placement of the patient's legs, such devices will decrease the surgeon's mobility and ability to place trocars. We have found devices such as Allen stirrups (Allen Medical Systems, Inc, Mayfield, OH) to offer maximal flexibility and range of motion for the surgeon. In the difficult case, such as the obese patient, such measures are even more important.

The bladder should be emptied prior to the initiation of surgery either by having the patient void immediately prior to surgery, by insertion of a straight catheter, or by placement of an indwelling Foley catheter for the duration of the procedure. Various philosophies exist on which of these are preferential; individual choices may be based on the type and length of a proposed procedure.

Once the patient has undergone anesthesia, an oral gastric or nasogastric catheter is placed in all cases. Multiple case reports have documented the risk of gastric perforation and injury resulting from Veress needle and trocar insertion (7,8). Unfortunately, oral gastric tube placement has yet to become standard practice in most operating rooms.

Trendelenburg's position may decrease the distance between the site of entry and the sacral promontory with overlying great vessels. Because of this change, we prefer the patient to be supine or in limited Trendelenburg's position for initial trocar insertion. It should be noted that in thin patients there is an even smaller margin of safety. Once the initial trocar has been placed, maximum Trendelenburg's position will generally facilitate ancillary trocar placement in gynecologic surgery.

CREATION OF A PNEUMOPERITONEUM

The need for a pneumoperitoneum prior to trocar insertion is a hotly contested area of endoscopy. Some feel the establishment of a pneumoperitoneum is critical to most safely placing a trocar, while opponents of preinsertion insufflation argue that morbidity is not increased with direct trocar insertion. Ultimately, the practitioner must choose which methodology in a particular patient is most appropriate.

Generally, the umbilical or periumbilical area has been chosen for needle placement. The anatomy of this region demonstrates a decreased amount of subcutaneous and preperitoneal tissue in most patients.

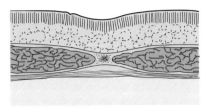

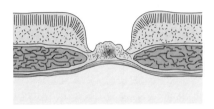

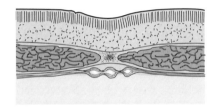

Three tissue cuts are demonstrated: cephalad to the umbilicus, through the umbilicus and caudad to the umbilicus. The diminution of tissue at the level of the umbilicus may inherently predispose this region to subsequent hernia formation.

Figure 7.1 demonstrates the tissue changes as the anatomic plane is advanced from cephalad to caudad of the umbilicus. It is the lack of significant tissue, especially fascia, that allows an optimal portal of entry but that is also predisposed to hernia formation.

The tissue may be stabilized by grasping with towel clips or lifting with the hands. However, it has been suggested that this does little to lift the important structures, such as the fascia or peritoneum, and only increases the distance that must be traversed prior to entry. The needle is opened to air so that on entry into the peritoneal cavity (which has a baseline negative pressure), air will flow into the cavity, allowing under-lying structures to fall away. In most instances, the needle is directed at an oblique angle toward the uterine fundus and away from the sacral promontory and great vessels. Care must be taken to avoid angling laterally toward the iliac vessels.

Once the needle is believed to be intraperitoneal, a syringe is used (1) to aspirate and check for return of blood or fecal matter and (2) to inject 10 to 20 mL of air or saline. If no air or fluid is returned, insufflation at a slow rate is begun. Should air or fluid be returned into the syringe, it is likely that misplacement of the needle has occurred preperitoneally or into a viscus. The needle is removed and the proce-dure repeated. At the time of insufflation, initial pressure readings are checked. Pressures lower than 7 to 8 mm Hg are compatible with intraperitoneal placement. Higher pressures might again indicate a malpositioned needle. It is best to stop at this point and reposition the needle rather than pressing forward and ending with a substantial preperitoneal insufflation that may markedly distort the anatomy. The abdomen is checked for tympany and distention during insufflation to assure an even spread of CO_2.

ALTERNATIVE SITES FOR VERESS NEEDLE INSERTION

Posterior Cul-de-sac

The posterior cul-de-sac is an excellent alternative site for Veress needle insufflation. At the Chicago Lying-in Hospital, this technique has been successfully used and taught by Dr Luis Cibils over the last 25 years. Cibils' mentor, Dr Raoul Palmer from France, routinely used the posterior cul-de-sac as an alternative to umbilical and periumbilical entry (9).

Ansari reported in the American literature the successful establish-ment of a pneumoperitoneum in 37 of 40 cases attempted (10). Others have reported similar success, including Neely et al, who routinely used the transvaginal approach (11) and found limited contraindications, including cul-de-sac obliteration, fixed retroversion, or previous vaginal vault surgery. Additional limitations include severe cervical or vaginal infections or a history of significant pelvic inflammatory disease. Neely et al reported entry difficulty in only four of 107 cases, and interestingly found extraperitoneal insufflation in several of the cases in which entry was not achieved. Mintz reported on the routine use of the cul-de-sac as an entry portal only after the initial examination under anesthesia demonstrated it to be free (12); this occurred in 80% of the cases in this series.

The technique for insertion via the pouch of Douglas is relatively simple. After placement of a weighted speculum and visualization of the cervix, the cervix is grasped with a tenaculum, a uterine elevator is placed, and the uterus is lifted anteriorly. A long Veress needle is useful in traversing the extra length. The cul-de-sac region is visualized by the traction on the cervix and the weighted speculum. Once the mucosa is taut over this area, the Veress needle is placed approximately 1 cm below the insertion of the vagina into the cervix. If properly performed, the Veress needle should readily pass through the thin tissues (which should be no more than 1 to 1.5 cm).

As with any entry technique into the peritoneal cavity, the needle is left open to room air. Aspiration/irrigation are performed and intraperitoneal pressures are checked. As suggested by Neely et al, the needle may be placed preperitoneally even with a transvaginal approach (11). Thus, if higher than expected pressures are seen, it is better to replace the needle.

Left Upper Quadrant

The left upper quadrant also has been used as an alternative site for Veress needle placement (13). We have previously reported on the use of this region for successful placement of both the Veress needle and 5-mm trocars (14). Cadavaric dissections have demonstrated the anatomic differences that exist between the left upper quadrant and the umbilicus. The Veress needle often will need to traverse both the anterior and posterior fascia prior to piercing the peritoneum.

The technique for left upper quadrant needle placement includes the previously discussed preparations and must include oral or nasogastric

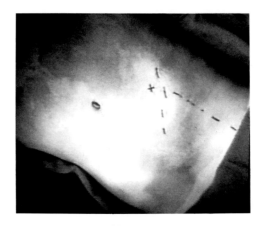

FIGURE 7.2

Localization for correct needle placement in the left upper quadrant. After identification of the midaxillary line, a line is drawn approximately 2 cm below the costal margin.

tube placement. The patient is positioned in a level position with little or no Trendelenburg's positioning. Prior to placement, the patient's spleen has to be palpated and noted not to be enlarged. A line is then drawn from the midclavicular point approximately 2 cm below the left costal margin (Fig 7.2). The needle, which is open to air, is then placed in the vertical position. It is relatively easy to sense the layers, as they tend to be better developed and more taut than at the umbilicus. Following placement, routine checks are made. At this level, the superior epigastric vessels begin to course more medially. Care should be taken to avoid pushing the needle medially or laterally, where epigastric vessel or splenic injury might occur. Contraindications to this approach include previous left upper quadrant surgery, splenomegaly, idiopathic thrombocytic purpura, or thrombocytic thrombotic purpura.

Impaling the Uterus

Several techniques have used the relatively safe position of the uterus in the pelvic cavity to aid in peritoneal entry with the Veress needle. Morgan used the Veress needle to pass through the cervical os, the endometrial canal, and the uterine fundus into the peritoneal cavity (15).

112   Laparoscopic Hysterectomy and Pelvic Floor Reconstruction

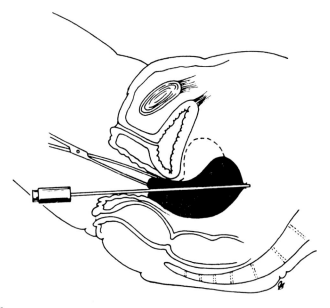

FIGURE 7.3

Transuterine insufflation. (Reprinted with permission from The American College of Obstetricians and Gynecologists. Wolf WM, Pasic R. Transuterine insertion of Veress needle in laparoscopy. Obstetrics and Gynecology, 1990;75:456–457.)

In 1500 cases he noted no complications with this novel transuterine technique. More recently, Wolfe and Pasic used a similar approach in difficult patients (Fig 7.3) (16). Their series of 100 patients comprised 86 who were defined as obese, with a body mass index (weight [kg]/height [m]^2) of more than 30, and 14 in whom a transabdominal attempt had been unsuccessful. In only two cases was there failure to achieve access. Wolfe and Pasic noted no significant intraoperative or follow-up complications.

The technique for transfundal Veress needle insufflation includes preoperative cervical cultures. The patient is placed in moderate Trendelenburg's position and a tenaculum is applied. A uterine sound may be used to ascertain uterine length and position, and may be left in place to guide the Veress needle. The uterus is anteverted during insertion. Following intraperitoneal placement, routine checks are performed. Contraindications include patients at risk for bowel adhesions to the uterus, those with a history of significant pelvic inflammatory disease, the presence of uterine fibroids, and patients undergoing infertility investigations since chromotubation may be difficult to perform.

OPEN LAPAROSCOPY

Open laparoscopy was developed as an alternative to blind entry and involves a layer-by-layer dissection down to the peritoneum. Harrith Hasson, the originator of this technique, first reported his series in 1971 (17). Hasson believed that by performing a "mini" laparotomy, in which all layers are exposed prior to incision, complications might be reduced. Multiple reports over the intervening years have demonstrated the ease with which open laparoscopy may be mastered and performed by surgeons of all skill levels (18).

It remains unclear whether complications are reduced by the performance of open laparoscopy (19). Critics maintain that the 1- to 1.5-cm incision made for an open laparoscopy is inadequate to allow and facilitate surgery in the difficult patient and cite references demonstrating similar rates of complications. These issues notwithstanding, all surgeons should be familiar with the technique of open laparoscopy should the occasion arise.

DIRECT TROCAR INSERTION

Review of the history of endoscopy reveals direct trocar insertion dating to endoscopy's infancy. This technique was abandoned in favor of pneumoperitoneum creation prior to trocar entry until 1978, when Dingfelder reported a series of patients undergoing trocar insertion without a prior pneumoperitoneum (20). Dingfelder suggested that some of the complications associated with the use of needles, such as preperitoneal insufflation, could be alleviated by direct trocar insertion techniques without increasing the morbidity of the procedure. Various investigators have subsequently published similar retrospective reviews of their cases (21–28).

Most recently, Byron et al reported a randomized comparison of Veress needle versus direct trocar insertion in 252 patients (29). There were no major complications in either arm of their study. These investigators noted seven cases of preperitoneal insufflation in the needle group versus one case in the direct application group. There was a statistically significant decrease in operative times with direct trocar insertion, although total operative time differed by less than 5 minutes. There also was a statistically significant increase in minor complications (preperitoneal insufflation, more than three attempts at entry, or failed entry) in the needle insertion group.

The technical aspects of direct trocar insertion are similar to Veress needle placement. One hand may be used to elevate the abdomen while the dominant hand is used to place the 10-mm trocar in a turning motion. As with the Veress needle, the trocar is pointed obliquely toward the uterus in the midline. Once placed, the laparoscope is placed to assure intraperitoneal entry prior to beginning insufflation.

DIFFICULTIES WITH NEEDLE AND TROCAR PLACEMENT

Preperitoneal Insufflation

Even in the most experienced hands, placement of the Veress needle is sometimes difficult. It cannot be stressed enough that if one does not believe they are intraperitoneal, either through the tactile sensation of entry, confirmation by the multiple syringe tests, or confirmation of insufflation pressures, it is much better to start over. Invariably, as the residency year begins, the following scenario occurs. The needle is placed by the junior resident, confirmation of placement cannot be made, and gas is insufflated. Pressures very quickly increase to more than 12 mm Hg. Unfortunately, by the time the problem is recognized, 1 to 2 liters of CO_2 may now be resting in the preperitoneal space. To make the situation even more difficult, this classically occurs in the obese patient, in whom all miscues are accentuated.

When the preperitoneal space expands from insufflation, the Veress needle will need to traverse an even greater distance prior to entry. Often, the laxity of the peritoneum that occurs as the peritoneum separates from the attached tissues makes piercing with the needle on subsequent attempts even more difficult.

Once this has occurred, several alternatives exist. Transvaginal placement of the Veress needle through the posterior cul-de-sac may be easily performed in a majority of patients. Once an adequate pneumoperitoneum has been established, the underlying pressure on the peritoneum will give adequate tension to allow placement of a 5- or 10-mm umbilical trocar. The left upper quadrant also may be used once preperitoneal insufflation has occurred. Unlike the umbilicus, where there is a greater degree of tissue flexibility, the left upper quadrant area is relatively immobile. It is near this point where the rectus muscle has insertions to the costal margin. This fixes the underlying peritoneum and may facilitate placement of the Veress needle or trocar even when a substantial amount of CO_2 has entered the periumbilical preperitoneal space.

An additional option would be the performance of an open laparoscopy. Although the tissue planes may be more difficult to dissect, this usually may be accomplished.

Kabukoba and Skillern reported using extraperitoneal insufflation to directly visualize Veress needle placement (30). When preperitoneal insufflation is recognized, instead of being removed the laparoscope is left in place and advanced 4 cm from the symphysis pubis. The Veress needle is then introduced suprapubically and, under direct visualization, is stabbed through the peritoneum. Kabukoba and Skillern found the technique to be successful in 11 consecutive patients (Fig 7.4).

The Patient With Previous Surgery

One of the classic relative contraindications to laparoscopy has been the patient with previous surgery. Because of the blind entry of the Veress needle or trocar, there has been appropriate concern regarding the risk of injury to an adherent underlying viscous in patients with previous abdominal surgery. Several studies have evaluated the risk of adhesions

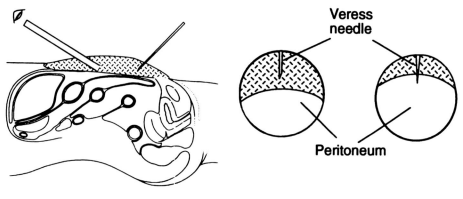

Veress needle

Peritoneum

FIGURE 7.4

(A) Extraperitoneal insufflation with the laparoscope and Veress needle in place. (B) Left view: the Veress needle through the laparoscope before insertion through the peritoneum. Right view: rising peritoneum and diminished extraperitoneal space following puncture of the peritoneum. (Reprinted with permission from The American College of Obstetricians and Gynecologists. Kabukoba JJ, Skillern LH. Coping with extraperitoneal insufflation during laparoscopy: a new technique. Obstetrics and Gynecology, 1992;80:144–145.)

based on the type of incision. Childers et al noted that 28 of 41 (68%) patients with a previous midline incision had anterior abdominal wall adhesions (31). Their cohort was composed of a number of patients who had undergone gynecologic oncologic procedures.

Levrant et al evaluated a nononcologic group and found that 59% of patients with a previous midline incision had significant anterior abdominal wall adhesions (32), compared with a 28% incidence of adhesions in a group of patients with a previous suprapubic transverse incision. In the collective group of patients, 96% of adhesions involved omentum and 28% involved bowel. In a group of 45 patients who had undergone previous laparoscopy and 91 patients with no previous surgery, no anterior abdominal wall adhesions were present.

In contrast to the studies of Childers et al and Levrant et al, Kaali and Bartafi reported direct trocar insertion in 416 women with a history of previous laparotomy (24). These investigators found an overall incidence of pelvic and abdominal adhesions of 11% of 1670 women undergoing laparoscopy, but no significant anterior abdominal wall adhesion in the higher risk group of 416 patients. These data suggest that appropriate caution is warranted in placing trocars in patients with previous surgery.

Several methods have been described to decrease the potential for viscous injury in the high-risk patient. Palmer advocated a syringe test prior to placement of the primary trocar (9). A spinal needle attached to a fluid-filled syringe may be placed in the same region as the primary trocar would be placed. If fluid or enteric contents were to be reaspirated after injection, underlying bowel or a loculated area of tissue may be present. The step is repeated until a free area has been located.

We have found placement of a 5-mm trocar in the left upper quadrant (in the same orientation as with the Veress needle) to be very useful in patients with previous surgery (14). This region tends to be adhesion free, even in patients with multiple surgeries. Contraindications exist for trocar placement in the left upper quadrant similar to those for Veress needle placement. The left upper quadrant also may be useful in cases in which large masses are present, filling the pelvis. In these cases, periumbilical placement of a primary trocar decreases visualization and will make operative cases difficult. In a similar fashion, for the patient with anterior wall adhesions, a decision can be made to either work around the adhesions or, if necessary, to lyse them, allowing safe placement of an umbilical trocar. In our own series, we often found this unnecessary and worked without difficulty through the 5-mm laparoscope in the left upper quadrant.

Childers et al found similar success with this technique in their high-risk population (31). In their series of patients, Childers et al noted that umbilical placement of a Veress needle or trocar would have resulted in bowel injury. They instead reported only one enterotomy in their group of extremely high-risk patients.

Reich suggested the use of the ninth intercostal space for needle and trocar placement (33). Hulka and Reich also noted that this region provides an excellent "panoramic view" in patients with potential for adhesions, and may be especially appropriate to check umbilical trocar placement and perform adhesiolysis if injury cannot be ruled out (34).

The Obese Patient

Obesity has been considered a relative contraindication to laparoscopy for decades. Unfortunately, the increased morbidity of laparotomy in such patients makes the performance of laparoscopy very appealing.

The evaluation of obesity may best be defined by the Quetelet index, also called the body mass index, which incorporates weight and height into the equation weight/height^2. Most clinicians are aware that taller patients will have a greater area in which to distribute their weight (35). In addition, patients may have great variability as to where fat deposits are concentrated (i.e., panniculus, thighs, buttocks, etc). This may markedly effect the successful performance of laparoscopy.

Loffer and Pent were two of the initial investigators to report difficulties in the obese patient (35) and suggested that the 45-degree angle routinely used to place a Veress needle at the umbilicus would often cause the needle to course through preperitoneal tissues and be unable to enter the peritoneal cavity. They instead recommended that both the Veress needle and trocar be placed at a 90-degree angle. Loffer and Pent were able to successfully perform laparoscopy in all of the 49 patients in their series weighing more than 200 pounds.

Hurd et al most recently evaluated 33 women by magnetic resonance imaging or computed tomography (36). Using sagittal views, they evaluated the relationship of increasing body mass index to the amount of tissue surrounding the umbilicus. Four specific distances were evaluated. point A, from the lower margin of the umbilicus to the anterior peritoneum at an angle 45 degrees from the horizontal (this is the standard insertion orientation that we and others have recommended); point B, from the base of the umbilicus at an angle 45 degrees to the peritoneum; point C, from the umbilical base to the peritoneum at a 90-degree angle; and point D, from the base of the umbilicus to the great vessels at a 90-degree angle (Fig 7.5). Patients were then stratified according to a body mass index less than 25 (normal), between 25 to 30 (overweight), and greater than 30 (obese). In their judgment, this roughly corresponded to weight ranges of less than 160 pounds (<73 kg) for their control group, 160 to 200 pounds (73 to 91 kg) for the

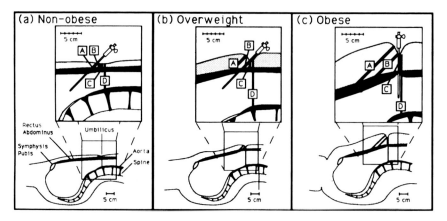

FIGURE **7.5**

Diagram of typical sagittal views from non-obese, overweight, and obese patients. A typical 11.5-cm Veress needle has been superimposed on each view for comparison. (Reproduced by permission from Hurd WH, Bude RO, Delancey JOL, et al. Abdominal wall characterization with magnetic resonance imaging and computed tomography: the effect of obesity on the laparoscopic approach. J Reprod Med 1991;36:473–476.)

overweight group, and over 200 pounds (>91 kg) for the obese group.

The results of this study are presented in Table 7.1. For the group of patients with a body mass index less than 25 (not overweight), the average A and B distances were 3 and 2 cm, respectively, with the distance to the aorta or vena cava being only 6 cm. This demonstrates why caution must be exercised when one places a standard 11.5-cm Veress needle. In evaluating the obese patients, the average length for distances A and B were greater than 16 cm and 12 cm, respectively, demonstrating the difficulty of achieving access with even an elongated needle when using an angle less than 90 degrees from the horizontal. It is of note that the average distance from the umbilicus to the aorta was 10 cm in the overweight group and 13 cm in the obese group.

Based on these results, Hurd et al concluded that it may be necessary to place Veress needles and trocars perpendicular through the base of the umbilicus to avoid preperitoneal insufflation (36). In overweight

TABLE 7.1

Comparison of distances between groups

GROUP	N	DISTANCE (cm)			
		A	B	C	D
		(LOWER MARGIN, 45°)	(BASE, 45°)	(BASE, 90°)	(UMBILICUS TO AORTA)
Nonobese	14	3 ± 2	2 ± 2[a]	2 ± 1[a]	6 ± 3
Overweight	9	6 ± 3	3 ± 2[a]	2 ± 1[a]	10 ± 2
Obese	10	>16 (M)[b]	12 (M)[ab]	4 ± 2[ab]	13 ± 4[b]

Data shown as mean ± SD or as median (M) where indicated.
[a] Versus distance A, $P < 0.01$ with the two-tailed Wilcoxon signed-rank test.
[b] Versus nonobese or overweight, $P < 0.05$ with the two-tailed Mann-Whitney U test.
Reproduced by permission from Hurd WH, Bude RO, Delancey JOL, et al. Abdominal wall characterization with magnetic resonance imaging and computed tomography: the effect of obesity on the laparoscopic approach. J Reprod Med 1991;36:473–476.

patients, they recommend the use of a 45-degree angle through the base instead of through the lower margin of the umbilicus.

In another study of interest, Toth and Graf reported placement of the Veress needle and trocar through the center of the umbilicus (37). They noted no episodes of false passage or preperitoneal emphysema in their series of 217 patients. While this report noted no postoperative hernia formation, we have had a case of omental herniation through a midumbilical trocar site. Loffer and Pent discourage placement of trocars through this site because of these same concerns (35).

Alternative sites for insufflation in obese patients include transfundal, posterior cul-de-sac, left upper quadrant, and open laparoscopy. Unfortunately, gaining access to create a pneumoperitoneum does not obviate the latter difficulties of trocar placement.

In selected patients, we have found placement of the 5-mm trocar in the left upper quadrant to be effective. Occasionally, patients will have "central obesity," in which there is a marked increase in tissue at or near the umbilicus to the lower pelvis but thinner tissue near the costal margin. In such cases, left upper quadrant placement of both the Veress needle and trocar may be performed more easily than at the level of the umbilicus.

The Patient With Previous Umbilical Surgery

Our studies demonstrate a very low risk for adhesions secondary to laparoscopy (32). This may be secondary to the limited closure or lack of peritoneal suturing in most cases.

The risk for patients with a previous umbilical hernia repair to undergo laparoscopy are less well defined. These cases may be especially difficult, since many are performed in infancy and often the clinician may believe that a subumbilical scar is secondary to a previous laparoscopy, when in fact it is the result of a remote hernia repair. Kaali and Bartafi noted no significant adhesions in 17 patients with previous herniotomy (24). In contrast, Bieber and Levrant found significant adhesions in seven of eight patients with a history of previous umbilical hernia repair (38). Using the left upper quadrant for both Veress needle and trocar placement allowed injury to be successfully avoided in this group of patients.

CONCLUSIONS

All endoscopic surgeons must be well versed in a multitude of entry techniques. Constant attention to detail, a thorough understanding of the endoscopic equipment, and knowledge of anatomy are critical to facilitate surgery. Nowhere is this more apparent than in the difficult patient. Endoscopists have discussed these issues in the literature and at meetings since the turn of the century. As we enter the 21st century, the goal remains the same: to safely enter the peritoneal cavity and provide the most efficacious surgery possible.

REFERENCES

1. Kelling G. Ueber Oesophagoskopie, Gastroskopie und Coelioskopie. Muench Med Wochenschr 1902;49:21.
2. Jacobaeus HC. Ueber die Moeglichkeit die Zystoskopie bei Untersuchung seroeser hoehlungen anzuwenden. Muench Med Wochenschr 1910;57: 2090–2092.

3. Orndoff BH. The peritoneoscope in diagnosis of diseases of the abdomen. J Radiol 1920;1:307–315.

4. Kalk H. Erfahrungen mit der Laparoskopie. Z Klin Med 1929;111: 303.

5. Kalk H, Lehrbuch WE. Und Atlas der Laparoskopie und leberpunktion. Stuttgart: Georg Thieme, 1962.

6. Frangenheim H. Die Laparoskopie und die Culdoskopie in der Gynaëkologie. Stuttgart: Georg Thieme, 1959.

7. Reynolds RC, Pauca A. Gastric perforation—an anesthesia induced hazard in laparoscopy. Anesthesiology 1973;38:84–85.

8. Ender GC, Moghissi KS. Gastric perforation during pelvic laparoscopy. Obstet Gynecol 1976:47(suppl 41):40–42.

9. Palmer R. Les explorations fonctionelles gyneologiques. Paris: Masson, 1963.

10. Ansari AH. The cul-de-cac approach to induction of pneumo-peritoneum for pelvic laparoscopy and pneumography. Fertil Steril 1970; 21:599–605.

11. Neely MR, McWilliams R, Makhlouf HA. Laparoscopy: routine pneumoperitoneum via the posterior fornix. Obstet Gynecol 1975;45:459–460.

12. Mintz M. Risks and prophylaxis in laparoscopy: a survey of 100,000 cases. J Reprod Med 1977;18:269–272.

13. Palmer R. Instrumentation et technique de la Celioscopie gyneologique. Gynecol Obstet (Paris) 1947;46:420–431.

14. Bieber EJ, Shangold G, Barnes RB. Closed laparoscopy through left upper quadrant access in patients with previous surgery. Fertil Steril 1991;suppl S139:48. Abstract.

15. Morgan HR. Laparoscopy: induction of pneumoperitoneum via transfundal puncture. Obstet Gynecol 1979;54:260–261.

16. Wolf WM, Pasic R. Transuterine insertion of Veress needle in laparoscopy. Obstet Gynecol 1990;75:456–457.

17. Hasson HM. Modified instrument and method for laparoscopy. Am J Obstet Gynecol 1971;110:886–887.

18. Hasson HM. Open laparoscopy: a report of 150 cases. J Reprod Med 1974;12:234–238.

19. Penfield AJ. How to prevent complications of open laparoscopy. J Reprod Med 1985;30:660–663.

20. Dingfelder JR. Direct laparoscope trocar insertion without prior pneumoperitoneum. J Reprod Med 1978;21:45–47.

21. Copeland C, Wing R, Hulka JF. Direct trocar insertion at laparoscopy: an evaluation. Obstet Gyneol 1983;62:656–659.

22. Pine S, Barke JI, Barna P. Insertion of the laparoscopic trocar without the use of carbon dioxide gas. Contraception 1983;28:233–239.

23. Saidi MH. Direct laparoscopy without prior pneumoperitoneum. J Reprod Med 1986;31:684–686.

24. Kaali SG, Bartafi G. Direct insertion of the laparoscopic trocar after an earlier laparotomy. J Reprod Med 1988;33:739–740.

25. Byron JW, Fujiyoshi CA, Miyazawa K. Evaluation of the direct trocar insertion technique at laparoscopy: Obstet Gynecol 1989;74:423–425.

26. Borgatta L, Gruss L, Barad P, Kaali SG. Direct trocar insertion vs Veress needle use for laparoscopic sterilization. J Reprod Med 1990;35:890–894.

27. Jarrett JC. Laparoscopy: direct trocar insertion without pneumo-peritoneum. Obstet Gynecol 1990;75:725–727.

28. Nezhat FR, Silfen S, Evans D, Nezhat C. Comparison of direct insertion of disposable and standard reusable laparoscopic trocars and previous pneumoperitoneum with Veress needle. Obstet Gynecol 1991;78:148–149.

29. Byron JW, Markenson G, Miyazawa K. A randomized comparison of Veress needle and direct trocar insertion for laparoscopy surgery. Surg Gynecol Obstet 1993;177:259–262.

30. Kabukoba JJ, Skillern LH. Coping with extraperitoneal insufflation during laparoscopy: a new technique. Obstet Gynecol 1992;80:144–145.

31. Childers JM, Brzechffa PR, Surwitt EA. Laparoscopy using the left upper quadrant as the primary trocar site. Gynecol Oncol 1993;50:221–225.

32. Levrant SG, Bieber EJ, Barnes RBB. Previous laparotomy or laparoscopy and the prevalence of anterior abdominal wall adhesions. Submitted for publication.

33. Reich H. Laparoscopic bowel injury. Surg Laparosc Endosc 1992;2:74–78.

34. Hulka J, Reich H, eds. Textbook of laparoscopy. Philadelphia: WB Saunders, 1994:9–101.

35. Loffer FD, Pent D. Laparoscopy in the obese patient. Am J Obstet Gynecol 1976;125:104–107.

36. Hurd WH, Bude RO, Delancey JOL, et al. Abdominal wall characterization with magnetic resonance imaging and computed tomography: the effect of obesity on the laparoscopic approach. J Reprod Med 1991;36:473–476.

37. Toth A, Graf M. The center of the umbilicus as the Veress needle's entry site for laparoscopy. J Reprod Med 1984;29:126–128.
38. Bieber EJ, Levrant S. The risk of anterior abdominal wall adhesions in patients with previous umbilical hernia repair. J Am Assoc Gynecol Laparoendosc 1994;1:54.

8

Identification and Dissection of the Pelvic Ureter

C.Y. Liu
Nicholas Kadar

E very gynecologist will encounter ureteral injury at some point during their practice. Ureteral injury occurs in 0.5% to 1.5% of all traditional gynecologic surgeries. The incidence of ureteral injury in gynecologic laparoscopic surgery is unknown at this time, although it is believed to be somewhat higher than that of traditional surgery. As gynecologists become more proficient in operative laparoscopy, the incidence of ureteral injury should diminish to a level comparable to or below that of traditional surgery. Ureteral injury seems most likely to occur in patients with distorted pelvic anatomy who are undergoing complicated gynecologic procedures, but studies reveal that most ureteral injuries occur during simple routine gynecologic surgeries, such as an uncomplicated hysterectomy.

It is more common to injure the ureter during a hysterectomy using the abdominal approach rather than the vaginal approach. This could be due to the possibility that surgeons performing routine pelvic surgeries develop a false sense of security and become neglectful of the fundamental techniques and surgical principles for avoiding ureteral injury. With rapid expansion in the field of operative laparoscopy, gynecologists are performing more video-guided surgeries, which provide better visibility of the operative field. However, there are two disadvantages to such surgeries: there is a loss of depth perception in the operative field and the surgeon is not able to palpate the various structures with his or her own fingers. Therefore, it is imperative that the surgeon has a thorough knowledge of the pelvic anatomy and strictly adheres to the fundamental principles and techniques that can prevent ureteral injury.

Only one third of ureteral injuries are detected during surgery, yet intraoperative recognition and treatment of ureteral injury is critical to prevent compromising renal function. Every pelvic surgeon must be skilled in identifying and, if necessary, dissecting the entire pelvic ureter. *Identification and dissection of the ureter is an acquired skill; as with any other type of surgery, this skill can be obtained by practice.* By routinely identifying the ureter in all pelvic surgeries, the surgeon will gain the confidence and experience that is required to deal with difficult situations as they arise. Because a surgeon who is familiar with all anatomic structures that might be encountered at an operation is best able to appreciate the distortions produced by disease and take advantage of the natural planes of cleavage when present, a thorough knowledge of the anatomy of the pelvis is crucial. In difficult pelvic surgery, the ureteral identification and dissection will almost always require a retroperitoneal approach. With a precise knowledge of the different fascial planes and various avascular spaces, the surgeon can perform a neat, effortless operation with a minimum of bleeding and intraoperative complications. The retroperitoneal anatomy and dissection are described in detail in Chapter 2.

With advanced video technology for laparoscopic surgery, the pelvic structures can be clearly magnified onto a television monitor, allowing visualization of microscopic details. The positive intra-abdominal pressure exerted against the peritoneum during laparoscopy pushes the peritoneum against the underlying ureter, resulting in remarkable visualization of a prominent ureter.

ANATOMY OF A URETER

The ureters vary between 25 and 30 cm in length, depending on the height of the individual. The abdominal and pelvic components are approximately equal in length. Following a straight, almost perpendicular line from the real pelvis to the pelvic brim, the ureters lie on the anterior surface of the psoas muscles. They are attached to the undersurface of the posterior parietal peritoneum, moving with the peritoneum when this is elevated. In their abdominal course, the right and left ureters are located approximately 4 to 5 cm lateral to the inferior vena cava and the aorta, respectively (Fig 8.1).

Approximately halfway between the pelvic inlet and the renal pelvis, the ovarian vessels cross the abdominal ureters, the left one at a higher level than the right, and laterally to them at the pelvic brim (Fig 8.1). At this point, the ovarian vessels enter the infundibulopelvic liga-

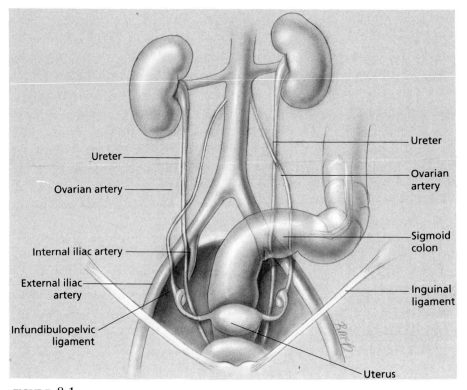

FIGURE 8.1

Retroperitoneal relationship of the ureter. (Reproduced by permission from Kadar N. Atlas of laparoscopic pelvic surgery. Boston: Blackwell Science, 1995:65.)

ment, then cross the ureters again, lying first above them and then medially to them as they run medially in the roof of the broad ligament from the pelvic brim to the ovaries. This anatomic relationship is significant because the ureter cannot be damaged if the pelvic side wall peritoneum is incised lateral to the anatomic position of the infundibulopelvic ligament. In addition, the infundibulopelvic ligament must be retracted medially to expose the ureter at the pelvic brim and on the medial leaf of the broad ligament.

THE PELVIC URETER

The ureters cross the iliac vessels as they enter the pelvic brim. The right ureter almost always crosses the external iliac artery, whereas the left ureter, lying closer to the midline, crosses the common iliac artery. On crossing the pelvic brim, the ureters run retroperitoneally along the lateral pelvic wall in close relationship to the internal iliac vessels and their tributaries. Throughout their pelvic course the ureters lie in a connective tissue sheath that is attached to the medial leaf of the broad ligament. Clear visibility is notable through the peritoneum until the ureter enters the region of the *ureteric canal*. At this point, the uterine artery crosses above the ureter and the dense cardinal ligament lies below it (Fig 8.2), obstructing visibility. The distance between the ureter and the cervix at the level of the ureteric canal is approximately 1.5 cm (Fig 8.3). After the ureter has passed through this canal, it continues forward anteriorly, passing onto the anterior vaginal fornix and entering the trigonal region of the bladder (Fig 8.4). The ureter actually lies closer to the cervix and vagina after it passes the ureteric canal, lying almost entirely in direct contact with the anterior vaginal wall. Within its loose areola sheath, the ureter is not fixed to the surrounding cardinal ligament. Spontaneous peristalsis is thus allowed, propelling the urine through this lumen. Although this is one of the most common sites of ureteral injury during gynecologic surgery, this loose areola sheath forms a convenient cleavage plane for use as a reference point when dissection of the ureter is required in this area.

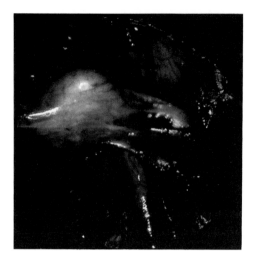

FIGURE 8.2

Ureter at the ureteric canal where the uterine artery crosses above the ureter and dense cardinal ligament lies below it.

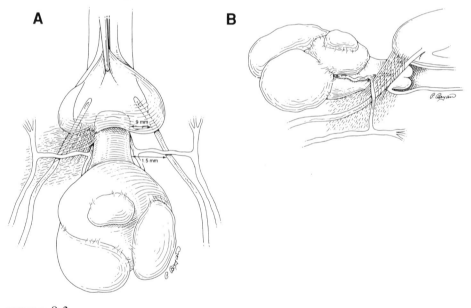

A

B

9 mm

1.5 mm

FIGURE 8.3

Relationship of the ureter to the cervix. (A) The distance between the ureter and the cervix at the level of ureteric canal is approximately 1.5 cm, which becomes 0.9 cm when the ureter is at the anterior vaginal fornix. (B) The relationship is shown between the ureter and the bladder pillar.

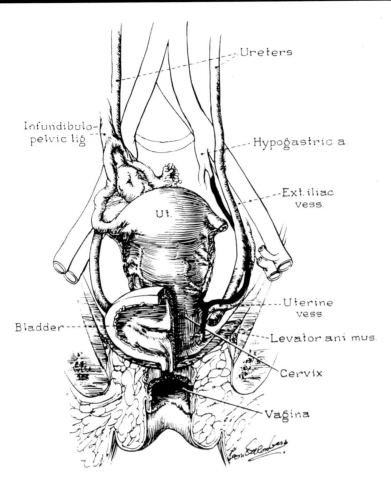

Ureters

Infundibulo-
pelvic lig.

Hypogastric a.

Ext. iliac
vess.

Ut.

Uterine
vess.

Bladder

Levator ani mus.

Cervix

Vagina

FIGURE 8.4

Normal anatomy of the ureters and their relationship to other pelvic organs encountered in gynecologic surgery. (Reproduced by permission from Wharton LR. In: Ridley JH, ed. Gynecologic surgery: errors, safegards, salvage. 2nd ed. Baltimore: Williams & Wilkins, 1981.)

The wall of the ureter consists of three distinct layers. The inner layer is comprised of transitional epithelium, the middle layer consists of circular and longitudinal smooth muscle fibers, and the outer layer is an adventitial sheath. Direct abrasion of the adventitial and muscular

Identification and Dissection of the Pelvic Ureter   131

layers of the ureter must be avoided during dissection as it may compromise the blood supply, resulting in ureteral stricture or fistula formation.

CONDITIONS REQUIRING URETERAL DISSECTION

Ureteral identification and dissection should be done in the face of any pelvic distorion, including extensive pelvic endometriosis, large ovarian and paraovarian cysts, cervical fibroids, pelvic inflammatory disease, and congenital anomalies. Any of these disease processes can increase the possibility of ureteral injury. This situation can be especially dangerous when there are pelvic masses expanding into the pelvic side wall, displacing the ureter's usual anatomic location. It may be pushed onto the anterior, posterior, medial, or lateral surface of the mass, with potential for injury during the resection of the mass. To prevent this from occurring, the surgeon must first identify the ureter, and only then proceed with the resection of the mass. With cases of severe endometriosis that involve the pelvic side walls and in cases of pelvic inflammatory disease, the pelvic peritoneum usually becomes thickened, rendering identification of the ureter by direct visualization impossible for the surgeon. These conditions require retroperitoneal dissection of the ureter. Once the ureter has been identified and dissected out, the surgeon can proceed with confidence, excising all pathologies while maintaining direct visualization of the ureter.

SURGICAL INJURIES TO THE URETER

From its anatomy, it should be evident that the ureter is particularly vulnerable to injury during pelvic surgery at three particular points: 1) at the pelvic brim as the infundibulopelvic ligament is being divided (vulnerability of the ureter increases with proximity of the division of infundibulopelvic ligament to the pelvic brim), 2) at the ovarian fossa, especially during resection of ovaries or ovarian remnants that are bound to the pelvic side wall by adhesions, and 3) lateral to the cervix during division or coagulation of the uterine artery, the uterosacral ligament, or the cardinal ligament, especially in the presence of endometriosis or pelvic inflammatory disease.

TECHNIQUE OF LAPAROSCOPIC
URETERAL DISSECTION

Laparoscopic surgery, with its magnified view of the pelvic structures, provides positive intraperitoneal pressure that pushes the covering peritoneum over the ureter. This makes ureteral identification much easier, especially at the point immediately after it has crossed the pelvic brim. Because the mesentery of the sigmoid colon often obscures the course of the left ureter, the right ureter is easier to identify. Visualization of the left ureter may necessitate separating the sigmoid colon from the pelvic wall and reflecting it medially. The ureter usually can be seen above the internal iliac artery near the pelvic brim, crossing the internal iliac artery as it turns medially toward the deep pelvis before reaching the ureteric canal in the region of the ovarian fossa.

Uncomplicated Ureteral Dissection

The purposes for performing simple uncomplicated ureteral dissection include first, ensuring that the ureteral locations are normal prior to hysterectomy (conditions that produce fibrosis and scarring in the cul-de-sac and pelvic side walls, such as endometriosis, previous pelvic inflammatory disease, and previous uterosacral ligament resection or plication, can pull the ureters closer to the cervix and the uterosacral ligaments); second, allowing visualization of the ureters throughout the entire hysterectomy procedure; and third, providing the pelvic surgeon with experience and confidence in handling the ureter.

Because the ureter is most easily identified at the level of the pelvic brim, ureteral identification should always start here. By lifting the tube and ovary anteriorly and upward away from the pelvic wall, the ovarian fossa is exposed and the ureter and its characteristic peristalsis can be

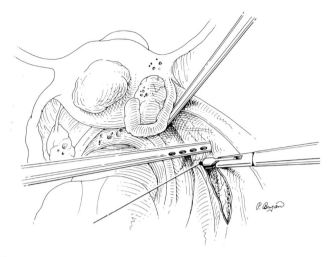

The peritoneum covering the ureter is opened with the CO_2 laser.

easily seen. The peritoneum covering the ureter is opened with scissors or laser (Fig 8.5). After this exposure is achieved, the blunt end of an atraumatic grasping forceps is used to gently tease the surrounding tissue away from the ureter (Plate 4). As the peritoneum covering the ureter continues to be opened, the ureter is dissected downward toward the deep pelvis.

The ureter is usually dissected down to the level of the ureteric canal where the uterine artery crosses the ureter, with the dense cardinal ligament lying below (Fig. 8.2). It is important to remember that under normal conditions, the ureter is surrounded by loose areolar tissue, which allows it to move freely and without restriction. This cleavage plane should be used to separate the ureter from adjacent structures to avoid injuring the ureter itself, dissecting in such a way that the ureter's blood supply is not compromised. Direct abrasion of the adventitia and muscular layers of the ureter can lead to troublesome bleeding, with overenthusiastic efforts to stop this bleeding resulting in compromising the blood supply, which could result in ureteral stricture or fistula formation.

Ureteral Dissection in the Presence of Cervical Fibroid and/or Adnexal Mass

With distortion of pelvic anatomy by such conditions as cervical fibroid or ovarian mass, the ureter may be displaced by lateral expansion. Particularly in these situations, it is crucial to visualize the entire course of the ureter relating to the mass. Initially, the ureter is identified cranially to the pelvic mass and dissected caudally towards it. Under direct visualization of the ureter, the pelvic mass is then dissected away from the pelvic wall. As the pelvic mass is peeled away from the pelvic side wall, the ureter is dissected further down caudally, continuing until the ureter is completely free of the mass. Ureteral dissection will frequently be required to go beyond the ureteric canal. Blunt-tip atraumatic forceps are most suited for this type of dissection. While carefully spreading the tip of the forceps inside the ureteric canal, the uterine artery is gently separated away from the ureter with the enlarging of the ureteric canal. The uterine artery is then ligated with suture or desiccated with a bipolar electrosurgical set and then divided to unroof the ureter (Plate 5). The process of coagulating and dividing the tissue above the ureter should be continued until the anatomy is clearly defined. With direct visualization of the ureter, the pelvic masses can then be excised. Large ovarian cysts may need to be decompressed, while a large myoma may need to be enucleated to improve the exposure of the operative field.

Ureteral Dissection in the Presence of Extensive Tubo-ovarian Endometriosis or Abscess

In cases of extensive ovarian endometriosis with tissues adhering tightly to the pelvic side wall, or with pelvic inflammatory disease involving tubo-ovarian abscess, the peritoneum covering the pelvic side wall may become so thickened that it is impossible to visualize the underlying ureter. The ureter then has to be identified and dissected out at a point directly on or above the pelvic brim. As the peritoneum covering the ureter is opened caudally and the ureter exposed, the tubo-ovarian complex can be dissected away from the pelvic side wall under direct visualization of the ureter. If a salpingo-oophorectomy is to be performed, the infundibulopelvic ligament can be desiccated or suture ligated and divided under direct visualization of the ureter.

Alternately, the retroperitoneal spaces can be opened and the ureter identified and dissected without peeling off the broad ligament for its entire pelvic course to be visible. The technique of retroperitoneal dissection is described below.

Retroperitoneal Dissection

Retroperitoneal dissection can be performed by first placing the peritoneum of the pelvic side wall on tension, with the uterus pushing upward and toward the contralateral side. The triangle of the pelvic side wall can be delineated and the peritoneum in the middle of the triangle opened longitudinally parallel to the external iliac vessels between the round ligament and the infundibulopelvic ligament. (The base of the triangle is the round ligament, the lateral border is the external iliac artery, and the medial border is the infundibulopelvic ligament; see Chapter 2.) The peritoneal incision is extended first to the round ligament, which is not divided at this time, and then toward and beyond the apex of the triangle, lateral to the infundibulopelvic ligament (Fig 8.6A), until the ligament has been sufficiently mobilized to allow it to be retracted

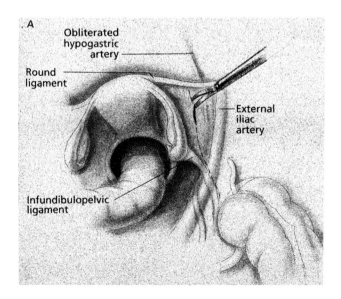

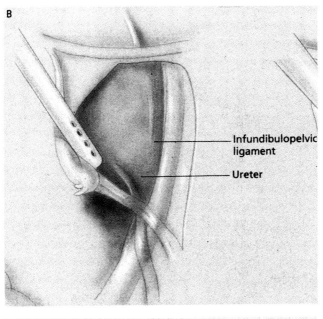

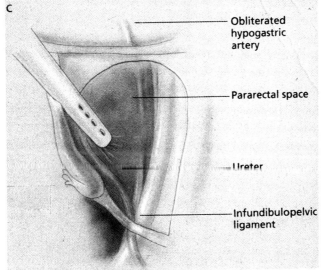

◀ FIGURE 8.6

(A) The peritoneum of the pelvic side wall triangle is opened to gain access to the retroperitoneum. (B) The infundibulopelvic ligament is mobilized and pulled medially to expose the ureter at the pelvic brim. (C) The pararectal space is opened by blunt dissection against the ureter in a medial direction. (Reproduced by permission from Kadar N. Atlas of laparoscopic pelvic surgery. Boston: Blackwell Science, 1995:68–69.)

medially, exposing the ureter at the pelvic brim (Fig. 8.6B,C). As this peritoneal incision is made, it is important not to displace the infundibulopelvic ligament from its anatomic position before the peritoneal incision is completed. If this displacement occurs, the natural anatomic relationship between the ureter and the infundibulopelvic ligament, which serves to protect the ureter from injury as it lies medial to this ligament, will be lost. The retroperitoneal dissections can then be performed as described below:

Step 1: The Ureter Is Identified at the Apex of the Pelvic Triangle: Using grasping forceps, the infundibulopelvic ligament is pulled medially to expose the ureter at the pelvic brim, at the point where it crosses the common or external iliac artery, a crucial step. It may be necessary to reflect the ureter off the medial leaf of the broad ligament for a short distance to aid its identification, although this is rarely required.

It is important to mobilize the infundibulopelvic ligament adequately to retract its proximal end sufficiently medially to expose the ureter at the pelvic brim. Failure to achieve adequate mobilization of the infundibulopelvic ligament is the most common error in carrying out dissection. The operator then searches for the ureter distal to the pelvic brim and lateral to the infundibulopelvic ligament, but frequently fails to find it because the ureter is covered at that point by fatty areolar tissue or, more distally, by the infundibulopelvic ligament itself, and cannot be seen except in especially thin patients. This error stems from the fact that the peritoneal incision has to be extended much further proximally than is required in an open case, frequently to the caecum on the right and the descending colon in the paracolic gutter on the left.

The dissection of the apex is more difficult on the left side, partly because the ureter is covered by the mesentery of the sigmoid colon, but especially because it crosses the iliac vessels higher (more proximally) and consequently lies more medially than the right ureter. As a result, it is more difficult to expose the left ureter by retracting the infundibulopelvic ligament medially. The peritoneal incision frequently has to be extended to the white line in the paracolic gutter to mobilize the sigmoid colon, and with it the infundibulopelvic ligament, which at this point lies extraperitoneally, under the mesentery. It also is frequently necessary to mobilize the medial leaf of the broad ligament from the pelvic brim and sacrum. To do this, the operator must dissect bluntly in a medial direction under the infundibulopelvic ligament, taking care not to perforate the medial leaf of the broad ligament or the right plane of dissection will be lost. Finally, the operator needs to be aware that the external iliac artery will be below the plane of dissection much of the time.

Step 2: The Obliterated Hypogastric Arteries are Identified Extraperitoneally: The dissection is carried bluntly underneath and caudad to the round ligament, until the obliterated hypogastric artery is identified extraperitoneally (Fig 8.7). Although the anatomy will be

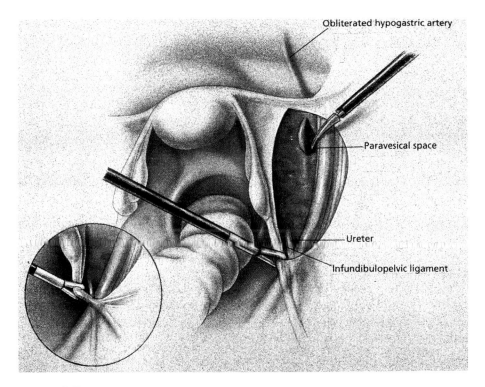

FIGURE 8.7

The obliterated hypogastric artery is identified extraperitoneally. (Reproduced by permission from Kadar N. Atlas of laparoscopic pelvic surgery. Boston: Blackwell Science, 1995:71.)

unfamiliar to most general gynecologists, this step is actually the most straightforward part of the dissection. If any difficulty is encountered, the artery should first be identified intraperitoneally where it hangs from the anterior abdominal wall, and then traced proximally to where it passes behind the round ligament. With both its intraperitoneal portion and the dissected space under the round ligament in view, the intraperitoneal portion of the ligament should be moved back and forth. It will almost always be possible to detect corresponding movements in the extraperitoneal portion of the ligament.

Step 3: The Paravesical Spaces Are Developed: Once the obliterated hypogastric arteries have been identified extraperitoneally, it is a simple matter to develop the paravesical space by bluntly separating the areolar tissue on either side of the artery. The dissection is started laterally to the artery, mindful that the external iliac vein is located laterally to this. The tips of the closed dissecting scissors are placed against the lateral edge of the artery and the artery is simply pulled medially, whereupon a bloodless plane will open laterally to this (see Fig 2.9). The medial border of the artery is then freed in an identical manner, but working in the opposite direction. During this maneuver the operator must take care not to press on the external iliac vein as the artery is displaced laterally (Fig 8.8). Ideally, dissection will be performed mostly medially, against the bladder, while the umbilical ligament is held fixed and deviated slightly laterally.

Step 4: The Pararectal Spaces Are Developed: The obliterated hypogastric arteries are next traced proximally to where they are joined by the uterine arteries, and the pararectal spaces are opened by blunt dissection proximal and medial to the uterine vessels, which lie on top of the cardinal ligaments. Once the pararectal spaces have been opened, the ureter on the ipsilateral side is easily identified on the medial leaf of the broad ligament, which forms the medial border of the space. The internal iliac artery on its lateral border also becomes clearly visible at this stage (see Fig 2.10).

We commonly use this technique of identification and dissection of the ureter when dealing with a markedly distorted pelvis.

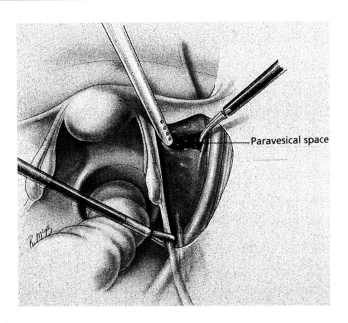

Paravesical space

FIGURE 8.8

The medial paravesical space is opened. (Reproduced by permission from Kadar N. Atlas of Laparoscopic pelvic surgery. Boston: Blackwell Science, 1995:72.)

RECOGNITION OF URETERAL INJURY

Ureteral injury needs to be recognized as early as possible, preferably before the patient leaves the operating room. Prompt repair of any ureteral damage is crucial if severe complications of renal damage and infection are to be prevented. The technique of ureteral identification and dissection in various gynecologic conditions has been described, but despite all precautions, ureteral damage can still occur. Any difficult pelvic surgery should prompt the surgeon to look for possible ureteral injury, even though no obvious sign of damage may have been recognized. A difficult ureteral dissection involving resection of infiltrating fibrotic endometriosis or scar tissue on or around the ureter are prime examples that the integrity of the ureter should be confirmed before concluding the surgery.

Whenever there is doubt about the possibility of ureteral injury, or when any pelvic surgery is especially difficult, we routinely perform a cystoscopic examination. Five milliliters of indigo carmine dye along with 10 to 20 mg of furosemide (Lasix [Hoechest-Roussel, Summerville, NJ]) is administered intravenously prior to cystoscopic examination. Within 5 to 10 minutes, the indigo carmine dye can be seen spurting out of ureteral orifices (Fig 8.9), thus assuring the patency of the ureter or ureters. Ureteral obstruction or injury is suspected if no dye effuses from the ureteral orifice within 15 minutes of the dye injection. A 6- or 8-Fr pediatric feeding tube or a small 4- or 5-Fr whistle-tip ureteral catheter can be used to pass up the ureter in retrograde fashion. If the catheter can be easily inserted up to the renal pelvis and there is free drainage of urine from the catheter, obstruction can be ruled out. It is crucial that urine comes out of the catheter, for it is possible to pass a catheter without resistance through a defect in the ureteral wall and deflect into the retroperitoneal space. If resistance is met or if the location of the catheter is uncertain, a retrograde pyelogram can be performed by injecting the contrast medium dye through the catheter.

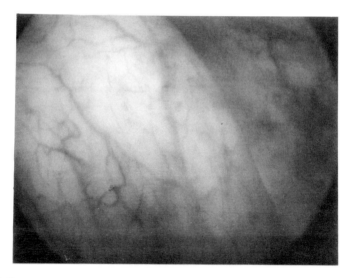

FIGURE 8.9

Cystoscopic view. Indigo carmine dye is seen ejecting out of the ureteral orifice.

An x-ray can then be used to determine the exact location of the obstruction.

Several different types of ureteral damage can occur during laparoscopic surgery. The ureter can have various degrees of laceration or thermal injury, be kinked, ligated, stapled, or even totally transected. If the wall of the ureter has been lacerated, the decision must be made as to whether this laceration can be repaired. If thermal injury has occurred, the decision must be made whether to treat conservatively. In both of the above cases, if the injury is too serious, the damaged area should be excised and ureteral reanastomosis or reimplantation performed. The ureteral kink or ligation can usually be relieved by removing the sutures; however, stapler injuries, such as ENDO-GIA (United States Surgical Corp, Norwalk, CT) or Lineal Cutter (Ethicon Endosurgery, Cincinnati, OH), are more difficult to handle because of the difficulty in removing the closed staples from the ureter. The completely transected ureter must be reanastomosed or reimplanted. Before attempting to repair any ureteral injury, one must be very cautious about one's own ability and experience with repairing an injured ureter through either a laparoscope or open surgery. Unless the surgeon is very knowledgeable and experienced in evaluating and managing such injuries, intraoperative consultation with an experienced urologist is advisable.

SUMMARY

With improved laparoscopic instrumentation and advanced video technology, the pelvic structures can be greatly magnified onto a high-resolution television monitor in minute detail. This facilitates proper identification of tissue planes and blood vessels and provides a neat, bloodless dissection for the identification of the ureter. Laparoscopic ureteral identification and dissection are acquired skills. Gynecologists who are interested in performing operative laparoscopy are encouraged to learn and practice ureteral identification and dissection, beginning with uncomplicated cases with clear anatomy. The skills obtained in identifying and dissecting the ureter under simple conditions will be invaluable when the anatomy is distorted by disease. Routine confirmation of the integrity of the lower urinary tract system prior to the conclusion of every difficult pelvic surgery is crucial in recognizing ureteral injury. If proper training and precautions are taken, injury to the ureter during laparoscopic surgery should rarely occur, and any injuries that do occur will be recognized and treated promptly before the patient leaves the operating room, thereby reducing the likelihood of long-term damage.

SUGGESTED READINGS

Beland G. Early treatment of ureteral injuries found after gynecological surgery. J Urol 1977;118:25.

Brudenell M. The pelvic ureter. Proc R Soc Med 1977;70:188–190.

Everett S, Mattingly RF. Urinary tract injuries resulting from pelvic surgery. Am J Obstet Gynecol 1956;71:502–507.

Gomel V, James C. Intraoperative management of ureteral injury during operative laparoscopy. Fertil Steril 1991;55:416–419.

Grainger DA, Soderstrom RM, Schiff SF, et al. Ureteral injuries at laparoscopy: insights into diagnosis, management and prevention. Obstet Gynecol 1990;75:839–843.

Hautrey CE. Surgical anatomy. In: Buschbaum HJ, Schmidt JD, eds. Gynecologic and obstetric urology. Philadelphia: WB Saunders, 1982:26–31.

Kadar N. Atlas of laparoscopic pelvic surgery. Boston: Blackwell Science, 1995.

Kane C, Drouin P. Obstructive uropathy associated with endometriosis. Am J Obstet Gynecol 1985;151:207–211.

Langmade CF. Pelvic endometriosis and ureteral obstruction. Am J Obstet Gynecol 1975;122:463–469.

Moore JG, Hibbard LT, Growdon WA, et al. Urinary tract endometriosis: enigmas in diagnosis and management. Am J Obstet Gynecol 1979;134:162–172.

St Lezin MA, Stoller ML. Surgical ureteral injuries. Urology 1991;38:497–506.

Symmonds RE. Ureteral injuries associated with gynecologic surgery: prevention and management. Clin Obstet Gynecol 1976;19:623–644.

Winslow PH, Kreger R, Ebbesson B, Oster E. Conservative management of electrical injury of ureter secondary to laparoscopy. Urology 1986;27: 60–62.

Witters S, Cornelissen J, Vereecken R. Iatrogenic ureteral injury: aggressive or conservative treatment. Am J Obstet Gynecol 1986;155:582.

PART TWO

Laparoscopic Hysterectomy

9

Laparoscopic-Assisted Vaginal Hysterectomy

D. Alan Johns

HISTORY

Since reports of the first laparoscopic hysterectomy by Reich et al in 1989 (1), the role of the laparoscope during hysterectomy has been radically redefined. Procedures ranging from total (and supracervical) laparoscopic hysterectomy to laparoscopical-assisted vaginal hysterectomy (LAVH) (2–5) have been described, and recently more unusual combined endoscopic/vaginal procedures (laparoscopic supracervical hysterectomy) (6) have been promoted.

Laparoscopical-assisted vaginal hysterectomy has been widely accepted in the medical community, but is only now being scientifically evaluated. Data on indications, contraindications, complications, cost-effectiveness, and outcomes of this relatively new approach will ultimately prove (or disprove) its worth, but LAVH likely will forever change the gynecologist's surgical approach to hysterectomy.

SURGEON PREREQUISITES

Laparoscopic techniques are required only when traditional vaginal hysterectomy would otherwise be impossible. This implies that the vaginal portion of the operation may be unusually challenging, even after the laparoscopic procedures have been completed. If the surgeon is not skilled and experienced in vaginal surgery, alternatives for vaginal completion of the procedure are limited. Conversely, the skilled vaginal surgeon with limited experience in operative laparoscopy will find the laparoscopic portion of the LAVH to be extremely time-consuming and frustrating. In either case, extended operative time and increased complications will likely result. Neither benefits the patient.

To safely and efficiently complete the LAVH, which would have otherwise required laparotomy, the surgeon must be experienced in both vaginal surgery and advanced operative laparoscopy. Previous experience in laparoscopic oophorectomy, adhesiolysis, and excisional techniques for endometriosis are mandatory, since adnexal masses, pelvic adhesive disease, and endometriosis are the most common indications for LAVH. The surgeon who is comfortable with laparoscopic treatment of extensive pelvic adhesive disease, endometriosis, and adnexal masses will be able to apply those skills to expand the indications for vaginal hysterectomy without significantly increasing complications or changing outcomes.

The ultimate cost of any surgical procedure is of increasing concern to all physicians. The laparoscopic surgeon who is able to take advantage of the most inexpensive techniques and technology to complete the appropriate surgical procedure in the shortest possible time with optimal outcomes and minimal complications will provide the most cost-effective care for his or her patients. It is therefore extremely important that the laparoscopic surgeon be familiar with multiple energy sources (electrosurgery, laser), techniques for hemostasis (sutures, staples, etc), and equipment (reusable, disposable, hybrid). The clinical situation can then dictate the most cost-efficient method for completion of the procedure. Given the multitude of options for completing an LAVH, cost and outcome considerations of each option must be carefully considered.

PATIENT SELECTION

Laparoscopic-assisted vaginal hysterectomy is not an acceptable substitute for vaginal hysterectomy. It is more expensive than simple vaginal hysterectomy, requires more operative time (2,5,7–9), and adds the risks inherent in trochar insertion to a relatively uncomplicated procedure. There is no evidence to date that LAVH decreases the incidence of postoperative bleeding or infection compared with simple vaginal hysterectomy. Although it may be reassuring to visually examine the pelvis following hysterectomy (as the laparoscope allows), there is no evidence that this offers any benefit to the patient sufficient to offset the risk of trochar insertion.

Because there is such variation in surgical skill and expertise between gynecologic surgeons, there will never be accepted contraindications to vaginal hysterectomy applicable to all gynecologists (10). Based on training and experience, each gynecologist must therefore determine which patients can safely undergo vaginal hysterectomy in his or her practice. Those patients whom the surgeon determines should undergo abdominal hysterectomy (for benign disease) based on his or her skill and experience become candidates for LAVH.

The gynecologist who is uncomfortable performing vaginal hysterectomy should not, however, view the laparoscope as a means to overcome deficiencies in vaginal surgery training. Laparoscopic techniques add to the capabilities of the vaginal surgeon; they do not replace them.

The most common indications for abdominal hysterectomy include pelvic pain of unknown etiology, uterine myoma, adnexal mass, endometriosis, and "minimal uterine mobility." The laparoscope allows an accurate diagnosis to be made in patients complaining of pelvic pain, but vaginal hysterectomy is rarely contraindicated once the diagnosis is known (11). Similarly, laparoscopic evaluation of adnexal masses often yields a diagnosis, allowing simple vaginal hysterectomy to be completed. Extensive laparoscopic surgery is often required however, to allow vaginal completion of the hysterectomy in the patient with adhesive disease, endometriosis, and large (>400 gm) myomatous uteri. The patient with "minimal uterine mobility" or a very small diameter vagina may be an ideal candidate for LAVH, but may be one of the few patients requiring total laparoscopic hysterectomy. These cases should be undertaken only by the most experienced endoscopic surgeons.

The patient found to be a candidate for LAVH must be thoroughly counseled concerning the potential benefits of the procedure as well as the risks. This discussion should include the risks and benefits of abdominal hysterectomy, allowing the patient to determine whether the risks unique to LAVH are offset by its advantages over abdominal hysterectomy.

EQUIPMENT

Equipment for all laparoscopic surgery should be simple, easy to use, clean and sterilized, inexpensive, and reusable. Unfortunately, it is difficult to sort through the bewildering array of available laparoscopic equipment to find the ideal instruments. Since the image on the video monitor is the surgeon's "eye," it is imperative that the best possible image be created. Once the laparoscopic surgeon is comfortable operating while watching the monitor (rather than looking directly through the laparoscope), assistants and operating room personnel are better able to assist and anticipate needs. Prolonged surgical cases are less tiring and the surgeon can take full advantage of the magnifying capabilities of the laparoscope. With all support personnel able to view the procedure with equal ease, the efficiency of the operating room is maximized.

The optimal video image requires the best available light source, laparoscope, camera, and monitor. This should be the first priority of the endoscopic surgeon. Inferior or outdated video equipment often produce blurry images on the television monitor. Operating under these circumstances would be equivalent to performing a laparotomy while wearing eyewear with opaque lenses. No surgeon would consider continuing a procedure under such conditions, yet endoscopic surgery is often attempted via a blurred image on a monitor.

Once an adequate video system is available, most other laparoscopic equipment is determined by the surgeon's preference. For LAVH using electrosurgical techniques, few instruments are required. Mandatory instruments include two 5-mm trochars, one 10-mm trochar, one irrigation/dissection probe, laparoscopic scissors, grasping forceps, and bipolar electrosurgical forceps (Fig 9.1). To minimize cost, all should be reus-

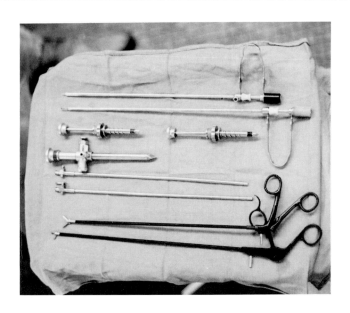

FIGURE 9.1

The basic set of reusable laparoscopic instruments necessary to complete most LAVH procedures.

able. An irrigation/suction control system is very helpful. Optional equipment includes unipolar electrosurgical scissors and needles, laparoscopic needle holders, a knot "pusher," and dissecting instruments. When deep, nodular endometriosis is encountered, the CO_2 laser offers distinct advantages in excision of these lesions prior to vaginal hysterectomy.

Continuous irrigation clears the operative field of blood and debris. "Aquadissection" (irrigation fluid passed through a dissection/irrigation probe under minimal pressure) aids in identification of tissue planes. If a nonelectrolyte solution is used for these purposes, electrosurgical instruments can be used in conjunction with the irrigation, since nonelectrolyte solutions will not interfere with electron flow. These solutions are also considerably less expensive than isotonic or buffered electrolyte solutions (12).

Stapling devices are available, but must be passed through 12-mm trochar sleeves and are expensive. Although these devices *may* shorten operative time, it is doubtful this will offset their cost. Their size

Laparoscopic–Assisted Vaginal Hysterectomy   153

(12 mm) often is a distinct disadvantage when dealing with large uteri. The surgeon should be familiar with all options for hemostasis (staples, sutures, and electrosurgery), and use the most efficient technique for the clinical situation.

TECHNIQUE

Prior to beginning the procedure, the patient should be optimally positioned for laparoscopic surgery. The arms should be tucked at the patient's sides and the legs should be positioned such that the thigh is level with the abdominal wall. The legs must be well supported with minimal pressure on the knee. After insertion of the umbilical trochar, the table is placed in full Trendelenburg's position. Shoulder braces may result in brachial plexus nerve injury and are unnecessary. The operating table should be lowered such that the surgeon's arms are at a comfortable level for operating. Commonly, the operating table is raised (rather than lowered), resulting in the surgeon holding his arms at an awkward angle. Longer cases are then more likely to produce fatigue and error.

Once the endoscopic portion of the case is completed, reposition the patient for vaginal hysterectomy (Fig 9.2), raising the patient's legs (changing stirrups if necessary) to a position adequate for vaginal hysterectomy. This will take no more than a few minutes, but will save the aggravation and frustration associated with attempting to operate vaginally with inadequate room for the surgeon or assistant.

Anesthesia should not be initiated until *all* laparoscopic equipment (including video cameras and monitors) is sterile, assembled, and tested. The most expensive portion of a surgical cost is operating room time. This time "on the clock" should not be spent searching for equipment, discovering and correcting problems, and assembling instruments. Electrosurgical instruments should be checked on a regular time schedule to avoid problems of insulation failure.

When all instruments and equipment are ready, anesthesia begins. The patient is prepared and positioned. The surgeon should always examine the patient prior to the procedure. From the vaginal examina-

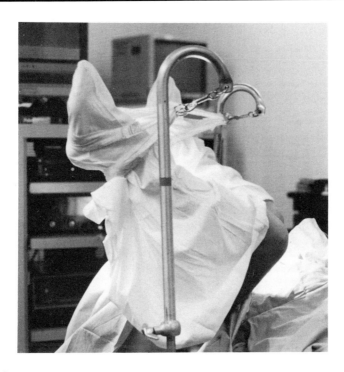

FIGURE 9.2

The patient's legs have been repositioned for the vaginal portion of the LAVH.

tion one should be able to ascertain the amount of the surgical procedure that can be performed vaginally. This information determines the extent of the endoscopic portion of the LAVH necessary. With this information in hand, one of the more important and risk-laden portions of the LAVH begins (trochar insertion).

Use of the Verres needle for insufflation prior to trochar insertion is a matter of surgeon preference. Whether Verres needle insufflation precedes trochar insertion or not, the incidence of bowel perforation and trochar injury to intra-abdominal structures has been shown to be identical (13–15). Likely the experience and skill of the *inserter* of the trochar is more important than the use of insufflation. To date, there are no data indicating that "shields" commonly used in disposable trochars offer any protection against intraperitoneal injury. Regardless, trochar injury to intraperitoneal structures is a known and occasionally unavoidable complication of laparoscopic surgery.

Two 5-mm reusable suprapubic trochars are placed medial or lateral to the inferior epigastric arteries. The precise placement of these trochars is determined by the pathology present. Larger uteri require more lateral secondary trochar placement to maximize access to adnexal structures. It is a rare circumstance when more than two accessory trochars are necessary to complete any LAVH.

The initial step in any laparoscopic procedure (including LAVH) is visual exploration of the abdomen. All areas of the peritoneal cavity are carefully evaluated, and any abnormalities are noted. The pelvis is then evaluated for any pathology unassociated with the indication for the surgery. A surgical "plan of action" is formed and the steps necessary to complete the procedure vaginally are formulated.

Endometriosis implanted on structures other than uterus, tubes, or ovaries should be excised. (Treatment of endometriosis in conjunction with LAVH is discussed in Chapter 11.) Adnexal and bowel adhesions should be lysed.

LAPAROSCOPIC-ASSISTED VAGINAL HYSTERECTOMY WITH SALPINGO-OOPHORECTOMY

If the ovaries are to be removed, identification and control of the ovarian vessels via a retroperitoneal approach is simple and quick. The round ligament is desiccated with bipolar electrosurgery and transected. The peritoneum overlying the pelvic side wall can then be opened and the medial leaf of the broad ligament dissected from the pelvic side wall structures (Plates 6 and 7).

The incision in the peritoneum is extended to the infundibulopelvic ligament. A blunt irrigation/dissection probe is used to dissect peritoneum from the ovarian vessels at the pelvic brim. After identification of the ureter, peritoneum overlying the ovarian vessels is opened around the infundibulopelvic ligament to the medial leaf of the broad ligament, thereby isolating the ovarian artery and vein. Connective tissue is dissected from the ovarian vessels and they are coaptated with bipolar electrosurgical forceps (Plate 8). A constant flow of nonelectrolyte irrigation fluid over the forceps limits lateral thermal injury and minimizes the risk of thermal injury to pelvic side wall structures.

An in-line ammeter measuring current flow between the blades of the bipolar forcep provides an objective end point of the desiccation and coaptation process. When there is minimal or no electron flow through the ovarian vessels, they are transected. Adequately coaptated vessels do not require sutures for severe hemostasis (16–18).

The incision in the medial leaf of the broad ligament is continued to the uterine artery. If the ovary is adherent to the pelvic sidewall, the peritoneum and ovary are simply dissected away from sidewall structures. Using a retroperitoneal approach, it is unnecessary to dissect the ovary from the peritoneum. The peritoneum and ovary are removed together. This approach also minimizes the risk of leaving an ovarian remnant and the subsequent problems associated with this entity.

If bleeding occurs after transection of the coaptated ovarian vessels, they are ligated with loop sutures or recoaptated. Because these vessels have been isolated and skeletonized, they can be easily identified and grasped when necessary.

The ovary and fallopian tube are now freed from the infundibulopelvic ligament and any attachments to the pelvic side wall. These structures remain attached to the uterus. The broad ligament is opened to the uterine artery (Plate 9).

LAPAROSCOPIC-ASSISTED VAGINAL HYSTERECTOMY WITHOUT BILATERAL SALPINGO-OOPHORECTOMY

When clinical circumstances require either or both adnexa to be retained, the procedure begins again at the round ligament. It is desiccated and transected approximately 2 to 3 cm from its insertion into the uterus. The anterior leaf of the broad ligament is opened and the medial leaf is identified.

An incision is made in the medial leaf of the broad ligament. The tube, utero-ovarian ligament, and remaining vessels in the broad ligament must now be controlled. Three methods of hemostasis are available to control these structures. A suture can be passed through one of the accessory trochar sleeves, through the "window" in the broad ligament, and back out the trochar sleeve. A knot pusher is used to tie the suture around this pedicle. The tube and ovary can then be detached from the uterus.

Stapling devices also can be passed through this opening in the broad ligament and the pedicle secured and cut in a single action. Creation of a window in the broad ligament prior to application of the stapler minimizes the risk of ureteral injury by creating a "pedicle" around which the jaws of the stapler are placed.

Electrosurgery provides the last option for detachment of the adnexa from the uterus. As mentioned previously, the round ligament is transected and the broad ligament opened. The fallopian tube is desiccated and transected. The utero-ovarian ligament is desiccated and transected. The jaws of the bipolar forceps are then positioned around the remaining broad ligament. It is desiccated and transected, using several small "bites." Veins in the broad ligament are large and occasionally difficult to coaptate. When using electrosurgery in this area, the surgeon must carefully dissect these vessels prior to coaptation and be prepared to control bleeding with sutures when necessary.

After the fallopian tube and ovary have been detached from the uterus, the broad ligament is opened to the uterine artery. Whether the ovaries are removed or retained, at this point the majority of hysterectomies can (and should) be completed vaginally. It is a rare circumstance when the uterosacral and cardinal ligaments cannot be controlled and transected vaginally. The skilled vaginal surgeon will be able to complete this portion of the procedure much more quickly using a vaginal rather than a laparoscopic approach. Because most gynecologic surgeons are more familiar with vaginal surgery techniques, it is likely (but unproven) that the risk of ureteral, bowel, and bladder injury is less when the operation is completed vaginally rather than laparoscopically. It must be remembered, the goal of LAVH is to complete the hysterectomy vaginally rather than abdominally, *not* to perform a "laparoscopic" hysterectomy.

THE UTERINE ARTERY

Rarely, based on a preoperative pelvic examination, the surgeon must control and transect the uterine artery to complete the hysterectomy vaginally. The uterine artery can be easily identified, but its control and transection can be treacherous. Since ureteral injury commonly occurs at this time, the surgeon must use skill and judgement in controlling this vessel endoscopically.

After the adnexal structures have been freed from the uterus or infundibulopelvic ligament and the broad ligament has been opened, the uterine artery is dissected with a blunt irrigation/dissection probe. The ureter is easily identified at this level by dissecting the uterine artery laterally.

The uterine artery should be dissected (prior to the cervical and uterine branches) from the ureter and pelvic sidewall. Only after a minimum of 2 cm of the vessel has been isolated should it be coaptated with electrosurgery or ligated. If electrosurgical coaptation is chosen, the bipolar forcep is placed next to the uterus (just as a clamp would be placed during vaginal or abdominal hysterectomy). Bipolar cutting current is used to coaptate the artery. Constant irrigation of the area will minimize lateral thermal injury and decrease the risk of thermal ureteral injury. After transection of the uterine artery, the surgeon may choose to place a loop suture around its proximal stump. The remaining cardinal ligamemt is coaptated or sutured and transected.

If the surgeon is unable to identify and dissect the uterine vessels or ureter, the endoscopic portion of the procedure should be abandoned. Laparoscopic attempts at coaptation or suturing without dissection and positive identification of the uterine artery may lead to uncontrollable bleeding or ureteral injury.

THE BLADDER

Opening of the peritoneum overlying the bladder during the laparoscopic portion of the LAVH simplifies dissection of the bladder from the lower uterine segment. Since this is done under direct vision, the bladder wall is more easily identified and avoided. When dense scarring is encountered (postcesarean section), dissection of the bladder from the lower uterine segment under laparoscopic control may minimize the risk of inadvertent bladder injury.

The vesicouterine fold is identified by pushing the uterus cephalad with the uterine manipulator. The peritoneum is lifted and the peritoneum incised at the appropriate location. If the bladder margin is not obvious, distention of the bladder with fluid (with or without dye) aids in identification of the limits of the bladder wall. After incision of the peritoneum, the bladder is dissected from the lower uterine segment with a blunt dissection/irrigation probe. Once the proper plane between the bladder and uterus is identified, this dissection becomes simple and relatively bloodless.

COLPOTOMY

In very rare circumstances the entire hysterectomy must be completed laparoscopically. This usually occurs when there is little or no space in the vagina through which one can clamp, cut, and suture. In these cases, the cardinal and uterosacral ligaments are transected and colpotomies performed. These steps are usually accomplished with electrosurgery. Specific techniques for total laparoscopic hysterectomy are outlined in Chapter 10.

LAPAROSCOPIC-ASSISTED VAGINAL HYSTERECTOMY

Based on the preoperative pelvic examination, the surgeon has completed only those laparoscopic procedures necessary to allow vaginal completion of the hysterectomy. The laparoscope and two secondary trochars are left in place and covered with a sterile drape.

The patient's legs are then repositioned in stirrups used for vaginal hysterectomy and redraped (Fig 9.2). This may take a few minutes, but provides optimal room for the surgeon and assistants. Leaving the legs positioned for laparoscopy or simply rotating the stirrups upward often leaves limited room in which to operate, leading to frustration and extended operating time.

The hysterectomy should be completed vaginally, using techniques familiar to the surgeon. It is likely that the surgeon is more skilled in vaginal than laparoscopic surgery techniques, allowing the vaginal portion of the case to be completed quickly and efficiently. After closure of the vaginal cuff, the abdomen is reinflated and inspected.

REINSPECTION

The more difficult the case, the more likely there will be bleeding in the pelvis at the conclusion of the procedure. The entire operative field should be carefully inspected for bleeding, ureteral damage, and bowel injury. Clots (which may conceal bleeding vessels) should be removed. Bleeding is controlled with electrosurgery or sutures. All coaptated vessels should be inspected and manipulated. Clots and debris are removed by copious irrigation.

The ureters are catheterized, filled with dye, and inspected if there is any question of injury. If integrity of the rectosigmoid wall is in doubt, a catheter with a 30-mL bulb is placed into the rectum and the bulb inflated. Betadine is injected through the catheter into the lumen of the bowel. Laparoscopic inspection will reveal leakage of betadine into the pelvis. Any defect thus identified can be appropriately corrected. As a final step, the upper abdomen is inspected for pathology or injury. Preoperative and postoperative photographs provide an excellent record of the appearance of the pelvis.

COMPLICATIONS

Laparoscopic-assisted vaginal hysterectomy *adds* the risks unique to laparoscopy to those associated with vaginal or abdominal hysterectomy. The risk unique to laparoscopy involves trochars. Trochar injuries to bowel, bladder, vessels, and other intra–abdominal structures account for the majority of complications of laparoscopic surgery. Conversely, puncture injuries to bowel and major vessels are *rare* complications of vaginal or abdominal hysterectomy. From this standpoint alone, it is unwise to perform LAVH when vaginal hysterectomy is possible.

There is no evidence to date that major complications associated with LAVH occur with any more frequency than with any other major laparoscopic procedure (2,4,5,8,9). Evaluation of large series of patients undergoing abdominal hysterectomy, vaginal hysterectomy, and LAVH should determine whether there is any advantage of one over the other when major complications are reviewed.

In an attempt to evaluate complications related to LAVH, a staging system has been devised to record the extent of the laparoscopic portion of the operation in a standardized format (Table 9.1). It is likely (although not proven) that ureteral injury most commonly occurs at the pelvic brim and at the level of the uterine artery. The frequency of

TABLE 9.1

Laparoscopic–assisted vaginal hysterectomy staging

Stage

   0 Laparoscopy done; no laparoscopic procedure performed prior to vaginal hysterectomy

   1 Procedure included laparoscopic adhesiolysis and/or excision of endometriosis

   2 Either or both adnexa freed laparoscopically

   3 Bladder dissected from uterus

   4 Uterine artery transected laparoscopically

   5 Anterior and/or posterior colpotomy or entire uterus freed

Subscript

   0 Neither ovary excised

   1 One ovary excised

   2 Both ovaries excised

If the extent of the procedure performed laparoscopically varied on the right and left pelvic side walls, the procedure is staged according to the most advanced side.

complications at each stage of LAVH will be recorded and evaluated. Hopefully this information will aid the surgeon in avoiding complications at these anatomic sites.

A review of current literature indicates the frequency of complications related to LAVH to be similar to or lower than traditional vaginal or abdominal hysterectomy. The frequency of complications also relates to the experience of the surgeon. As the gynecologic surgeon becomes more skilled in laparoscopic techniques, the combination of traditional and laparoscopic surgery will greatly expand surgical capabilities without a concurrent increase in complications.

POSTOPERATIVE CARE

Postoperative care of the patient following LAVH is identical to that for vaginal hysterectomy. Since these patients have had little manipulation of the bowel, postoperative ileus is extremely unusual. The patients are allowed oral fluids as soon as they desire. Regular diets follow as soon as possible. Oral analgesics are begun when the postoperative nausea has subsided. Indwelling urinary catheters are unnecessary and may increase the risk of urinary tract infection. Intermittent catheterization is used when urinary retention is encountered. Patients requiring repeated catheterization are instructed in self-catheterization, eliminating the necessity for dismissal with indwelling catheters.

Using this postoperative regimen, the average hospital stay for 346 patients undergoing LAVH (with and without bladder repairs) at Harris Hospital–Ft Worth (Ft Worth, TX) was 34 hours (19). A comparable length of stay was found in a corresponding group of patients undergoing vaginal hysterectomy.

Patients dismissed from hospital care this quickly after a major surgical procedure must be evaluated regularly by the surgeon either in person or by telephone. Any unusual complaints must be immediately evaluated. When followed carefully and conscientiously, these patients can be expected to recover as uneventfully as if they remained hospitalized.

ECONOMICS OF LAVH

To evaluate the medical economic impact involved with laparoscopy on the surgical approach to hysterectomy for benign disease, all hysterectomies performed for benign disease at Harris Hospital–Fort Worth were reviewed over a 3-year period (20). During this time, 58 gynecologists performed 2272 hysterectomies (without vaginal repairs). Disposable laparoscopic instruments and stapling devices were not used by any physician during this period. Electrosurgery and sutures were used for hemostasis. Records of each case were reviewed for surgical approach (total abdominal hysterectomy, vaginal hysterectomy, LAVH, and failed LAVH), operative time, postoperative diagnosis, operative blood loss, length of stay, complications, uterine weight, and hospital charges. Trends of each parameter were analyzed in 6-month blocks. During this study period, the percentage of procedures performed abdominally declined from 59% to 38%. The percentage of vaginal hysterectomies remained stable and the percentage of LAVH increased from 20% to 40%. It is obvious that these physicians were not converting vaginal hysterectomy to LAVH, but converting total abdominal hysterectomy to LAVH. During this time period the average operating time for LAVH was 102 minutes, exceeding that of total abdominal hysterectomy (82 minutes) and vaginal hysterectomy (65 minutes). The average hospital charge for LAVH ($6500) was consistently below that for total abdominal hysterectomy ($6990) and above that for vaginal hysterectomy ($6250).

A brief review of this study, in contrast to other published data (3,5,7,8,21) concludes that LAVH is a safe alternative to abdominal hysterectomy in a significant number of patients. Using reusable equipment and electrosurgical techniques, LAVH can be performed at a cost comparable to or less than abdominal hysterectomy. Other studies have shown the cost of LAVH to significantly exceed that of abdominal hysterectomy when disposable laparoscopic instruments are used (3,5,7,8,21). A constant improvement in endoscopic skills associated with an improved knowledge of electrosurgical energy sources maximize the cost-effectiveness of LAVH. Proper patient selection allows the most cost-effective alternative (vaginal hysterectomy) to be performed when possible.

CONCLUSION

There is no "correct" method for completing hysterectomy in any given patient. Clinical indications, potential complications, and circumstances encountered in the operating room should always dictate the safest and most cost-effective method for each patient.

The gynecologic surgeon must be knowledgeable in the use of all endoscopic energy sources as well as sutures and stapling devices. The cost of all instruments and devices used in the operating suite should be well known to every surgeon. The possibilities for cost savings can then be intelligently evaluated.

The advantages of vaginal over abdominal hysterectomy are unquestioned. The possibility of converting what would otherwise be an abdominal procedure to a vaginal hysterectomy using laparoscopic techniques is also obvious. The safest and most cost-effective method for converting the abdominal hysterectomy to a vaginal procedure remains to be determined. Is LAVH more cost-effective and safer than total laparoscopic hysterectomy? Is supracervical hysterectomy better than LAVH or vaginal hysterectomy? With LAVH in its infancy, answers to these questions are yet to be determined.

REFERENCES

1. Reich H, DeCaprio J, McGlynn F. Laparoscopic hysterectomy. J Gynecol Surg 1989;5:213–226.
2. Boike GM, Elfstrand EP, DelPriore G, et al. Laparoscopically assisted vaginal hysterectomy in a University Hospital: report of 82 cases and comparison with abdominal and vaginal hysterectomy. Am J Obstet Gynecol 1993;168:1690–1701.
3. Davis GD, Wolgamott G, Moon J. Laparoscopically assisted vaginal hysterectomy as definitive therapy for stage III and IV endometriosis. J Reprod Med 1993;38:577–581.

4. Phipps JH, John M, Hassanaien M, Saeed M. Laparoscopic and laparoscopically assisted vaginal hysterectomy: a series of 114 cases. Gynaecol Endosc 1993;2:7–12.

5. Boike GM, Efstrand EP, Lurain JR. Laparoscopically assisted vaginal hysterectomy in a university hospital: report of 50 cases with comparison to vaginal and abdominal hysterectomy. Presented at the Central Association of Obstetricians and Gynecologists, Chicago, IL.

6. Semm K. Presented at the American Association of Gynecologists and Laparoscopists Annual Meeting. San Francisco, November, 1993.

7. Nezhat F, Nezhat C, Gordon S, et al. Laparoscopic versus abdominal hysterectomy. J Reprod Med 1992;37:247–250.

8. Summitt RL Jr, Stovall TG, Lipscomb GH, Ling FW. Randomized comparison of laparoscopy assisted vaginal hysterectomy with standard vaginal hysterectomy in an outpatient setting. Obstet Gynecol 1992;80:895–901.

9. Johns DA, Diamond MP. Laparoscopically assisted vaginal hysterectomies. J Reprod Med 1994;6:424–428.

10. Stovall T. A clinical continuum of obstetrics and gynecology, laparoscopic-assisted vaginal hysterectomy: pros and cons. ACOG Update 1994;K(8). Audiotape.

11. Kovac SR, Cruikshank SH, Retto HF. Laparoscopy assisted vaginal hysterectomy. J Gynecol Surg 1990;6:185–193.

12. Soderstrom RM. Glycine as an irrigant during microsurgical hemostasis. A microsurgeon's observations. J Reprod Med 1991;36:265–256.

13. Yuzpe AA. Pneumoperitoneum needle and trocar injuries in laparoscopy. A survey on possible contributing factors and prevention. J Reprod Med 1990;35(5):485–490.

14. Jarrett JC. Laparoscopy: direct trocar insertion without pneumoperitoneum. Obstet Gynecol 1990;75(4).

15. Kaali SG, Bartfai G. Direct insertion of the laparoscopic trocar after an earlier laparotomy. J Reprod Med 1988;33:739–740.

16. Harrison JD, Morris DL. Does bipolar electrocoagulation time effect vessel weld strength? Gut 1991;32:188–190.

17. Dunn MR, Sigel B. The mechanism of blood vessel closure by high frequency electrocoagulation. Surg Gynecol Obstet 1965:823–831.

18. Odell RC. Electrosurgery in laparoscopy. Infertil Reprod Med Clin North Am 1993;4:289–304.

19. Johns DA. LAVH—cost, complications, outcomes in 356 patients. 1994 (submitted for publication).
20. Johns DA, Diamond M. The medical and economic impact of laparoscopically-assisted vaginal hysterectomy (LAVH) in a large metropolitan not-for-profit hospital. Am J Obstet Gynecol 1995;6:1709–1719.
21. Leibert MA. The most expensive hysterectomy. J Gynecol Surg 1992;11:57.

10

Surgical Techniques of Total Laparoscopic Hysterectomy

C.Y. Liu
Harry Reich

Approximately 1.7 million women in the United States underwent a hysterectomy between 1988 and 1990. Seventy-five percent of hysterectomies were done abdominally and 25% were done vaginally (1). In the United States from 1965 to 1987, according to one major insurance company's report, the most common indications for hysterectomy, were leiomyomata (30%), endometriosis (19%), genital prolapse (16%), gynecologic malignancies (10%), and endometrial hyperplasia (6%). The remaining 19% of hysterectomies were due to other causes, such as dysfunctional uterine bleeding or adnexal diseases (2). There are three objectives of hysterectomies: 1) to save a life, 2) to relieve symptoms, and 3) to restore normal anatomy and function. Vaginal hysterectomy has the advantages of a shorter operating time, a more comfortable and quicker postoperative recovery period, fewer complications, and cosmetic appeal to the patient. Since vaginal hysterectomy is much more cost effective and acceptable for the patient compared with the abdominal hysterectomy, it seems logical that all hysterectomies should be performed vaginally. However, certain conditions render a vaginal hysterectomy difficult and, in some instances, dangerous. Some of the conditions are listed below:

1. Narrow vagina with lack of mobility of the uterus
2. Massively contracted pelvis
3. Myomatous uterus greater than 18 weeks' gestational size
4. Extensive pelvic endometriosis involving the cul-de-sac and the rectovaginal septum and space
5. Adnexal mass in which malignancy is suspected
6. Congenital abnormalities, such as double uterus, double cervix, and double vagina
7. History of multiple previous major pelvic surgeries and/or pelvic inflammatory disease
8. Severe arthritis that prohibits placement of the patient in sufficient lithotomic position for vaginal exposure
9. Stage 1 ovarian, cervical, or endometrial cancer.

With technologic advancements in laparoscopic instrumentation and improved skill in operative laparoscopy, the gynecologist, when confronted with the above-mentioned conditions, should first evaluate the patient's pelvis laparoscopically prior to making a large abdominal incision. In the vast majority of cases, with the aid of operative laparoscopy, a difficult or contraindicated vaginal hysterectomy can be converted into a relatively easy vaginal hysterectomy (3). However, in certain cases (including poor mobility of the uterus; massively contracted pelvis; double uterus and double cervix; stage 1 endometrial, ovarian, or cervical cancer; extensive endometriosis involving cul-de-sac and uterosacral ligaments; and rectovaginal septum requiring concomitant excision of infiltrating fibrotic endometrial nodules) a total laparoscopic hysterectomy is advisable. To perform a total laparoscopic hysterectomy, the surgeon must be familiar with various fascial planes and avascular spaces in the pelvis and be proficient in performing various complicated operative laparoscopy procedures, including retroperitoneal dissection, ureteral and bladder dissections, and laparoscopic suture techniques. However, the reader is reminded that when a hysterectomy is indicated, the transvaginal approach should first be considered. If a vaginal hysterectomy is not feasible after thorough evaluation, a laparoscope should be inserted and the pelvis re-evaluated before making a large abdominal incision. In the majority of cases, a laparoscopic-assisted vaginal hysterectomy can be performed. A total laparoscopic hysterectomy is indicated and performed only in rare cases.

DEFINITION AND CLASSIFICATION

The term "laparoscopic-assisted vaginal hysterectomy" is confusing. The same term is used to describe a number of completely different procedures, ranging from a minimum amount of surgery performed laparoscopically with a fairly standard vaginal hysterectomy (3) to most or all of the hysterectomy being performed laparoscopically with minimal vaginal surgery (4–8). To have statistically significant series-to-series comparison of the results and complication rates, a generally accepted definition and classification of the laparoscopic-assisted hysterectomy must be standardized and used by the gynecologist.

We propose the following classification system (9). We regard securing and dividing the uterine artery as the most critical step in the procedure. If the laparoscopic component of the operation is completed above the uterine artery and the uterine arteries are subsequently ligated vaginally, we suggest that such a procedure be called "laparoscopic-assisted vaginal hysterectomy." If, however, the uterine arteries are secured laparoscopically and the remaining cardinal and uterosacral ligaments are secured vaginally, we suggest the procedure be termed "laparoscopic hysterectomy." If, in addition, the uterosacral and cardinal ligaments are also secured laparoscopically and the cervix is completely freed from the vagina by laparoscopic technique, the procedure is analogous to a total abdominal hysterectomy and should be called a "total laparoscopic hysterectomy." The complete descriptive classification of laparoscopic-assisted hysterectomy is thus:

1. Diagnostic laparoscopy with vaginal hysterectomy
2. Laparoscopic-assisted vaginal hysterectomy (LAVH)
3. Laparoscopic hysterectomy (LH)

4. Total laparoscopic hysterectomy (TLH)
5. Laparoscopic supracervical hysterectomy (LSH or CASH)
6. Laparoscopic hysterectomy with lymphadenectomy (LHL)
7. Laparoscopic hysterectomy with lymphadenectomy and omentectomy (LHL + O)
8. Radical laparoscopic hysterectomy (RLH)

CONTRAINDICATIONS

The contraindications for the laparoscopic hysterectomy are the same as those for operative laparoscopy. Certain medical conditions, including severe anemia, diabetes, pulmonary disorders, cardiac disease, and bleeding diathesis, must be carefully evaluated before surgery. Age should rarely be a deterrent.

Laparoscopic hysterectomy may be indicated for postpartum hysterectomy; however, postpartum bleeding due to placenta accreta, uterine atony, uterine rupture, or other unspecified bleeding is at present considered a relative contraindication for laparoscopic hysterectomy. Cesarean hysterectomy is an absolute contraindication for this type of surgery.

We consider that a pelvic mass too large to fit intact into an impermeable sack is a contraindication for laparoscopic surgery. The largest sack currently available for removal of intraperitoneal masses is the LapSac (Cook Ob/Gyn, Spencer, IN), which measures 8 × 11 in. While some investigators advocate laparoscopic fluid aspiration of a large ovarian cyst (10), we feel that postmenopausal cystic ovaries should not be subjected to fluid aspiration before oophorectomy. The inevitable spillage changes the diagnosis from a stage "Ia ovarian cancer" to a stage "Ia with spill." Its effect on survival is unknown, but it may be detrimental. It must be emphasized that small-gauge needles, placed through thickened portions of the ovary, and cyst aspiration devices with surrounding suction and endoloop placement do not prevent spillage. Ovaries should be removed intact through a culdotomy incision (11).

IMPORTANT INSTRUMENTS

A high-flow CO_2 insufflator, capable of delivering up to 10 to 15 L/min of CO_2, is necessary to compensate for the rapid loss of gas during suctioning. The ability to maintain a relatively constant intra-abdominal pressure between 10 and 15 mm Hg during laparoscopic hysterectomy is essential.

A sturdy uterine mobilizer, capable of extreme anteversion and movement of the uterus in an arc of 45 degrees to the right and left, is important. There are several excellent uterine mobilizers available commercially, including the Valtchev, Pelosi, and Blairden uterine manipulators. Unfortunately, these uterine mobilizers are all expensive. An alternative method is to insert a uterine sound into the uterine cavity and secure it with sterile rubber bands to two single-toothed tenaculums, which are attached to the anterior and posterior cervical lips. This excellent uterine mobilizer, available in every operating room, has served one of the authors well.

An operating room table capable of placing the patient in steep Trendelenburg's position is invaluable for operative laparoscopy. For years, we have been performing complicated operative laparoscopy with the patient in steep Trendelenburg's position with shoulder braces and the arms at the patient's sides without adverse effects.

Bipolar forceps use high-frequency, low-voltage cutting current (20 to 50 W) to coagulate vessels as large as the ovarian and uterine arteries. The Kleppinger bipolar forceps (Richard Wolf, Rosemont, IL) is excellent for large-vessel hemostasis and is preferable to disposable stapling devices because of much lower costs and reduced risks of hematoma formation.

SUTURING

A special technique is required when suturing with large curved needles through a 5-mm trocar abdominal incision into the peritoneal cavity.

During the laparoscopic hysterectomy, all the 5-mm trocars are placed lateral to the deep inferior epigastric vessels and rectus abdomini muscle in the lower abdomen. The trocar sleeve penetrates the skin, external and internal oblique transversalis, and peritoneum. The trocar sleeve, after removal, leaves an obvious tract for easy re-entry. Suturing with a CT-1 or CTX needle is performed as described below.

1. The trocar sleeve is taken out of the abdomen and loaded by grasping the end of the suture with a needle holder, pulling it through the trocar sleeve, and letting the suture loose.
2. The needle holder is reinserted into the sleeve and the suture is grasped approximately 1 in from the needle.
3. The needle driver is inserted into the peritoneal cavity through the original tract, as visualized on video; the needle follows.
4. At this stage, an atraumatic grasping forceps from the opposite side is used to grasp the needle and place it on the needle driver at the desired angle and position, ready for suturing.
5. After suturing has been completed, the needle is anchored in the parietal peritoneum on the anterior abdominal wall to prevent losing it during the procedure. The suture is cut adjacent to the needle, after which the cut end of the suture is pulled out of the peritoneal cavity through the 5-mm trocar sleeve.
6. Then, while holding both strands of the suture, the surgeon makes a simple half-hitch, but not a surgeon's knot, which will not slip down through the trocar sleeve as well.
7. The Clarke knot pusher is put on the suture that is held firmly across the index finger, and the throw is pushed down to the tissue. A square knot is made by pushing another half-hitch down to the knot to secure it, while exerting tension from above.
8. To retrieve the needle, the trocar sleeve is unscrewed, after which the needle holder inside it pulls the needle through the soft tissue. The trocar sleeve is replaced easily with or without another suture (12).

SURGICAL TECHNIQUE OF TOTAL LAPAROSCOPIC HYSTERECTOMY

Under general anethesia with endotracheal intubation, the patient is placed in low dorsolithotomic position with both legs and feet supported by Allen's Stirrups (Allen Medical, Mayfield, OH) (Fig 10.1). A single dose of first-generation cephalosporin is given intravenously as a prophylactic antibiotic (13). After the bladder is emptied, 20 to 30 mL of concentrated indigo carmine dye is instilled into the bladder as a precautionary measure to facilitate recognition of any potential bladder injury during the procedure. A uterine sound inserted into the uterine cavity is tied to two single-toothed tenaculum, which are attached to the anterior and posterior lips of the cervix. This acts as a uterine manipulator during surgery. A 10-mm laparoscope is inserted through a 12-mm trocar sleeve in a vertical intraumbilical incision. Four 5-mm puncture sites are made in the lower abdomen, all of which are lateral to the deep inferior epigastric vessels and the rectus abdominus muscles (Fig 10.2). The location of these trocar sites varies with the size of the uterus and the pathology in the pelvis. Careful inspection is made of the internal viscus, including the pelvic organs. Corrective measures are done by using

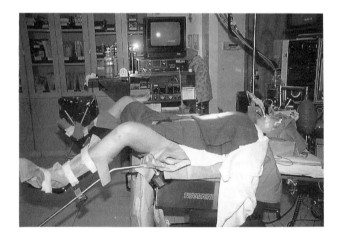

FIGURE 10.1

Patient's position for laparoscopic procedure.

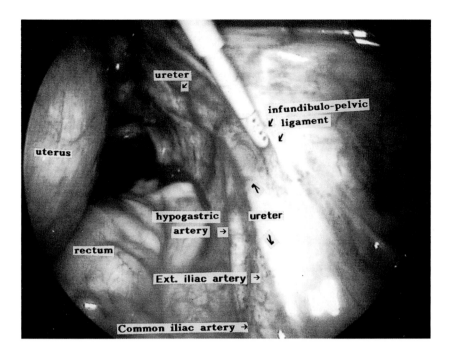

PLATE 1: Pelvic course of the ureter. (Reproduced by permission from Kadar N. Atlas of laparoscopic pelvic surgery. Boston: Blackwell Science, 1995:52.) See page 15.

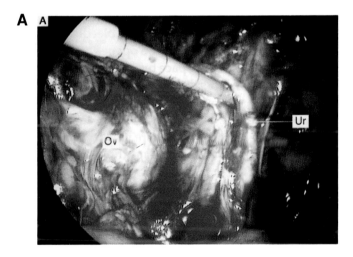

PLATE 2: Resection of a residual ovary after identifying the ureter and freeing it from the ovary. Ur, Ureter; Ov, ovary; PRS, pararectal space; EIA, external iliac artery; EIV, external iliac vein; OvnR, ovarian remnant; Ps, psoas muscle. (Reproduced by permission from Kadar N. Atlas of laparoscopic pelvic surgery. Boston: Blackwell Science, 1995:61.) See page 27.

B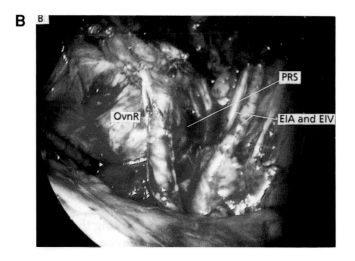

C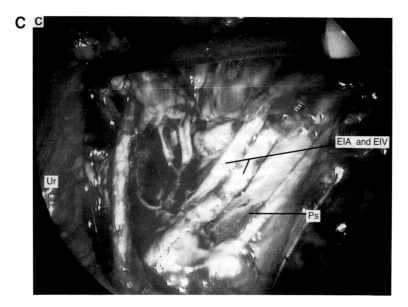

PLATE 2: (continued)

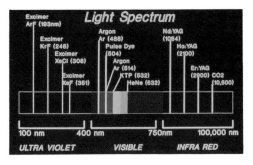

PLATE 3: Lasers currently used in surgery and medicine. See page 72.

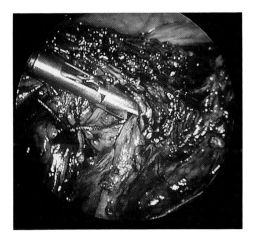

PLATE 4: The blunt end of an atraumatic grasping forceps is used to gently tease the surrounding areola tissue away from the ureter. See page 134.

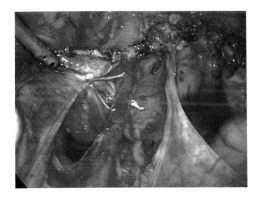

PLATE 5: The uterine artery is ligated and divided to unroof the ureteric canal. See page 135.

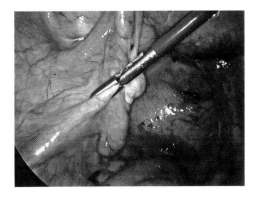

PLATE 6: Medial traction is applied to allow entry into the retroperitoneal space. See page 156.

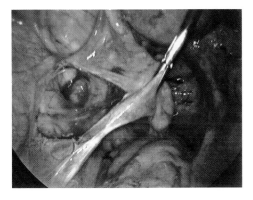

PLATE 7: The ovarian artery and vein are skeletonized and isolated. See page 156.

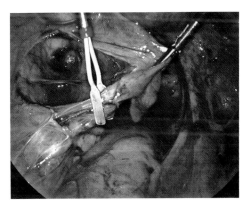

PLATE 8: Coaptation of the ovarian artery and vein. See page 156.

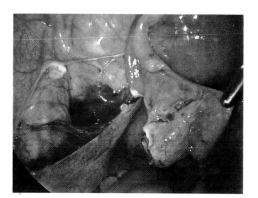

PLATE 9: After control of the infundibulopelvic ligament, the broad ligament is opened and dissected to the uterine artery. See page 157.

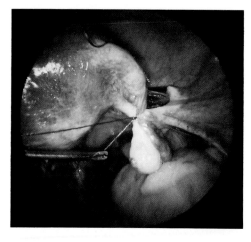

PLATE 11: The right uteroovarian junction is ligated. See page 180.

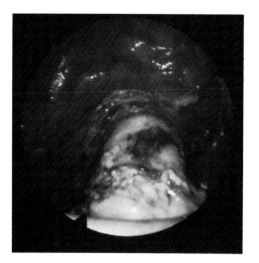

PLATE 10: The bladder has been dissected to the upper part of vagina. The glistening white surface of the vesicocervical space is clearly seen. See page 178.

A

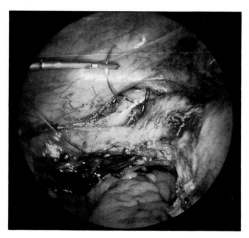

PLATE 12: The left uterine artery and cardinal ligament are suture ligated with O-vicryl suture. See page 181.

B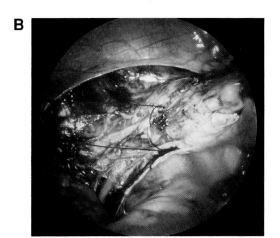

A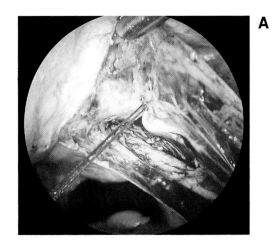

C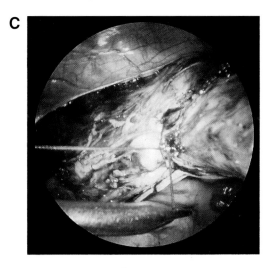

B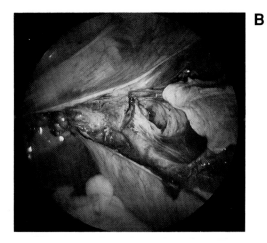

PLATE 12: (continued)

PLATE 13: (A) The left uterine artery is suture ligated prior to its crossing over the left ureter. (B) The same patient at the end of the procedure. See page 181.

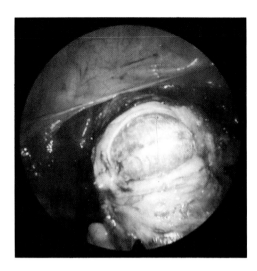

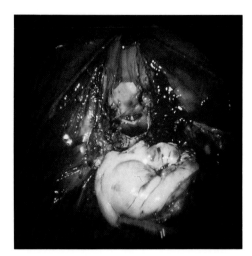
B

PLATE 14: The anterior culdotomy is performed with a high-power density CO_2 laser. To facilitate the identification, a 4 × 4 sponge, which is grasped by the tip of a sponge forceps to tent the anterior cul-de-sac, is stained blue with methylene blue dye. See page 183.

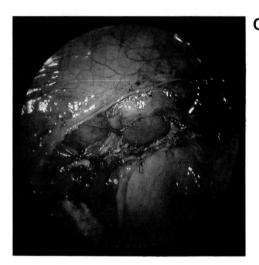
C

A
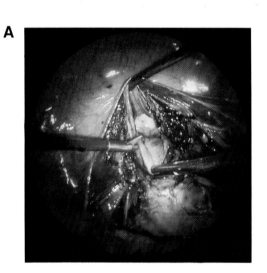

PLATE 15: Circumferential culdotomy is performed with scissors. The uterus is pushed into the vagina and is left there to maintain the pneumo-peritoneum for the laparoscopic suturing of the vaginal cuff. See page 183.

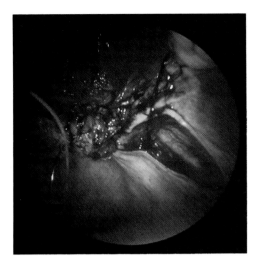

PLATE 16: Under direct visualization of the left ureter, the uterosacral ligament is sutured to the left corner of the vaginal cuff laparoscopically. See page 183.

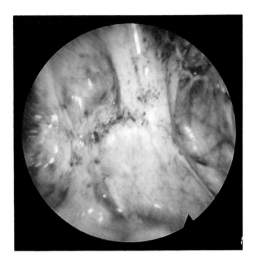

PLATE 18: Complete obliteration of the cul-de-sac. The rectum is adherent to the posterior cervix and cul-de-sac. Invasive nodular endometriosis is obvious as indurated yellowish tissue in the uterosacral ligaments and anterior rectal wall. See page 211.

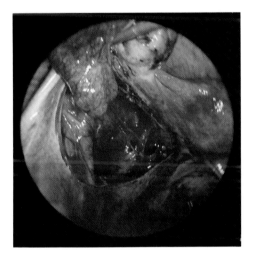

PLATE 17: The peritoneum beneath the left ovary has been incised anterior to the ureter, and the involved peritoneum has been stripped off of the lateral pelvic wall. Some of the peritoneum has been separately excised, while some remains attached to the left ovary, which will be removed. See page 206.

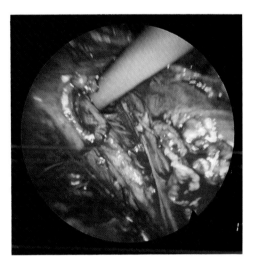

PLATE 19: Blunt dissection is useed to begin the isolation of the right ureter from the right uterine vessels. Here the blunt suction-irrigator is dissecting the space between the uterine vessels (above the shaft) and the ureter (running diagonally below the shaft). See page 216.

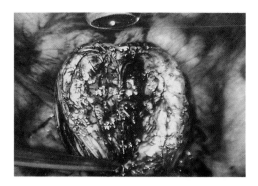

PLATE 20: Hemostatic myoma bed following complete enucleation. Uterine arteries have not been ligated. See page 232.

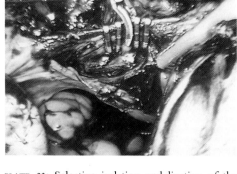

PLATE 23: Selective isolation and ligation of the left uterine artery with vascular clips. See page 235.

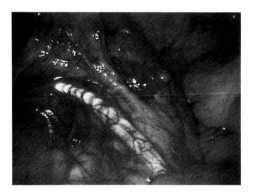

PLATE 21: The right ureter is visualized by placement of a lighted ureteral stent. See page 234.

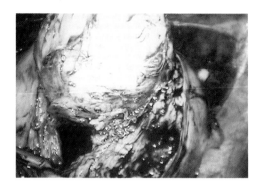

PLATE 24: Morsellation of a large anterior wall fibroid after securing both uterine arteries. See page 235.

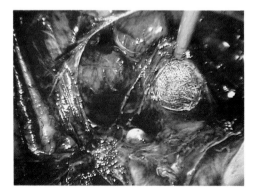

PLATE 22: A sponge placed in the plane between the bladder (above) and cervix (below) greatly facilitates bladder mobilization and reduces inadvertent entry into the bladder. See page 234.

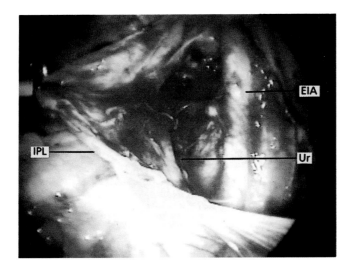

PLATE 25: The infundibulopelvic ligament has been pulled medially to expose the ureter at the pelvic brim. EIA, external iliac artery; IPL, infundibulopelvic ligament; Ur, ureter. (Reproduced by permission from Kadar N. Atlas of laparoscopic pelvic surgery. Boston: Blackwell Science, 1995:106.) See page 270.

A
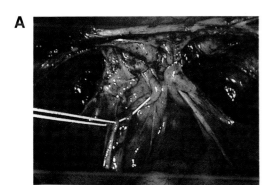

B
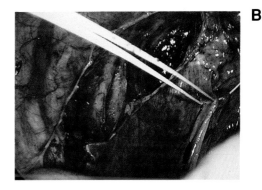

PLATE 26: The cul–de–sac is obliterated with 2-0 permenant suture. A pursestring Moschcowitz McCall technique is used. (A) Both ureters are identified and dissected out before the procedure begins. (B) The left ureter is clearly seen lateral to the suture. See page 319.

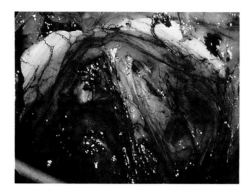

PLATE 27: Laparoscopic view of the Retzius's space. The right paravaginal fat has been removed. See page 319.

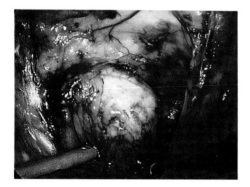

PLATE 28: The bladder is mobilized medially and glistening white pubocervical fascia is identified. See page 320.

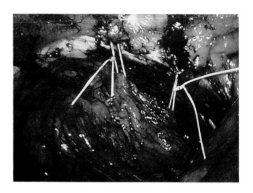

PLATE 29: Two sutures are placed on each side of the urethra, one at the midurethral level and the other at the level of the urethrovesical junction. Both sutures are sutured through the ipsilateral side of Cooper's ligament. Both sutures are double looped and sutured deep into the anterior vaginal wall, avoiding the vaginal mucosa. See page 320.

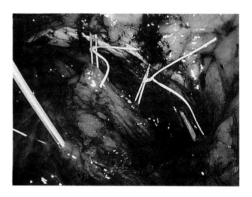

PLATE 30: A suprapubic catheter is placed at the end of the procedure. The obturator nerve is visible lateral to the sutures. See page 321.

A

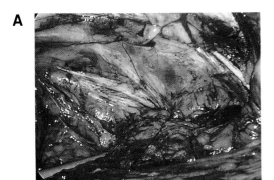

B

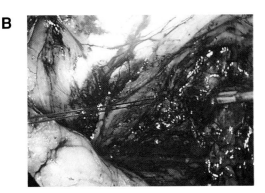

PLATE 31: Laparoscopic view at the end of paravaginal suspension. See page 336.

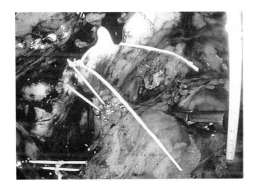

PLATE 32: A combination of Burch and paravaginal suspension in a patient with stress urinary incontinence and a not well-supported urethrovesical junction even after paravaginal suspension. See page 336.

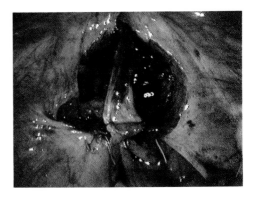

PLATE 33: View of the cul-de-sac after resection of the hernia sac. The vaginal skin graft has been attacheed to the sacrouterine ligaments. See page 346.

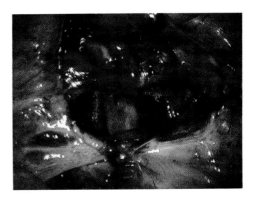

PLATE 34: Vicryl mesh is draped over the skin graft, underneath the posterior wall of the vagina. See page 346.

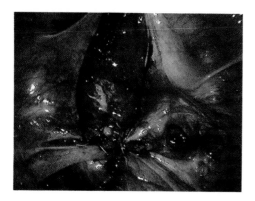

PLATE 35: The vaginal vault is attached to the sacrouterine ligaments. In this case, the bladder was previously dissected off the vaginal vault. See page 346.

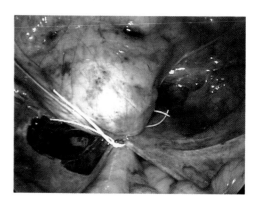

PLATE 37: Laparoscopic view at the completion of high McCall vaginal vault suspension. See page 359.

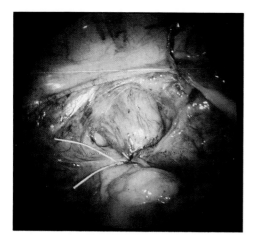

PLATE 36: The suture should be tied without leaving any gap between the sacrospinous ligament and the vagina. See page 356.

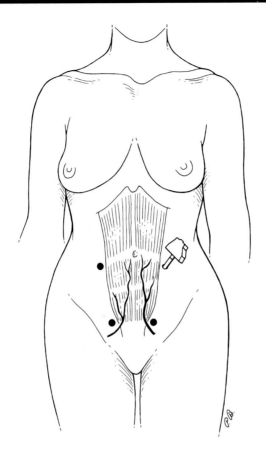

FIGURE 10.2

The trocar puncture sites for complicated laparoscopic procedures. The lower 5-mm trocar sites are lateral to the deep inferior epigastric vessels. The upper trocar sites are lateral to the abdominal rectus muscles.

various laparoscopic instruments. CO_2 laser, whenever used, is delivered into the abdomen through a 10-mm operative laparoscope. As with any other surgery, the operative techniques for total laparoscopic hysterectomy may vary from case to case, but the following description outlines the standard technique.

Step 1

Both pelvic ureters are identified and dissected to at least the level of the ureteric canal, where the uterine artery crosses above the ureter and the cardinal ligament lies below the ureter. This step is accomplished by opening the peritoneum covering the ureter with CO_2 laser or scissors (Fig 8.5). If there is pelvic side wall pathology, such as ovarian endometrioma, dense tuboovarian–pelvic side wall adhesion, or ovarian tumor, the ureters need to be identified and dissected cephalad to the pathology. Often, the dissection of the ureter will start at or above the pelvic brim. This is usually easier on the right side, where the ureter can be readily visualized just beneath the bifurcation of the iliac artery. It is more difficult to identify the ureter on the left side, where its course is usually obscured by the sigmoid colon. The sigmoid colon should be freed and reflected from the left iliac fossa to expose the ovarian vessels, the mesocolon vessels, and the iliac artery. In most cases, the left ureter is located above the internal iliac artery in the area of the pelvic brim. Under direct visualization of the ureter the adnexal organs are then dissected and freed from the pelvic sidewall. The ureter then continues to be dissected downward to the deep pelvis. The uterosacral ligaments, at this point, are dissected away from the ureters. The detailed technique of ureteral dissection is described in Chapter 8.

Step 2

The purpose of this step is to reflect the bladder to the upper part of the vagina. First, both round ligaments are coagulated with bipolar Kleppinger forceps and divided with scissors. This can also be achieved with the closed tips of a laparoscopic scissors using coagulate current. A transverse incision is made on the vesicouterine peritoneal fold. The upper junction of the vesicouterine fold is identified as a white line when viewed laparoscopically (Fig 10.3A). The peritoneum attaches to the broad ligament tightly above this white line. There is a distance of 2 to 2.5 cm between the white line and the dome of the bladder. The peritoneum is attached to the cervix loosely, which forms the vesicouterine pouch. The initial incision should be made below the white line to avoid difficult and bloody dissection of the bladder (Fig 10.3B). After the transverse incision below the white line is made, the peritoneum below the incision is elevated. Three condensations of the connective tissues can be seen (Fig 10.4A). The middle band of the loose connective tissue is the vesicocervical ligament, which does not contain

A 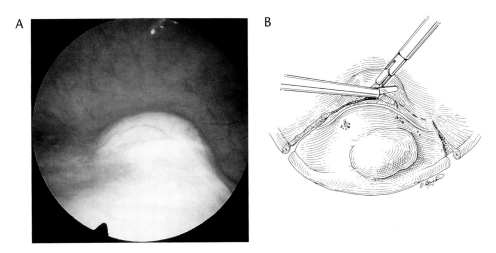 B

FIGURE 10.3

(A) The upper border of the vesicouterine fold appears as a white line when viewed laparoscopically. (B) A transverse incision is made below the white line.

A 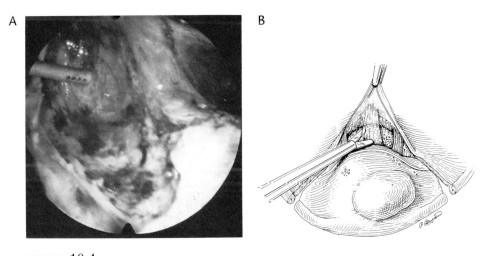 B

FIGURE 10.4

(A) Lifting the peritoneum covering the vesicouterine fold after it has been opened transversely, three condensations of connective tissue bands can be seen. Vesicocervical ligaments are seen in the middle and bladder pillars are seen on both sides of the cervix. (B) The vesicocervical ligaments can be transected with scissors without incurring bleeding.

blood vessels and can be divided bloodlessly (Fig 10.4B). Thus, the vesicocervical space is entered with its characteristic glistening white surface. The lateral bands of connective tissue on both sides of the cervix are the bladder pillars, which are part of the endopelvic fascia and extend from the cardinal ligaments and connect between the pubovesical fascia and the bladder base. The bladder pillars hold the bladder to the cervix and contain blood vessels from the cervix. The bladder pillars are coagulated (Fig 10.5) and divided either with scissors or laser, after which the bladder can be easily dissected down to the upper part of vagina (Plate 10). This also pulls the ureters laterally and away from the cervix. If the cul-de-sac is obliterated partly or completely because of endometriosis or previous pelvic inflammatory disease, the rectosigmoid colon is dissected away from the cervix and the endometriosis nodules in that area are resected.

If dense fibrosis and scarring between the bladder and low uterine segment is encountered, due to endometriosis, pelvic inflammatory disease, or previous multiple cesarean sections or other surgeries, the white line of the upper border of vesicouterine junction is obscured. Two-hundred milliliters of fluid instilled into the bladder will distend the

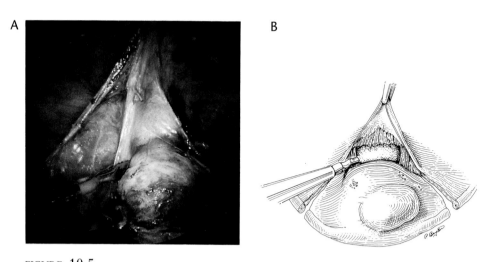

A   B

FIGURE 10.5

The bladder pillar contains blood vessels from the cervix and requires electrocoagulation before transection.

bladder and delineate the upper margin of the bladder, providing a guide for the incision.

The hysterectomy should *not* start until both ureters are identified and dissected, and the bladder and rectosigmoid colon are reflected all the way to the upper vagina.

Step 3

The anterior leaf of the broad ligaments is opened downward and toward the cervix, and the uterine artery is identified. An opening is usually made on the avascular portion of the posterior leaf of the broad ligament above the uterine vessels.

Step 4

If the tube and ovary are to be removed, the infundibulopelvic ligament is first mobilized, and Kleppinger bipolar forceps are used to compress and desiccate the vessels (Fig 10.6), which are divided with the scissors or laser

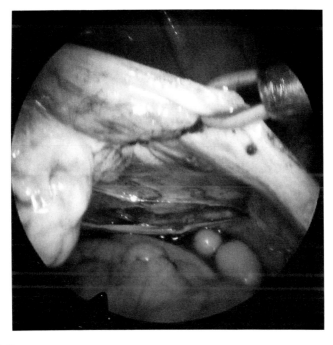

FIGURE 10.6

The left infundibulopelvic ligament is desiccated with a Kleppinger bipolar forceps. The left ureter can be clearly seen below on the pelvic side wall.

Surgical Techniques of TLH   179

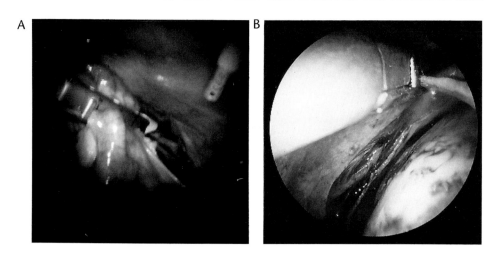

A   B

FIGURE 10.7

(A) An automatic laparoscopic stapling device is used to staple and transect the left utero-ovarian junction. (B) An automatic laparoscopic stapling device is applied to the left infundibulopelvic ligament.

with direct visualization of the ureter. This is followed by desiccation and division of mesosalpinx and meso-ovarian. If the ovary is to be preserved, the utero-ovarian junction, which includes the proximal part of the fallopian tube, utero-ovarian ligament, and mesosalpinx (the round ligament has already been divided as described in step 3), is desiccated with Kleppinger bipolar forceps and then divided. An automatic laparoscopic stapling device (MULTI-FIRE ENDO GIA-30 [United States Surgical Corp, Norwalk, CT] or Lineal Cutter-35 [Ethicon Endo-surgery, Cincinnati, OH]) may be time-saving for this portion of the procedure (Fig 10.7). This device can be inserted into the peritoneal cavity through the 12-mm umbilical trocar sleeve and guided by a 5-mm laparoscope through a left upper 5-mm trocar sleeve. This step also can be achieved using ligatures through an opening in the broad ligament and tying the infundibulopelvic ligament or the utero-ovarian junction with the extracorporal knot-tying technique, using the Clark knot pusher (Fig 10.8 and Plate 11).

Step 5

At this point the posterior leaf of the broad ligament is divided to the

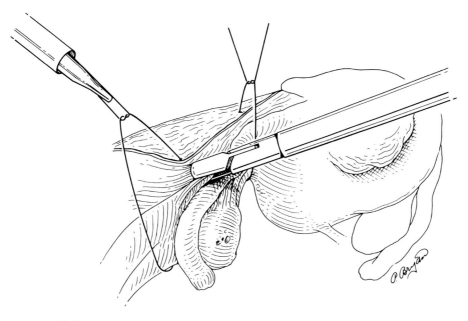

FIGURE 10.8

The left infundibulopelvic ligament is ligated with an O-vicryl suture.

uterine artery, which is skeletonized laterally to the ureteric canal where the uterine artery crosses above the ureter (Fig 8.2). With the ureter in direct view, the uterine artery is desiccated with Kleppinger bipolar forceps and divided. This also can be achieved by using suture technique with 0-vicryl on a CT-1 needle. The suture can include both uterine artery and cardinal ligament (Fig 10.9 and Plate 12). The uterine artery also can be suture ligated prior to its crossing over the ureter at the area of the ureteric canal (Plate 13). An automatic laparoscopic stapling device also can be used effectively in this step. However, before firing the stapling device, both the ureter and the bladder must be carefully monitored, making sure that nothing is inside the jaws of the stapling device except the uterine artery and the cardinal ligament (Fig 10.10).

Step 6

With direct visualization of both ureters, the remaining cardinal ligament and both uterosacral ligaments are desiccated with bipolar forceps and divided with scissors or laser.

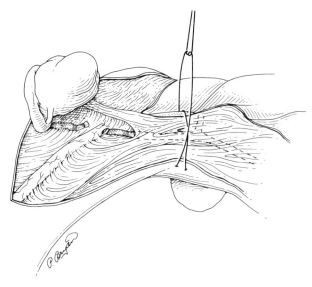

FIGURE 10.9

The left uterine artery and cardinal ligament are suture ligated with an O-vicryl suture.

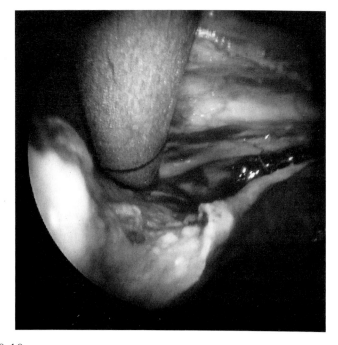

FIGURE 10.10

The right ureter is found to be inside the jaw of an automatic stapling device.

Step 7

At this point the surgical assistant puts a wet 4×4 sponge on the tip of a sponge forceps and places it in the anterior vaginal fornix, tenting the vagina from below. The anterior culdotomy is performed laparoscopically using a high-power density CO_2 laser, such as 80 W, 200 mJ (Plate 14). With the sponge in the vagina as a guide and the suction-irrigator probe as the backstop, circumferential culdotomy is performed and the cervix is completely detached from the vagina. This step requires careful coordination between the surgeon and the assistants, because the CO_2 gas leaks rapidly as soon as the anterior cul-de-sac is opened. This step can be performed more easily by removing the uterine manipulator from the cervix as soon as the anterior culdotomy is done. A small sponge pad in a surgical glove, with its opening tied and placed inside the vagina, can maintain positive pneumoperitoneum. The anterior lip of the cervix and the anterior vaginal wall are then grasped laparoscopically with toothed grasping forceps, and the circumferential culdotomy is performed with scissors (Fig 10.11 and Plate 15) or a monopolar needle electrode. The uterus is then pulled or pushed into the vagina to maintain the pneumoperitoneum. For the large fibroid uterus, morcellation through the vagina can be done.

Step 8

The vagina is then closed either transversely or vertically, with special emphasis on suturing both uterosacrocardinal ligaments to the vaginal vault to ensure adequate vaginal support. Three interrupted figure-of-eight or continuous sutures with O-vicryl are used to close the vaginal cuff laparoscopically. Under direct visualization of the left ureter, a suture is placed deeply through the left uterosacrocardinal ligament and into the vagina; the suture then exits the vagina through the anterior vaginal wall, including the pubocervical fascia. The suture then goes through the same steps again to ensure closure of the vaginal corner (Fig 10.12 and Plate 16). The suture is tied with an extracorporal knot-tying technique using a knot pusher. The same procedure is then performed on the right side of the vaginal corner, including the right uterosacrocardinal ligament, and the posterior and anterior vaginal walls. An additional figure-of-eight or continuous suture is placed between

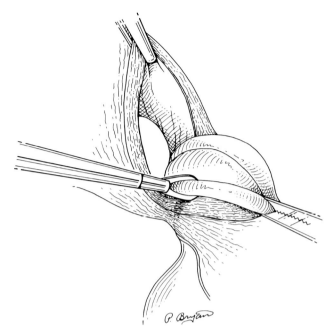

FIGURE 10.11

Circumferential culdotomy is performed with scissors.

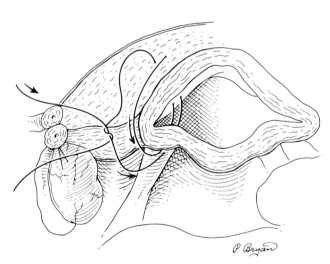

FIGURE 10.12

Under direct visualization of the left ureter, the uterosacral ligament is sutured to the left corner of the vaginal cuff laparoscopically.

184   Laparoscopic Hysterectomy and Pelvic Floor Reconstruction

these two lateral sutures to close the middle portion of the vagina (Fig 10.13). If an enterocele or vaginal prolapse is present, it is repaired at this step.

Step 9

The entire pelvic cavity is carefully inspected laparoscopically and irrigated with copious amounts of Ringer's lactate solution. All debris and blood clots are removed and the pelvis is viewed underwater (Fig 10.14) to ensure satisfactory hemostasis. Both ureters are inspected carefully. If ureteral injury is suspected, 5 mL of indigo carmine dye and 20 mg of furosemide (Lasix) are injected intravenously, and a cystoscopic examination is performed. Visualization of the normal peristalsis of the intramural portion of the ureters and ejection of the indigo carmine dye from the ureteral orifices (Fig 8.9) reassures that the integrity of ureters has not been compromised.

POSTOPERATIVE CONSIDERATIONS

Postoperative care for total laparoscopic hysterectomy is essentially the same as for LAVH, which is described in Chapter 9. The vaginal cuff is checked for granulation tissue at 6 and 12 weeks postoperatively. Sexual activity may be resumed when the vaginal incision has healed, usually after 6 weeks.

RESULTS

As of July 1992, we have performed 518 laparoscopic hysterectomies (14). The patient's age, body weight, uterine weight, operating time, hospital stay, and blood loss are presented in Table 10.1. Pathologies and indications are presented in Table 10.2 and concomitant procedures are presented in Table 10.3.

The overall complication rate was 5.7%. One patient, a heavy smoker, developed bilateral pneumonia on the third postoperative day after an otherwise uncomplicated hysterectomy. She subsequently

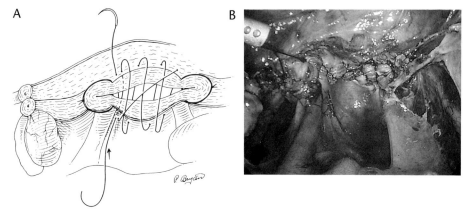

FIGURE 10.13

A continuous suture is placed between two corner stitches to close the middle portion of the vagina.

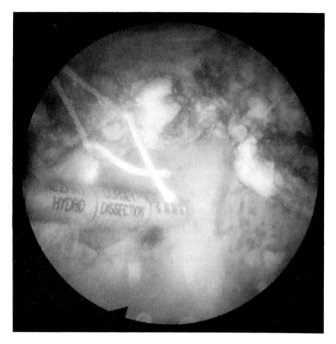

FIGURE 10.14

Underwater viewing of the pelvic pedicles to ensure complete hemostasis. The peritoneal cavity is deflated and filled with irrigation solution before performing the underwater examination.

186   Laparoscopic Hysterectomy and Pelvic Floor Reconstruction

TABLE 10.1

518 Laparoscopic hysterectomies and concomitant surgeries

	PATIENT CHARACTERISTICS					
	AGE (yr)	BODY WEIGHT (lb)	UTERINE WEIGHT (gm)	OPERATING TIME (min)	HOSPITAL STAY (d)	BLOOD LOSS (mL)
Range	26–79	106–328	48–1000	45–390	1–7	25–1000
Mean	42	142	175	120	1.4	115

TABLE 10.2

Pathologies in 518 laparoscopic hysterectomies and concomitant surgeries

PATHOLOGY	NO. OF PATIENTS
Leiomyoma	289
Endometriosis[a]	211
Adenomyosis	185
Ovarian cysts (>6 cm)[b]	7
Postmenopausal uterine bleeding with endometrial polyp/submucosal fibroids[c]	5
Benign pathology[d]	37
Endometrial adenocarcinoma (stage I)	5
Ovarian cancer (stage I)	2
Cervical cancer (stage I)	2
Total	743

[a] Fifty-eight patients had stage IV endometriosis; 49, stage III (AFS classification).
[b] Five cysts were hemorrhagic cysts, one was a dermoid cyst, and one was a benign serous cystadenoma.
[c] All five patients had previous major pelvic surgery.
[d] Surgery performed for extensive adhesions, hydrosalpinx, etc.

Table 10.3

Procedures concomitant with 518 laparoscopic hysterectomies

Procedures[a]	No. of Patients
Vaporization/excision of endometriosis	211
Lysis/excision of adhesions	240
Appendectomy	158
Retropubic colposuspension (Burch procedure)	58
Repair of bowel injury[b]	4
Repair of bladder injury	5
Pelvic lymphadenectomy	3
Lymphadenectomy and omentectomy	2
Radical hysterectomy with lymphadenectomy	2
Total	683

[a] Procedures exclude salpingo-oophorectomy.
[b] Two small bowel injuries and two rectal injuries.

developed adult respiratory distress syndrome and died 9 days after surgery. The autopsy attributed her death to massive bilateral pneumonia.

Complications included febrile morbidity (2.1%), injuries to the urinary tract system (1.3%), injuries to the bowel (1.1%), vaginal cuff bleeding (0.5%), unanticipated blood transfusions (0.3%), and pulmonary embolism (0.2%) (Table 10.4). Four patients who developed pelvic hematoma also had postoperative fever; two of these patients required a second-look laparoscopy to evacuate a hematoma and the other two hematomas were resolved gradually with conservative measures. In each of these cases, MULTI-FIRE ENDO GIA-30, an automatic laparoscopic stapling device that had just appeared on the market, was used. We were led to believe that there was a built-in mechanism to preserve the microcirculation and thus to promote healing of the stapling sites.

When an automatic stapling device is used, careful underwater examination of the stapler line for complete hemostasis at the end of

TABLE 10.4

The complications of 518 laparoscopic hysterectomies and concomitant surgeries

COMPLICATION	NO. OF PATIENTS	RATE (%)	RATE PER 100 WOMEN[a]
Febrile morbidity	11		2.12
Pneumonia[b]	1	0.19	
Pelvic hematomas[c]	4	0.77	
Dehydration	1	0.19	
Transient febrile episodes	5	0.96	
Urinary tract system	7		1.35
Bladder injury	5	0.96	
Vesicovaginal fistula	1	0.19	
Ureterovaginal fistula	1	0.19	
Intestinal complications	6		1.15
Small bowel enterotomy	2	0.38	
Thermal injury of sigmoid colon	1	0.19	
Partial bowel obstruction	1	0.19	
Richter's hernia[d]	2	0.38	
Vaginal cuff bleeding	3		0.57
Unanticipated blood transfusion	2		0.38
Pulmonary embolism	1		0.19
Total	30		5.76

[a] Rate per 100 women who underwent hysterectomy and concomitant surgery.
[b] This patient later developed adult respiratory distress syndrome and died.
[c] Two of the patients had second-look laparoscopy and the hematomas were evacuated.
[d] Richter's hernia occurred at the 12-mm trocar puncture sites.

surgery after discontinuation of the pneumoperitoneal pressure is important for hematoma prevention. Any bleeding, including oozing, detected at this time requires bipolar coagulation behind the stapler line. No hematoma formation occurred in either group using electrosurgery or sutures for large vessel hemostasis.

Six bladder injuries occurred in our series, five of which were detected intraoperatively and successfully repaired. Early recognition of bladder injury during surgery can be facilitated by routine installation of concentrated indigo carmine dye into the bladder preoperatively. One patient developed a vesicovaginal fistula 4 weeks postoperatively. This late occurrence of vesicovaginal fistula is unusual. We reviewed the operative videotape and were unable to detect any evidence of bladder injury. We postulate that the fistula formation might have been due to a suture penetrating the bladder wall during the vaginal cuff closure. One case of ureterovaginal fistula that was unrecognized during surgery occurred early in our experience. Subsequently, we routinely identify and dissect the ureters before initiating the hysterectomy in all our cases, and we have had no further ureteral injuries. Ureteral identification is critically important before laparoscopic ligation of the uterine artery and cardinal ligaments. On several occasions the ureters were inside the jaws of the automatic stapling device and would have been injured if the dissection of the ureters had not been done before applying the stapling device. We were also surprised, on many occasions, at the close proximity of the ureters to the cervix. When a hysterectomy is performed laparoscopically, the surgeon must rely on ureteral visualization to avoid injury.

Bowel injury during the hysterectomy is usually associated with extensive adhesions and endometriosis (15). In our series, two small bowel injuries occurred during enterolysis due to extensive adhesions. If laparoscopic repair of small bowel laceration is intended, special care must be taken to avoid narrowing the intestinal lumen and compromising the vascular supply of the intestine during the repair (16,17). Two intentional rectal wall resections were performed for full-thickness infiltration of endometriosis in our series, and the rectal defect was repaired laparoscopically (17,18). It is important that bowel preparation be done in all patients suspicious for cul-de-sac pathology. The regimen for bowel preparation has served us well over the years, both in open and laparoscopic surgeries. This consists of 1) administering erythromycin 250 mg every 6 hours and neomycin 1 gm every 4 hours starting 48 hours before surgery; 2) a clear liquid diet at least 36 hours before surgery; and 3) PEG-3350 and electrolytes for oral solation (Golytely [Braintree Laboratories, Braintree, MA]) 4 liters by mouth beginning the afternoon prior to surgery. We also have had two patients develop Richter's hernia in the 12-mm trocar sites, which emphasizes the need to suture the fascia when the trocar size exceeds 8 mm (19–21).

CONCLUSION

In reviewing the literature and from our own experience in performing laparoscopic hysterectomies, we conclude that even with experience, laparoscopic hysterectomy is not an innocuous procedure. Gynecologists who are interested in performing laparoscopic hysterectomy must know their limits and select patients accordingly. The high cost of laparoscopic-assisted hysterectomy has been criticized (22). The two primary reasons for increased operative costs are exclusive use of disposable instruments and the surgeon's inexperience in performing the surgery, thus prolonging the operating time. It is imperative that gynecologists become as cost-effective as possible without compromising safety or efficacy. The transition from open surgery to video-guided surgery requires considerable adjustment. Knowledge of laparoscopic instrumentation, suturing techniques, physics and clinical applications of electrosurgery and laser, and avoiding/managing laparoscopic complications are required. Assisting and precepting with surgeons proficient in laparoscopic hysterectomy are critical, for we are convinced that one cannot learn the operation outside the operating room. Conversion to abdominal hysterectomy should never be considered a complication; rather, it is a prudent surgical decision when the surgeon becomes uncomfortable with the laparoscopic approach.

REFERENCES

1. Wilcox LS, Koonin LM, Pokras R, et al. Hysterectomy in the United States, 1988–1990. Obstet Gynecol 1994;83:549–555.

2. Pokras R. Hysterectomy: past, present, and future. Stat Bull Metrop Insur Co 1989;70:12.

3. Kovac SR, Cruikshank SH, Retto WF. Laparoscopic assisted vaginal hysterectomy. J Gynecol Surg 1990;6:185–193.

4. Liu CY. Laparoscopic hysterectomy, a review of 72 cases. J Reprod Med 1992;37:351–354.

5. Liu CY. Laparoscopic hysterectomy. Report of 215 cases. Gynecol Endoscopy 1992;1:73–77.

6. Liu CY. Laparoscopic hysterectomy. Gynecol Endoscopy 1993;2:73–75.

7. Reich H. Laparoscopic hysterectomy. Surg Laparoscopy Endoscopy 1992;2:85–88.

8. Reich H, McGlynn F, Sekel L. Total laparoscopic hysterectomy. Gynecol Endoscopy 1993;2:59–63.

9. Garry R, Reich H, Liu CY. Laparoscopic hysterectomy—definitions and indications. Gynecol Endoscopy 1994;3:1–3. Editorial.

10. Parker WH, Berek JS. Management of selected cystic adnexal masses in postmenopausal women by operative laparoscopy: a pilot study. Am J Obstet Gynecol 1990;163:1574–1577.

11. Mann WJ, Reich H. Laparoscopic adnexectomy in postmenopausal women. J Reprod Med 1992;37:254–256.

12. Reich H, Clarke HC, Sekel L. A simple method for ligating in operative laparoscopy with straight and curved needles. Obstet Gynecol 1992;79:143–147.

13. Hirsch HA. Prophylactic antibiotics in obstetrics and gynecology. Am J Med 1985;78(suppl 6B):170–176.

14. Liu CY, Reich H. Complications of total laparoscopic hysterectomy in 518 cases. Gynecol Endoscopy 1994;3:203–208.

15. Wheeless CR Jr. Gastrointestinal injuries associated with laparoscopy. In: Phillips JM, ed. Endoscopy in gynecology. Downey, CA: Am Assoc Gynecol Laparosc, 1978.

16. Reich H. Laparoscopic bowel injury. Surg Laparoscopy Endoscopy 1992;2:74–78.

17. Reich H, McGlynn F, Budin R. Laparoscopic repair of full thickness bowel injury. J Laparoendoscop Surg 1991;1:119–122.

18. Harder F, Vogelbach P. Single layer end-on continuous suture of colonic anastomosis. Am J Surg 1988;155:611–614.
19. Kadar N, Liu Cy, Reich H, Gimpelson R. Incisional hernias following major laparoscopic gynecological procedures. Am J Obstet Gynecol 1993;168:1493–1495.
20. Schiff I, Naftolin F. Small bowel incarceration after uncomplicated laparoscopy. Gynecology 1974;43:674.
21. Bourke JB. Small intestinal obstruction from a Richter's hernia at the site of a laparoscope. BMJ 1977;2:1393–1394.
22. Baggish MS. The most expensive hysterectomy. J Gynecol Surg 1992;8: 578. Editorial.

11

Laparoscopic Hysterectomy for Extensive Endometriosis

David B. Redwine

Endometriosis is the occurrence outside the uterus of tissue that somewhat resembles native endometrium. Endometriosis cannot be considered simplistically as ectopically placed endometrium since it differs fundamentally with respect to hormone receptor content (1–4), hormone response (5,6), and visual appearance (7–11).

THEORIES OF ETIOLOGY

Sampson's Theory

Sampson's theory of reflux menstruation and implantation (12) remains popular, but the initial attachment of single or multiple endometrial cells to the peritoneal surface has not been conclusively demonstrated. Additionally, the time-related geographic spread of endometriosis throughout the pelvis that would be predicted to occur with repeated seeding of the peritoneum by refluxed endometrium has not been demonstrated. Several studies measuring disease extent across advancing age by number of pelvic areas involved (13), surface area (14), and revised American Fertility Society classification system (15) have failed to find evidence that older age groups of patients with endometriosis have more disease than younger age groups. Pelvic endometriosis can occur in areas that are unexplainable by Sampson's theory (16–19). This theory of origin also implies a high and progressively increasing rate of recurrence after complete surgical destruction. However, the actual rate of persistent or recurrent disease is surprisingly low after aggressive conservative surgical excision at laparotomy (20) or laparoscopy (21) and the rate of recurrent or persistent disease does not appear to increase with the passage of time following excision (21). Because of these deficits, Sampson's theory is losing favor to more modern concepts.

Embryonically Patterned Metaplasia or Rests

During organogenesis, cells migrate caudally across the dorsal coelomic epithelium while undergoing differentiation to form the pelvic organs. Embryogenesis is directed by a sophisticated but incompletely understood fetal system. This system presumably acts in part by detecting and manipulating cell surface antigens. Such a fetal developmental control system may be the fetal anlage of the adult immune system.

If a developmental or heritable defect in this controlling system existed, then differentiation and migration of cells may be aberrant or incomplete. Cellular morphology and functionality might be expressed overabundantly or inadequately. Such cells or tracts of cells are laid down in the migratory pathway of fetal organogenesis across the posterior pelvic floor, although location anywhere might be possible, depending on the degree of aberrant differentiation or migration. These cells may be endometrium-like initially or may possess the ability to undergo metaplasia into endometriosis after puberty. Arrest of migration across the posterior pelvis would conveniently explain the observation that endometriosis is most commonly and predictably found in the cul-de-sac, uterosacral ligaments, and medial broad ligaments. Abnormalities of the fetal development control system may be preserved into adult life, giving rise to detectable abnormalities of the adult immune system. In adult patients with endometriosis, such abnormalities might be interpreted as being contemporaneously associated with the cause of the disease rather than as echoes of a "big bang" that may have occurred in utero. The degree of residual abnormality of the adult immune system may control the virulence of the endometriosis that develops, with the result that some patients may develop invasive disease or adhesions while most do not. The competence of the adult immune system might be impaired by exposure to environmental toxins, with endometriosis emerging as a possible result, as occurs in primates (22–25). Incomplete müllerian regression in fetal life in males could give rise to the potential for development of endometriosis of the male bladder (26) or prostate (27) in later life during estrogen treatment of advanced prostatic cancer.

Other Theories

Hematogenous metastasis of endometriosis has been proposed to explain remote occurrence of the disease. According to this theory, exfoliated endometrial cells are swept into the venous drainage of the uterus, with subsequent deposition possible anywhere in the body. Venous blood draining the uterus must pass through the capillary bed of the lungs. Therefore, hematogenous spread should also result in a high rate of secondary pulmonary endometriosis unless there exists a high rate of occurrence of atrial or ventricular septal defects among patients with extrapelvic endometriosis. Since neither pulmonary endometriosis nor cardiac atrial or ventricular septal defects have been reported to be more frequent in patients with endometriosis, hematogenous spread remains speculative.

The theory of lymphatic spread has been supported by the finding of endometriosis in lymph nodes (17–19), although the number of reported cases is quite small compared with the number of women with endometriosis. However, endometriosis in lymph nodes could equally plausibly be explained by a developmental process that resulted in embryonic deposition of endometriosis in lymph nodal tissue.

SYMPTOMATOLOGY, DIAGNOSIS, AND TREATMENT DECISIONS

Pelvic pain may arise from primary and secondary effects of endometriosis or from pathology or dysfunction of the uterus, tubes, or ovaries. Nongynecologic pelvic pain also may occur from musculoskeletal or intestinal origins. It is important to try to determine the source of pain so that appropriate surgery can be applied. Simply put, complete removal of endometriosis will relieve pain caused by that disease so long as it does not recur, while pain originating in the female pelvic organs may require removal of some or all of those organs. Simply because conservative surgical techniques exist for the complete eradication of endometriosis does not make such surgery appropriate for all patients.

Gynecologic pain syndromes are somewhat predictable by virtue of the affected anatomy (28). The geographic distribution of pelvic endometriosis, which is predictable and unchanging over several decades (29), leads to characteristic symptom patterns related to affected anatomy. The distribution of pelvic areas of occurrence of endometriosis is shown in Table 11.1, while the most common areas of intestinal

TABLE 11.1

Distribution of endometriosis in the pelvis among 1277 patients with histologically proven endometriosis in the author's practice

PELVIC AREA	NO. OF PATIENTS (%)
Cul–de–sac	892 (69.8)
Left broad ligament	660 (51.7)
Right broad ligament	551 (43.1)
Left uterosacral ligament	524 (41.0)
Right uterosacral ligament	478 (37.4)
Bladder	406 (31.8)
Left ovary	214 (16.8)
Fundus	203 (15.9)
Right ovary	199 (15.6)
Left fallopian tube	104 (8.1)
Right fallopian tube	73 (5.7)
Vagina	12 (0.9)
Scar	3 (0.23)
Umbilicus	1 (0.08)

Endometriosis patients with previous hysterectomy with (N = 93) or without (N = 45) bilateral salpingo-oophorectomy are excluded.

endometriosis are shown in Table 11.2. The mechanism by which endometriosis causes pain is not known. Cyclic bleeding of endometriosis with menses is unpredictable (5), and many lesions are nonhemorrhagic (7–11). Therefore, some other mechanism must be responsible for pain, such as a paracrine secretion by endometriotic glands resulting in local pain and possibly systemic effects.

Since the cul-de-sac, uterosacral ligaments, and medial broad ligaments are the most commonly involved pelvic areas, it is logical that symptoms will arise from immediately adjacent organs. Therefore, dyspareunia, painful bowel movements, tenderness on examination, and chronic pelvic pain are common complaints. In the occasional patient with an ovarian endometrioma, lateral pain may occur. Rectal pain, rectal pain with passage of flatus, or rectal pain with each bowel movement may occur with intestinal endometriosis. Nodular deformation of the bowel wall may produce symptoms of partial intestinal obstruction. Pain due to endometriosis may occur at variable times of the menstrual cycle. Many patients may begin to experience pain around ovulation with a crescendo pattern of pain up to menses, during which the pain may be severely aggravated. While such severe pain with menses is correctly termed "dysmenorrhea," such pain may be different from uterine cramps. Many patients can distinguish uterine cramping superimposed on top of the already existing pain of endometriosis. Careful questioning may allow the examiner to determine whether pain is likely

TABLE 11.2

Distribution of intestinal endometriosis among 370 patients with intestinal disease in the author's practice

INTESTINAL AREA	NO. OF PATIENTS (%)
Sigmoid	243 (65.7)
Rectal nodule	163 (44.0)
Ileum	56 (15.1)
Appendix*	35 (9.5)
Cecum	22 (5.9)

*Some patients had undergone previous appendectomy.

due to endometriosis, the uterus, or perhaps both. Some patients may experience chronic pain that may be exacerbated prior to and during menses.

Physical Examination for Endometriosis

The physical examination is limited by finger length, technique, and psychic expectations. It is fortunate that most gynecologists can easily palpate the pelvic and intestinal areas most commonly involved, since tenderness in these areas is frequently the only positive sign suggesting the presence of endometriosis. Tender nodularity is considered by many to be pathognomonic for endometriosis (30), although nodularity is less common than tenderness. When tenderness is found on examination, pathology is usually present in that location. Although a palpable adnexal mass may be endometriosis, some higher pelvic areas cannot be reached on examination. Digital rectal examination may reveal nodularity of the anterior bowel wall and adjacent cul-de-sac. Since intestinal endometriosis almost never penetrates to the bowel lumen, the mucosa will usually be felt to slide across a nodule in the bowel wall.

The technique of the pelvic examination is important, and obvious signs may be missed, even on speculum examination. The posterior blade of the vaginal speculum normally comes to rest behind the cervix, obscuring the posterior fornix. If endometriosis is invading the vaginal mucosa, it can remain hidden behind the posterior blade, and thus be missed (Fig 11.1). On bimanual examination, after determining the position, size, and tenderness of the uterus and ovaries, special attention must be paid to the presence or absence of tenderness in the uterosacral ligaments and cul-de-sac. This can be best elicited by performing the second part of the examination with "one hand tied behind your back." Without the use of the external examining hand, the fingers of the internal hand are used to gently palpate separately the uterosacral ligament on one side, followed by the cul-de-sac, then the other uterosacral ligament. The facial expression of the patient should be noted as each area is palpated. A normal pelvic examination is not associated with tenderness, while the tenderness associated with endometriosis will usually produce at least a grimace. Some patients will arch the back, cry out,

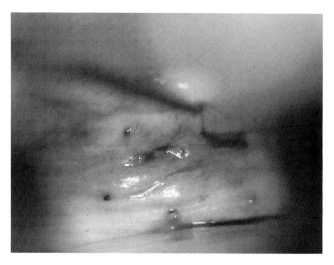

FIGURE 11.1

View of the posterior vaginal fornix through a speculum. A tenaculum is grasping the posterior cervix and retracting it anteriorly so that the fornix can be visualized. The posterior blade of the speculum may hide this area.

and push away on the table. A doctor's psychic expectations can bias clinical diagnosis. Many clinicians believe that pelvic inflammatory disease is more common than endometriosis, while actually the reverse is true. Pelvic pain and tenderness with or without nodularity on examination, particularly in the absence of fever or elevated white blood cell count or sedimentation rate, should lead to a diagnosis of endometriosis in most patients. Likewise, a diagnosis of uncomplicated pelvic infection not responding to appropriate antibiotics should raise the suspicion of endometriosis.

Diagnostic Testing

Laboratory and imaging tests are not as helpful as the history and physical examination in diagnosing endometriosis. Indeed, since most patients do not have ovarian involvement and since endometriosis is frequently present as a peritoneal process with varying degrees of local invasion, tests such as pelvic ultrasound, computed tomography, and magnetic resonance imaging will routinely be misleading when endometriosis is present. Even among patients subsequently requiring full-thickness or segmental bowel resections for intestinal endometriosis, barium enema and sigmoidoscopy are usually interpreted as negative.

Deciding on Conservative Versus Radical Surgery

Several factors help determine a patient's candidacy for conservative or radical surgery. The most obvious is that a patient who desires to bear a child will be a candidate for conservative surgery. In women not desiring future childbearing, radical surgery may be chosen by the patient if uterine or ovarian symptoms or pathology is present. The more common uterine conditions that might prompt consideration of radical surgery include symptomatic uterine fibroids, menorrhagia, endometrial or cervical pathology, or painful uterine cramps. Although imaging tests may suggest the presence of uterine pathology, the decision to perform surgery is best made primarily on the basis of symptoms.

Ovarian conditions that may prompt consideration of removal of the ovaries include cysts, lateral pelvic pain, ovulation pain, or premenstrual syndrome. A borderline or low serum estradiol level may prompt a decision to remove the ovaries at the time of hysterectomy.

Although hysterectomy with castration is thought of as curative of endometriosis, there is no scientific evidence that endometriosis is destroyed by low levels of estrogen. Symptomatic endometriosis persisting after castration has been well documented (31) and pain relief occurs in most such patients after excision (32). Hysterectomy with castration and retention of endometriosis may relieve pelvic pain, but it should not be presented to patients as curative of the disease. Endometriosis can remain symptomatic even in postmenopausal patients who are not on estrogen.

Patients with known obliteration of the cul-de-sac, known disease of the colon, suggestive bowel symptoms, or significant nodularity of the cul-de-sac or uterosacral ligaments should undergo bowel preparation. Oral colonic lavage (4 liters the afternoon before surgery) followed by two enemas the evening before surgery results in a superb bowel preparation. Tolerance to this bowel preparation can be increased by the addition of flavor crystals, chilling, or use of a nose plug. Clear liquids are allowed by mouth the day before surgery. An alternate oral bowel preparation is magnesium citrate. Some patients may give a history of total intolerance to all known oral bowel preparations. In such patients,

3 days of clear liquids followed by enemas until clear the evening before and again the morning of surgery is a satisfactory alternative. It is fortunate that the lower colon usually can be cleansed by enemas, since this is the area of the intestinal tract that is most commonly involved by endometriosis. If full-thickness bowel resection is anticipated, prophylactic intravenous antibiotics are given.

PRINCIPLES OF SURGICAL TREATMENT OF ENDOMETRIOSIS

Since no medicine eradicates endometriosis, it is the responsibility of the surgeon to identify and remove all disease. The identification of endometriosis at surgery is as much an art as a science, and past errors in the identification of endometriosis have contributed to the misunderstanding of this disease (33). In simple terms, the surgeon must be suspicious that any abnormality of the peritoneal surface is endometriosis unless proven otherwise by biopsy. This presupposes that the surgeon can also identify normal peritoneum by its cardinal criteria (34). Although the visual diagnosis of endometriosis may be correct in many instances, not all abnormalities of the peritoneal surface are endometriotic.

Invasive endometriosis presents other problems. In the mechanical practice of surgery, it is sometimes difficult to judge the depth of invasion of endometriosis by its visual appearance alone (35,36). Invasive endometriosis is associated with pain, and the surgical treatment of endometriosis must be adequate to deal with invasive disease without undue risk of damage to surrounding vital structures. The surgical technique also must be adequate for treatment of superficial or invasive intestinal endometriosis. Fortunately, even in a referral practice, lower stages of endometriosis are more common than advanced disease (Table 11.3).

Demonstrating the efficacy of a surgical technique in treating endometriosis requires two surgeries to measure objectively the extent of disease: the initial therapeutic surgery and a follow-up surgery. A randomized controlled trial is not necessary to demonstrate efficacy of a

TABLE 11.3

Extent of endometriosis in 103 patients undergoing laparoscopic hysterectomy with or without castration by the author.

rAFS Stage	No. of Patients (%)	No. of Patients with Gastrointestinal Endometriosis (%)
0	41 (39.8)	0 (0)
I	33 (32.0)	1 (1.0)
II	20 (19.4)	3 (2.9)
III	4 (3.8)	1 (1.0)
IV	5 (4.8)	3 (2.9)

All laparoscopic cases had control and transection of the uterine vessels and laparoscopic vaginal entry with vaginal closure from below. Cases without laparoscopic culdotomy are not included. Three cases converted to laparotomy are not included. rAFS = revised American Fertility Society.

surgical treatment of endometriosis because each patient must serve as her own control to answer the question: Is the disease reduced or eradicated by a certain surgical technique? Postoperative medical treatment of endometriosis will obscure surgical results and is unnecessary since it does not eradicate endometriosis.

TECHNIQUE

The principles of safe surgery include 1) identification of a surgical goal that is scientifically valid and therapeutically feasible, 2) development of a surgical strategy based on excellent knowledge of anatomy to achieve this goal in an efficient fashion, and 3) sufficient physical separation of normal tissue and structures from diseased tissue before application of surgical energy. Separation of normal tissues and structures from diseased tissue is accomplished primarily by blunt dissection and retraction. My technique for laparoscopic hysterectomy is directed at maximum safety, efficiency, and economy, as well as removal of all disease.

For laparoscopic hysterectomy in patients with extensive endometriosis, the surgical goal is removal of the uterus (and perhaps the tubes and ovaries) for relief of symptoms related to these structures, and removal of all endometriosis as well. The surgical strategy is accomplished most efficiently in the following order: 1) initiation of laparoscopy, 2) creation of all peritoneal incisions, 3) isolation of all vascular pedicles, 4) transection of all vascular pedicles, 5) culdotomy, and 6) completion of surgery vaginally. This sequence reduces instrument changes.

INITIATION OF LAPAROSCOPY

After induction of general anesthesia, the patient is placed in low lithotomy position with the edge of the buttocks well down over the end of the table. This allows full range of motion of the intrauterine manipulator. If knee stirrups are used, they should be well padded to avoid peroneal nerve injury during a prolonged surgery. The vulva, vagina, and abdomen are prepared in the usual fashion, and a retention catheter is placed in the bladder. With a speculum in the vagina, the cervix is grasped with a tenaculum and the vaginal mucosa is injected circumferentially with a dilute solution of xylocaine and epinephrine, as is frequently done during the performance of a vaginal hysterectomy. The scissors or scalpel is now used to create a mucosal incision around the cervix, with care taken not to create an anterior or posterior colpotomy at this time, since this would make maintenance of a pneumoperitoneum difficult. In addition, a sharp incision in the vaginal mucosa closed with interrupted absorbable sutures heals more cleanly and with less chance of granulation than does an electrosurgical burn that is later closed with interlocking absorbable sutures. The rectovaginal septum should be developed bluntly yet cautiously, with digital dissection ceasing when the fibrosis or nodularity associated with obliteration of the cul-de-sac is encountered. This not only reduces the risk of blunt trauma to the bowel wall, but also keeps the distorted anatomy unaltered until it can be visualized and handled in the systematic fashion discussed below. If endometriosis is noted to be invading the posterior vaginal wall adjacent to the cervix, the injection is made in the normal mucosa around the invasive nodule, and the mucosal incision is altered slightly on the posterior vaginal wall to allow the involved mucosa to remain attached to the cervix when the uterus is finally removed. An intrauterine manipulator is placed, and the tenaculum and speculum are removed.

A small vertical incision is created within the elevated umbilicus and a 10-mm, all-metal, reusable trocar is inserted directly. The all-metal sheath allows any electrical charge induced in the laparoscope and sheath to be discharged harmlessly at low current density in the abdominal wall. The reusable trocar and sheath is economical and environmentally friendly. The point of the trocar is typically somewhat dull from repeated use, which decreases the likelihood of sharp perforation of the bowel during insertion. A previous Pfannensteil incision is no guarantee against omental or intestinal adhesions reaching to the umbilicus. Prior insufflation with a Verres needle is not used, since this would increase the number of blind instrument insertions from one to two. A 10-mm operating laparoscope is passed through this umbilical port and, if intraperitoneal placement is confirmed, carboperitoneum is established. The inferior epigastric vessels are visualized behind the parietal peritoneum and two 5.5-mm reusable trocars with fiberglass shafts are inserted lateral to these vessels. To make insertion of these trocars easier and safer, the abdominal wall is elevated with the tip of the shaft of the already-inserted laparoscope placed just lateral to the epigastric vessels. The 5.5-mm trocars are then inserted toward midline while held in a horizontal position, sliding underneath the shaft of the laparoscope and entering the pocket of pneumoperitoneum beyond. This avoids directing the trocars toward the iliac vessels during insertion. A 5-mm–shafted, atraumatic grasper is inserted in the left lower quadrant and a suction-irrigator is inserted on the right. There are many reported variations of trocar and laparoscope placement, but I use only the three ports outlined above.

By operating while looking down the laparoscope rather than at a video monitor, no assistant surgeon is needed to hold a camera. Although a skilled assistant can be helpful, an inexperienced assistant will hinder surgery by inattention or misdirected retraction. A surgical scrub technician can provide uterine manipulation and retraction as directed.

Laparoscopic Hysterectomy for Extensive Endometriosis   205

CREATION OF ALL PERITONEAL INCISIONS

Peritoneal incisions are created around the endometriosis and pelvic organs to be removed, using between 70 and 90 W of pure cutting current passed down the 3-mm scissors in the operating channel of the laparoscope. Since the peritoneal incisions are not created mechanically, the scissors need not be extremely sharp. The peritoneum must be under great tension during electrosurgical cutting, otherwise loose peritoneum will pillow around the tip of the active electrode, resulting in a coagulation effect instead of a smooth cutting effect. Peritoneal tension is maintained most often by grasping the peritoneum with the atraumatic graspers and drawing the tissue medially, combined with manipulation of the uterus.

The peritoneal incisions remain shallow, cutting just through the peritoneum into the loose areolar tissue beneath. The logical placement of the peritoneal incisions is important, not only to ensure that all endometriosis is removed, but also in dealing with the ovaries efficiently. In most patients undergoing hysterectomy and bilateral salpingo-oophorectomy (BSO), it is helpful to make the first peritoneal incisions lateral to the infundibulopelvic ligaments, proceeding from a point roughly adjacent to the bifurcation of the iliac vessels to the round ligament anteriorly. Endometriosis rarely involves this area and it is reasonably distanced from major blood vessels to serve as a site of safe retroperitoneal entry (Figs 11.2 and 11.3).

If an ovary is adherent to the lateral pelvic peritoneum, the first incision will allow retroperitoneal dissection to proceed posteriorly past the adjacent ovaries and to separate the peritoneum, with the ovary still attached, from the underlying sidewall structures. This will decrease the likelihood of ovarian remnant syndrome or retained endometriosis. If the ureter is encased by fibrosis and lies hidden beneath the adherent ovary, the normal peritoneum over the ureter cephalad to the ovary is located. The peritoneum is opened here and blunt retroperitoneal dissection along the ureter down behind the adherent ovary is begun to free the ureter completely (Plate 17). Atraumatic graspers can safely pull on the ureter to assist the dissection (Fig 11.4). After the ureter has been

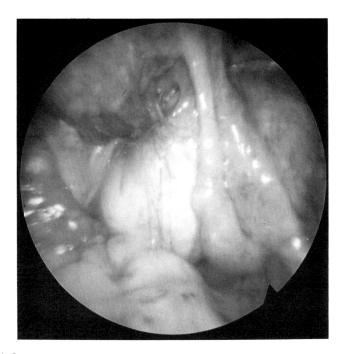

FIGURE 11.2

Stage IV endometriosis. The right ovary is enlarged by an endometrioma cyst that is adherent to the posterior uterine fundus. The cyst also can be seen distending the tissue lateral to the right infundibulopelvic ligament. Obliteration of the cul-de-sac is more common in patients with large endometriomas and was present in this case, although in this frame the cul-de-sac cannot be seen beneath the enlarged ovary.

sufficiently freed, the peritoneum is incised in a normal area posterior to the adherent ovary, again seeking to encompass all disease in the vicinity. The line of incision then proceeds medially toward the base of the uterosacral ligament, again incorporating endometriosis in the vicinity.

If the ovary is nonadherent, the initial peritoneal incision is made lateral to the infundibulopelvic ligament, as discussed above. Next, the peritoneum is incised posterior to the ovary, beginning near the region of the bifurcation of the common iliac vessels and working medially toward the uterosacral ligament. If an area of endometriosis lies over the ureter, the peritoneal incision is made through normal peritoneum posterior to the ureter. The endometriosis can then be separated from the ureter by blunt dissection. The atraumatic graspers can be used to grasp and pull the ureter to allow better retraction. If there is no endometriosis in the vicinity of the ureter, the peritoneal incision can be made anterior to the ureter, allowing the ureter to fall to safety posteriorly, still attached to the peritoneum.

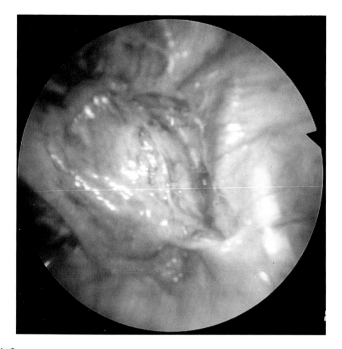

FIGURE 11.3

A peritoneal incision has been created lateral to the right infundibulopelvic ligament using 90 W of pure cutting current. The right round ligament has been transected with 50 W of coagulation current, and the peritoneal incision has been extended down the anterior broad ligament. Notice that the retroperitoneal space has been opened lateral to the peritoneum of the right sidewall. The bulge of the right ovary can be seen medial to the iliac vessels. Blunt dissection is easy in the retroperitoneal space, and although the ovary is confluently adherent to this peritoneum, the peritoneum can be separated from the lateral sidewall structures and will remain attached to the ovary as oophorectomy is performed. This will reduce the possibility of ovarian remnant syndrome.

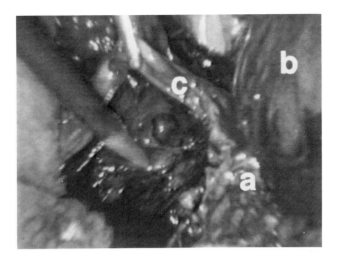

FIGURE 11.4

Pelvic side wall dissection during treatment of obliteration of the cul-de-sac. The obliterated cul-de-sac (a) is seen with the rectum adherent to the posterior uterine fundus (b). Traction on the ureter (c) with an atraumatic grasper allows the enveloping fibrosis to be stripped away by blunt dissection with the 3-mm scissors.

In dealing with the anterior pelvic peritoneal surfaces, the round ligament is placed on stretch and severed with 50 W of coagulation current. The coagulation waveform has a higher peak-to-peak voltage, so it is more powerful than cutting current at similar wattage settings. This makes it very useful for cutting parenchymal tissue, such as the round and uterosacral ligaments. The anterior leaf of the broad ligament is grasped and elevated, then incised alongside the uterus with cutting current. It is important not to make this incision too close to the uterus, since this may lead the dissection which follows into the vessels coursing along the lateral uterine body. This peritoneal incision is then carried across the anterior cervix, once again grasping and elevating the peritoneum to enhance tissue tension. This incision across the bladder peritoneum should be made in a fashion to incorporate all endometriosis onto the peritoneum, which will remain attached to the uterus (Fig 11.5). Otherwise, any endometriosis should be excised separately. If an incision

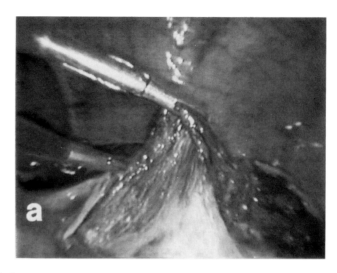

FIGURE 11.5

The peritoneal incision has been carried transversely across the bladder. The grasper above is elevating the edge of the bladder while the 3-mm scissors below are used to begin blunt dissection of the areolar tissue between the bladder and the anterior cervix. The peritoneal incision has been created to incorporate all endometriosis onto the peritoneum (a), which remains attached to the uterine fundus.

already has been created in the vagina, care should be taken not to dissect too much at this point, since pneumoperitoneum can be lost.

If the posterior cul-de-sac is free with no obliteration, the peritoneal incisions frequently can be created so that most of the endometriosis will be removed with the peritoneum attached to the uterus, tubes, and ovaries. This strategy leads to a somewhat predictable line of incision, particularly in the region of the posterior cul-de-sac, where an incision resembling an elongated W is created to surround disease that may invade along much of the length of each uterosacral ligament. The peritoneal incision of the posterior leaf of the broad ligament, followed by blunt dissection, has begun the lateral isolation of the uterosacral ligament. The peritoneal incision is carried around any endometriosis near the base of the ligament, then anteromedially toward the central cul-de-sac. This allows the ligament to be isolated on three sides by peritoneal incisions. The parenchyma of the ligament has not been approached yet. The cut edge of the base of the ligament can then be grasped and drawn forcefully anteriorly toward the cervix, and the ligament can be "shaved" off of the pelvic floor using electrosurgery to remove all invasive disease. Blunt palpation with the scissors and graspers will allow the surgeon to judge the depth of invasion accurately. Occasionally, it may be desirable to remove an area of involved peritoneum separately. Separate peritoneal resections, in fact, will increase the likelihood that the pathologist will diagnose endometriosis, since even extensive areas of peritoneal endometriosis may be hidden by peritoneal shriveling following fixation in formalin.

Obliteration of the cul-de-sac (Plate 18) presents a special challenge to the surgeon since it suggests the presence of invasive endometriosis of the uterosacral ligaments, cul-de-sac, and anterior wall of the rectum. Failure to treat such significant disease may cause continuing symptoms despite removal of the uterus, tubes, and ovaries. One third of patients with previous castration and persistent endometriosis had obliteration of the cul-de-sac identified at the time of their castration procedure, and intestinal involvement is increased in this group also (32). Unfortunately, many patients may undergo hysterectomy and castration without bowel preparation, so when intestinal endometriosis is encountered, it remains untreated. Some also advocate performance of a supracervical hysterectomy if obliteration of the cul-de-sac is encountered to reduce the risk of damage to the bowel (37). This strategy allows invasive endometriosis of the pelvic floor and bowel wall to remain behind. Persistent invasive endometriosis associated with obliteration of the cul-de-sac may continue to cause symptoms after hysterectomy with or without castration, so clinicians should not assume that symptoms will abate when disease is left behind after removal of the ovaries.

In the conservative laparoscopic en bloc resection of the pelvic floor technique for treatment of the obliterated cul-de-sac (34), the uterosacral ligaments are isolated then amputated from the posterior cervix, and an intrafascial dissection is carried down the posterior cervix until the fatty tissue of the rectovaginal septum is encountered and developed bluntly. After severing the lateral fibrofatty attachments of the rectum to the lateral pelvic walls sufficiently, the invasive, nodular endometriosis that had been invading the posterior cervix, uterosacral ligaments, and cul-de-sac is progressively isolated onto the anterior wall of the bowel. The importance of developing the normal rectovaginal septum distal to the obliterated cul-de-sac must be emphasized, since this represents a point of application of one of the principles of safe surgery: diseased tissue is completely physically isolated on all sides from the normal tissue that is to remain behind. This increases the likelihood that all disease will be removed. After all nodular disease has been isolated, it will be realized that the cul-de-sac remains obliterated, but now lies displaced and isolated onto the anterior bowel wall (Fig 11.6). The

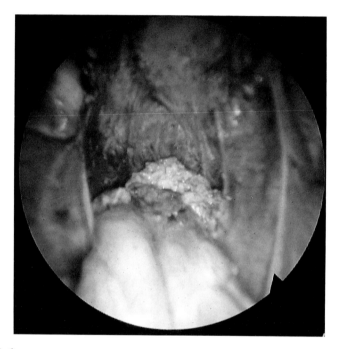

FIGURE 11.6

The obliterated cul-de-sac remains obliterated, but the nodular, invasive endometriosis of the uterosacral ligaments, posterior cervix, and cul-de-sac has been isolated to the anterior wall of the rectum. This technique is preferred when the likelihood of a significant rectal nodule is high, since it gives the clearest view of the normal bowel wall proximal and distal to the nodular mass. This allows the surgeon to judge the necessity for a partial-thickness, full-thickness, or segmental bowel resection. Notice the clean retroperitoneal tissue in the background.

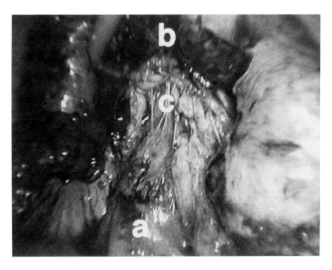

FIGURE 11.7

Alternate method of treatment of the obliterated cul-de-sac when the likeli-hood of nodular intestinal disease is low. A transverse incision has been created across the rectosigmoid colon (a), and the obliterated cul-de-sac (b) has been reflected anteriorly and lies still connected to the uterine fundus. The rectovaginal septum (c) is developed bluntly.

decision of whether to perform a partial-thickness, full-thickness, or segmental bowel resection to remove this nodular mass from the bowel wall is then made.

While these steps also may be performed in the above order prior to a laparoscopic hysterectomy, the technique may be altered slightly when a hysterectomy is concurrently performed in patients who have only serosal or outer muscularis involvement of the bowel wall. In such patients, the dissection may begin on the anterior bowel wall adjacent to the obliterated cul-de-sac, with the involved serosa and/or outer muscularis dissected off the deeper bowel wall until the dissection leads back out of the bowel wall and into the rectovaginal septum (Fig 11.7). Although this will increase surgical efficiency, the technique requires great experience to accurately judge the minimal degree of superficial bowel wall involvement that makes a patient a candidate for this varia-tion. In addition, the layers of the bowel wall separate bluntly quite easily, with the result that the dissection in the bowel wall can quickly go beyond the involved area, with greater damage than necessary resulting to the bowel. To avoid this, the surgeon must anticipate the need to dissect sharply back out to the surface of the bowel and back into the rectovaginal septum after the superficial disease has been passed, thus reflecting the superficial bowel disease onto the peritoneum that remains attached to the uterus rather than vice versa. Many surgeons otherwise might become lost in the bowel wall. Therefore, it may be preferable to perform the en bloc resection of invasive pelvic floor endometriosis as a separate procedure just before the later stages of the hysterectomy are begun, since the deranged anatomy is more likely to be restored to normal by this technique. The bowel wall can be suture repaired easily through the open vaginal cuff after the uterus is removed. If the mucosa has been penetrated, it is closed with running 3-0 chromic, while the seromuscular layer is closed with interrupted 3-0 silk sutures. The integrity of the bowel wall can be checked by filling the pelvis with irrigation fluid, then injecting air through a sigmoidoscope. Bubbles will reliably indicate any leaks.

Some patients with obliteration of the cul-de-sac also will have invasion of the posterior vaginal fornix (Fig 11.1) by endometriosis extending directly from an adjacent rectal nodule. In such a case, the dissection down the posterior cervix toward the rectovaginal septum will necessarily cut through the gristly fibrosis of this invasive disease, which can be momentarily disorienting even to an experienced surgeon. However, a vaginal mucosal incision and preliminary blunt dissection of the rectovaginal septum should already have been performed, as discussed above. If so, disorientation is only temporary, since once the rectovaginal septum is encountered, the dissection immediately enters the vagina. The vagina is tamponaded with a wet lap sponge to maintain pneumoperitoneum. At this point, the invasive endometriosis has been divided into two parts: one part includes the posterior vaginal fornix still attached to the cervix and the other part includes the uterosacral ligaments and nodular disease of the bowel wall still attached to the bowel. Laparoscopic dissection is then used to complete the isolation of the disease of the bowel wall, which can then be removed by laparoscopic bowel resection. The mucosal disease attached to the cervix now becomes simply an extension of the cervix that will be removed with the specimen.

ISOLATION OF ALL VASCULAR PEDICLES

Before transection of any vascular pedicles, it is most efficient to isolate all vascular pedicles. This avoids instrument changes until necessary and reduces the potential for back bleeding. There usually will be four pedicles to be isolated: 1) the right infundibulopelvic ligament if the right tube and ovary are to be removed (or right utero-ovarian ligament if the right tube and ovary are to remain in place), 2) the left infundibulopelvic ligament if the left tube and ovary are to be removed (or left utero-ovarian ligament if the left tube and ovary are to remain in place), 3) the left uterine artery/vein, and 4) the right uterine artery/vein. The grasper, 3-mm scissors, and suction–irrigator already in use to create the peritoneal incisions are the only instruments needed for these next steps.

If the ovaries are to be removed, the infundibulopelvic ligaments should already have peritoneal incisions anterior and posterior to them (Fig 11.3 and Plate 17). Each ligament is retracted medially and retroperitoneal dissection is carried out to strip the areolar tissue lateral to it. A blunt probe can then be passed beneath the ligament and swept anteriorly and posteriorly to completely isolate the ligament.

The technique is different if the ovaries are to be retained. The peritoneal incisions should already have been created. Posteriorly, the peritoneal incisions will lie adjacent to the body of the uterus, with some variation possible to incorporate endometriosis of the broad ligament. Monopolar coagulation current at 50 W passed down a 3-mm scissors is used to transect the utero-ovarian ligament and the adjacent fallopian tube. Care is taken not to enter the underlying vessels at this point. The peritoneal incision immediately anterior to the fallopian tube has been carried somewhat laterally toward the midportion of the round ligament, which is then similarly transected with coagulation current. If the round ligament were transected near the uterus, the subsequent dissection may enter the tortuous path of the ascending uterine vessels, increasing the risk of bleeding. By working laterally, the subsequent dissection of the uterine vessels is facilitated. The utero-ovarian vessels have now been exposed, and the broad ligament beneath has been perforated by the peritoneal dissection. These steps are repeated on the opposite side.

Once all the peritoneal incisions surrounding the uterus and endometriosis have been made, the areolar tissue surrounding the uterine vessels and ureter can be stripped bluntly away. This can be facilitated by simply grasping small amounts of the areolar tissue and pulling it away from the vessels. Once the uterine artery comes into view, it can be grasped and drawn slightly anteriorly. Blunt dissection is then used posterior to the uterine artery to begin to identify the ureter (Plate 19). The ureter is progressively physically isolated from the uterine vessels, using traction on the ureter if necessary (Fig 11.4). During this dissection, a tiny branch of the uterine artery supplying the wall of the adjacent ureter will be seen. This vessel can be coagulated without risk of damage to the ureter, and this usually will be required to physically isolate the two structures. If retroperitoneal fibrosis related to endometriosis is present, it will rarely encroach on the uterine vessels as they cross over the ureter. However, the ureter may be involved by investing fibrosis extending from invasive disease of the uterosacral ligament or broad ligament, requiring ureterolysis by blunt dissection.

TRANSECTION OF ALL VASCULAR PEDICLES

After creation of all peritoneal incisions and isolation of all vascular pedicles, the atraumatic grasper is replaced with a bipolar coagulator. This represents the first instrument change during the procedure. All four exposed vascular pedicles are now sequentially desiccated with bipolar coagulation, then transected with 50 W of monopolar coagulation current using the 3-mm scissors (Fig 11.8).

The uterine vessels may be coagulated and transected directly over the ureter (Fig 11.9) or alongside the body of the lower fundus. If taken over the ureter, the stump of the vessels can be grasped and drawn

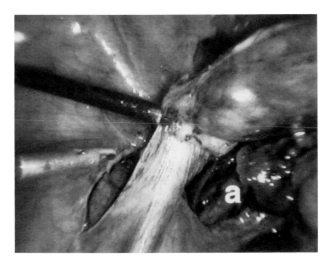

FIGURE 11.8

The left uterosacral ligament has been isolated by peritoneal incisions lateral and medial to it. A bipolar coagulator is passed across the vascular pedicle, which is then coagulated completely. The left ureter (a) lies posteriorly, well out of harm's way.

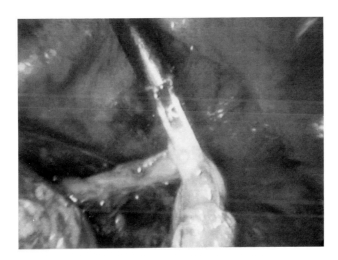

FIGURE 11.9

The left uterine artery has been physically completely isolated from the adjacent ureter. It is grasped and elevated away from the ureter during bipolar coagulation.

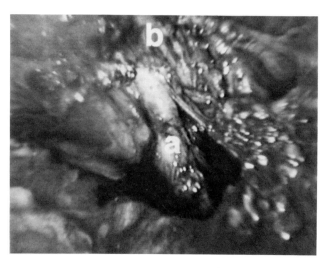

FIGURE 11.10

The right ureter (a) is seen entering the base of the bladder (b).

medially toward the uterus and peeled off of the paracervical tissue with monopolar electrosurgery at 50 W. This completely exposes the course of the ureter into the bladder (Fig 11.10), ensuring maximum safety for the ureter at this step.

In an alternate technique, the bipolar coagulator is directed across the uterine vessels at the level of the internal os and bipolar desiccation followed by monopolar transection performed. While this action occurs well away from the ureter, the ureter is not fully exposed and the surgeon must now anticipate the hidden course of the ureter as it passes medially toward the bladder. After transection of the pedicle, it is necessary to dissect immediately alongside the cervix with monopolar and bipolar coagulation to free the cervix without damage to the ureter.

Sizable vessels frequently ascend the posterior vaginal wall toward the posterior uterus. These vessels lie medial to the ureter and lateral to the uterosacral ligaments. The ureter usually can be separated sufficiently from these vessels to allow bipolar coagulation to control the vessels before monopolar transection.

VAGINAL ENTRY AND COMPLETION OF
SURGERY FROM BELOW

The bladder can now be completely advanced off of the cervix and the upper vagina using monopolar electrosurgery and blunt dissection. If a sponge has been inserted beneath the vaginal mucosa at the start of the case, vaginal entry anteriorly usually occurs at this point. If sufficient pneumoperitoneum remains, a posterior culdotomy can be created over a sponge stick inserted in the posterior vaginal fornix (Fig 11.11).

With the escape of pneumoperitoneum, the surgeon now operates vaginally. The last mucosal and areolar attachments of the vagina to the cervix are severed and the specimen removed with endometriosis-laden peritoneum still attached. Since the endometriosis may be difficult for the pathologist to find on the shriveled attached peritoneum, it may be

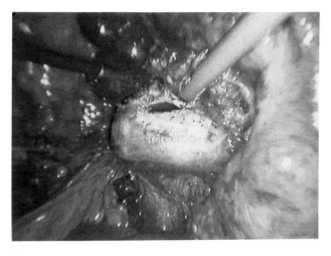

FIGURE 11.11

After complete development of the rectovaginal septum, a sponge stick is used to stretch the posterior fornix. The 3-mm scissors with 90 W of pure cutting current is used to create a posterior culdotomy incision immediately adjacent to the cervix. With the escape of pneumoperitoneum, the procedure is terminated from below.

helpful to tag areas of peritoneal disease with sutures. The vaginal cuff is closed in the surgeon's routine fashion, but with a special difference in mind. Complete ureteral dissection during transection of the uterine arteries eliminates much of the cardinal ligament, which is frequently incorporated into the angles of the vaginal cuff. Therefore, care must be taken not to incorporate the exposed ureter into the sutures across the anterior vaginal cuff, which can lead to urinary fistulas following surgery (38).

RESULTS

There is no scientific evidence that removal of the uterus, tubes, and ovaries will make endometriosis go away. Although symptom relief may occur, the symptoms relieved may be of uterine, tubal, or ovarian origin. A literature review found that removal of the uterus, tubes, and ovaries with retention of endometriosis will relieve pain in between 56% and 100% of patients (39), while total abdominal hysterectomy/BSO without treatment of obliteration of the cul-de-sac resulted in pain relief in 71% of patients. In most patients with continuing pain after total abdominal hysterectomy/BSO with retention of endometriosis, later excision of residual endometriosis will result in pain relief (32).

It makes better clinical sense to remove endometriosis at the time of hysterectomy and castration than to depend on eradication of a disease by removal of something else. Laparoscopic-assisted vaginal hysterectomy (LAVH), BSO, and excision of all endometriosis have been shown to carry good symptomatic results (40). Such surgery will have an additive effect, relieving pain due to endometriosis as well as pain from uterine, tubal, or ovarian causes.

In my series, two of 106 patients undergoing laparoscopic hysterectomy required conversion to abdominal hysterectomy due to fibroids that made visualization of the pelvis impossible.

While some may criticize the lack of randomized controlled trials demonstrating superiority of laparoscopic techniques over laparotomy techniques (41), such criticism is premature. Laparotomy treatments have been developed over the course of decades, while laparoscopic procedures are still under development. Only when mature laparoscopic techniques have been agreed on will comparison with laparotomy techniques be rational.

COMPLICATIONS

The urinary tract, particularly the ureters, is at risk during any hysterectomy. Techniques for laparoscopic hysterectomy continue to evolve, and certain strategies for avoidance of ureteral damage are emerging. Although complete exposure of the ureters with full development of the ureteral tunnel will reduce the risk of ureteral damage while controlling the uterine vessels, this is no guarantee against ureteral damage during suture of the vaginal cuff or coagulation of bleeders of the vaginal cuff. These injuries are not necessarily related to the amount or invasiveness of endometriosis present, and most are likely to occur in patients with minimal or mild disease, since these patients will be more common than patients with extensive disease. In 104 LAVHs with or without BSO that I performed (62 of which were in association with endometriosis), two patients had urinary tract injury. In one, a cystotomy was created by making the transverse peritoneal incision across the cervix lower than anticipated. The cystotomy was immediately identified and repaired laparoscopically without difficulty. However, this brought the subsequent dissection lower than usual in the pelvis, creating the potential for unrecognized injury to the ureter. After uneventful removal of the uterus, the right ureter was burned during bipolar coagulation of a bleeder near the vaginal cuff. The injury was unrecognized and the patient presented 10 days later with a ureterovaginal fistula that required reimplantation. The fact that almost 70 previous laparoscopic hysterectomies had been performed without urinary tract damage shows that experience is no guard against unanticipated injury. In the second patient, the left ureter was partially lacerated during vaginal clamping of the cardinal ligaments. The injury was recognized and repaired at laparotomy over a stent and the patient did well. The ureter had been completely unroofed laparoscopically and therefore hung lower in the pelvis than usual.

OPERATING TIMES

Laparoscopic-assisted vaginal hysterectomy has been criticized for taking much more time than abdominal hysterectomy. This leads to increased hospital charges. Slow surgery is a result of inefficient techniques and possibly the use of video monitors. My operating times for LAVH with or without BSO compared with abdominal hysterectomy with or without BSO by rAFS stage are shown in Figure 11.12. In this series of patients, laparoscopic hysterectomy with removal of both ovaries and excision of endometriosis was chosen more frequently than hysterectomy and excision of endometriosis alone, and the women selecting LAVH/BSO were older (mean age, 40.5 years) than those selecting LAVH (mean age, 35.0 years). Median operating times for laparoscopic procedures compare favorably with operating times for the equivalent abdominal approach for disease-matched patients.

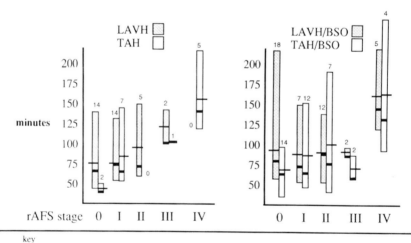

key

- rAFS: revised American Fertility Society classification of endometriosis
- numbers above bars represent number of patients
- all laparoscopic hysterectomies included transection of uterine arteries and culdotomy

FIGURE 11.12

Operating times: laparoscopic versus abdominal hysterectomy with or without BSO by rAFS stage.

In the group undergoing LAVH/BSO, the median operating time was similar for rAFS stages 0 through III, increasing significantly with stage IV. These operating times were very similar to those in patients undergoing LAVH alone. Two points may explain this. First, the peritoneal excision required for removal of endometriosis is similar in the lower stages (even when the ovaries are enlarged and adherent), while stage IV disease was more likely to be associated with intestinal endometriosis, which would lead to longer surgery. Second, it is easier to isolate and control the infundibulopelvic ligament than it is to control the utero-ovarian ligament, so the time saved with oophorectomy can be used to deal with the more invasive peritoneal disease that may be present in stages II and III.

CONCLUSION

Hysterectomy is indicated for the treatment of uterine symptoms, while removal of the ovaries is indicated for the relief of ovarian symptoms. In patients with extensive endometriosis, the surgery should include excision of endometriosis to reduce the potential for continued symptoms from this disease. The surgeon can excise endometriosis laparoscopically and prepare the uterus, tubes, and ovaries for vaginal removal. When logical steps are followed in sequence, the procedure can be accomplished in a timely fashion with a slightly increased risk of ureteral injury and good relief of symptoms. Laparoscopic hysterectomy in patients with endometriosis will not be rational for every gynecologist, owing to prolonged operating times in the hands of some. More important than completion of the procedure laparoscopically and vaginally is complete excision of endometriosis. A surgeon need not apologize if this is done by laparotomy.

REFERENCES

1. Bergqvist A, Rannevik G, Thorell J. Estrogen and progesterone cytosol receptor concentration in endometriotic tissue and intrauterine endometrium. Acta Obstet Gynecol Scand Suppl 1981;101:53–58.

2. Gould SF, Shannon JM, Cunha GR. Nuclear estrogen binding sites in human endometriosis. Fertil Steril 1983;39:520–524.

3. Janne O, Kauppila A, Kokko E, et al. Estrogen and progestin receptors in endometriosis lesions: Comparison with endometrial tissue. Am J Obstet Gynecol 1981;141:562–566.

4. Tamaya T, Motoyama T, Ohono Y, et al. Steroid receptor levels and histology of endometriosis and adenomyosis. Fertil Steril 1979;31:396–400.

5. Metzger DA, Olive DL, Haney AF. Limited hormonal responsiveness of ectopic endometrium: histologic correlation with intrauterine endometrium. Hum Pathol 1988;19:1417–1424.

6. Metzger DA, Szpak CA, Haney AF. Histologic features associated with hormonal responsiveness of ectopic endometrium. Fertil Steril 1993;59:83–88.

7. Jansen RPS, Russell P. Nonpigmented endometriosis: clinical, laparoscopic, and pathologic definition. Am J Obstet Gynecol 1986;155:1154–1159.

8. Nezhat F, Allan CJ, Nezhat C, Martin DC. Nonvisualized endometriosis at laparoscopy. Int J Fertil 1991;36:340–343.

9. Redwine DB. Age related evolution in color appearance of endometriosis. Fertil Steril 1987;48:1062–1063.

10. Stripling MC, Martin DC, Chatman DL, et al. Subtle appearance of pelvic endometriosis. Fertil Steril 1988;49:427–431.

11. Martin DC, Hubert GD, VanderZwaag R, et al. Laparoscopic appearances of peritoneal endometriosis. Fertil Steril 1989;51:63–67.

12. Sampson JA. The development of the implantation theory for the origin of peritoneal endometriosis. Am J Obstet Gynecol 1940;40:549–557.

13. Redwine DB. The distribution of endometriosis in the pelvis by age groups and fertility. Fertil Steril 1987;47:173–175.

14. Koninckx PR, Meuleman C, Demeyere S, et al. Suggestive evidence that pelvic endometriosis is a progressive disease, whereas deeply infiltrating endometriosis is associated with pelvic pain. Fertil Steril 1991;55:759–765.

15. Marana R, Muzii L, Caruana P, et al. Evaluation of the correlation between endometriosis extent, age of the patients and associated symptomatology. Acta Eur Fertil 1991;22:209–212.

16. Moore JG, Binstock MA, Growdon WA. The clinical implications of retroperitoneal endometriosis. Am J Obstet Gynecol 1988;158:1291–1296.

17. Javert CT. The spread of benign and malignant endometrium in the lymphatic system with a note on coexisting vascular involvement. Am J Obstet Gynecol 1952;64:780–806.
18. Javert CT. Pathogenesis of endometriosis based on endometrial homeoplasia, direct extension, exfoliation and implantation, lymphatic and hematogenous metastasis. Including five case reports of endometrial tissue in pelvic lymph nodes. Cancer 1949;62:477–487.
19. Russell HB. Decidual reaction of endometrium ectopic in an abdominal lymph node. Surg Gynecol Obstet 1945;81:218–220.
20. Wheeler JM, Malinak LR. Recurrent endometriosis. Contrib Gynecol Obstet 1987;16:13–21.
21. Redwine DB. Conservative laparoscopic excision of endometriosis by sharp dissection: life table analysis of reoperation and persistent or recurrent disease. Fertil Steril 1991;56:628–634.
22. Rier SE, Martin DC, Bowman RE, et al. Endometriosis in rhesus monkeys (*Macaca mulatta*) following chronic exposure to 2,3,7,8-tetrachlorodibenzo-*p*-dioxin. Fundam Appli Toxicol 1993;21:433–441.
23. Fanton JW, Golden JG. Radiation-induced endometriosis in *Macaca mulatta*. Radiat Res 1991;126:141–146.
24. Wood DH, Yochmowitz MG, Salmon YL, et al. Proton irradiation and endometriosis. Aviat Space Environ Med 1983;54:718–724.
25. Wood DH. Long term mortality and cancer risk in irradiated rhesus monkeys. Radiat Res 1991;126:132–140.
26. Oliker AJ, Harris AE. Endometriosis of the bladder in a male patient. J Urol 1971;106:858–859.
27. Beckman EN, Pintado SO, Leonard GL, Sternberg WH. Endometriosis of the prostate. Am J Surg Pathol 1985;9:374–379.
28. Renaer M, Guzinski GM. Pain in gynecologic practice. Pain 1978;5:305–331.
29. Fallon J. Endometriosis. Evidence of tubal origin in the distribution of lesions. Arch Surg 1951;62:412–418.
30. Fallon J, Brosnan JT, Moran WG. Endometriosis. Two hundred cases considered from the viewpoint of the practitioner. N Engl J Med 1946;235:669–673.
31. Kempers RD, Dockerty MB, Hunt AB, et al. Significant postmenopausal endometriosis. Surg Gynecol Obstet 1960;3:348–356.
32. Redwine DB. Endometriosis persisting after castration: clinical characteristics and results of surgical management. Obstet Gynecol 1994;83:405–413.

33. Redwine DB. The visual appearance of endometriosis and its impact on our concepts of the disease. Prog Clin Biol Res 1990;323:393–412.

34. Redwine DB. Is "microscopic" peritoneal endometriosis invisible? Fertil Steril 1988;50:665–666.

35. Redwine DB. Laparoscopic en bloc resection for treatment of the obliterated cul de sac in endometriosis. J Reprod Med 1992;37:695–698.

36. Koninckx PR, Martin DC. Deep endometriosis: a consequence of infiltration or retraction or possibly adenomyosis externa? Fertil Steril 1992;58: 924–928.

37. Hasson H. Cervical removal at hysterectomy for benign disease: risks and benefits. J Reprod Med 1993;38:781–790.

38. Kadar N, Lemmerling L. Urinary tract injuries during laparoscopically assisted hysterectomy: causes and prevention. Am J Obstet Gynecol 1994; 47–48.

39. Redwine DB. Treatment of endometriosis-associated pain. Infertil Reprod Med Clin North Am 1992;3:697–720.

40. Davis GD, Wolgamott G, Moon J. Laparoscopically assisted vaginal hysterectomy as definitive therapy for stage III and IV endometriosis. J Reprod Med 1993;38:577–581.

41. Richardson DA. Ethics in gynecologic surgical innovation. Am J Obstet Gynecol 1994;170:1–6.

12

Laparoscopic Hysterectomy for Large Myomatous Uteri

Howard C. Topel

A pproximately 75% of the 650,000 hysterectomies performed in the United States are accomplished through a large abdominal skin incision. A major indication for almost half of these abdominal hysterectomies is the presence of symptomatic uterine leiomyomas. Although abdominal hysterectomy has been associated with higher morbidity and mortality rates than vaginal hysterectomy, surgeons are inclined to remove a myomatous uterus with a more invasive laparotomy technique. In many cases, the vaginal approach is often precluded by significant technical limitations and spatial constraints imposed by a large uterus.

The often-stated goal of laparoscopic-assisted vaginal hysterectomy is to convert a potential abdominal hysterectomy into a less morbid vaginal operation. If this goal is to be achieved, then a significant percentage of the abdominal hysterectomies performed for uterine leiomyomas must be evaluated and ultimately converted to a laparoscopic technique. However, laparoscopic removal of a large myomatous uterus is a complex operation that challenges both the cognitive and technical skills of the surgeon. Although much attention has been focused on learning and developing laparoscopic techniques, it is the cognitive aspects of an operation, the mental planning and preparation, that often facilitate the technical execution and determine the difference between success or failure.

It is important to thoroughly study the true uterine size, as well as to determine the location and number of myomas. Careful preoperative assessment of these variables will help to establish an operational plan, to anticipate potential problems, and to minimize intraoperative complications. It also helps to determine whether the laparoscopic option is indeed a viable alternative. In some cases, this evaluation may convince the surgeon to abandon a laparoscopic attempt, and instead recommend a conventional laparotomy operation.

A simple bimanual examination can be misleading since the uterine size is often underestimated and the complexity of the pathology not fully appreciated. Therefore, every patient with a large uterus who is a candidate for a laparoscopic hysterectomy should undergo a pelvic sonogram with a combined transvaginal and abdominal study. This imaging technique is reliable, readily available, and well tolerated by the patient. For most cases ultrasound scanning can accurately identify the nature and extent of large pelvic masses. Although more sensitive and accurate, magnetic resonance imaging usually is reserved for more complex uterine pathology or inconclusive ultrasound studies.

Patients with a uterus greater than 12 weeks' gestational size or with a large lateral fibroid can be treated for 3 to 4 months with a gonadotropin-releasing hormone agonist. Although a 30% to 50% re duction in total uterine volume has been reported, the clinical results are quite variable and inconsistent. However, in selected cases, preoperative gonadotropin-releasing hormone agonists are administered in an effort to reduce the uterine size, minimize vaginal bleeding, and gain a mechanical advantage at the time of surgery. For patients who experience heavy bleeding, have anemia, or must postpone surgery for several months, a gonadotropin-releasing hormone agonist can be used as an effective temporizing method.

For this complicated surgery, each patient must be thoroughly counseled as to the nature of the pathology, the type of operation proposed, the possible complications, and the potential for conversion to open laparotomy. All patients are offered the option to arrange for autologous or donor-directed blood donations. Each patient takes a Fleet's enema the night before surgery; in some cases a bowel preparation may be indicated.

TECHNIQUE

The technique for laparoscopic removal of a large myomatous uterus involves many of the same surgical steps described for performing a standard laparoscopic-assisted vaginal hysterectomy. However, the large uterine size, associated with the complexities of myomatous pathology, requires specific modifications in technique as well as special attention to planning and execution. This complicated operation cannot be performed in a singular or rote manner, always using the same instrumentation and the same techniques for every patient. To avoid poor outcome and minimize complications, a well-planned, multidimensional approach involving a variety of energy sources, multiple instrumentation choices, and different methods of ligation must be used. The approach must include a cognitive selection process that is based on the surgeon's experience and surgical judgment.

With the patient in the lithotomy position, great care is taken to keep the legs well supported and in a low profile position. The legs are positioned so that the wide range of motion required by the laparoscopic instrumentation is not limited. A strong uterine manipulator is needed to move a heavy uterus, not only anteriorly, posteriorly, and from side to side, but it must also rotate the uterus along its long axis. This rotational movement is essential to help enucleate a key myoma and for the proper exposure of vital structures.

With a large pelvic mass extending up toward the umbilicus, great care should be exercised to avoid trauma when inserting a Verres needle and a 10-mm umbilical trocar. For a uterus of 16 weeks' gestational size or smaller, the standard umbilical placement is commonly used with a modified vertical direction for insertion. If a larger uterus is present, the left upper quadrant can be used for creation of the pneumoperitoneum and for positioning of the laparoscope.

For secondary trocars, I prefer to use three 12-mm ports with reducer caps. These large trocars allow greater flexibility in technique by using a variety of instrument sizes from any port and from either side of the patient. The position of the secondary trocars will be determined by the uterine pathology and size. Following the initial inspection of the pelvis, these trocars may be placed more lateral and more cephalad than usual to maximize the best angles for dissection and ligation. Before placement of the secondary trocars it is crucial to pause for a moment to establish a surgical plan. This will ensure that each trocar will be in the most optimal position and will help maximize the chances of a successful operation.

A large myomatous uterus presents a series of unique problems when attempting to perform a laparoscopic hysterectomy. The increased uterine size may create serious spatial constraints that technically limit the laparoscopic approach. A uterus with myomas extending laterally into the broad ligament may prevent adequate exposure and ligation of the uterine arteries. In addition, the ureters may be difficult to identify or may be displaced into an atypical position. An anterior fibroid could obstruct visualization of the bladder reflection and inhibit dissection of the bladder off the cervix, while a posterior wall fibroid at the level of the cervix may obstruct access to the posterior vaginal fornix.

To proceed with the hysterectomy, it may be necessary to first enucleate one or more of the key myomas from the uterus. A large pedunculated or broad-based subserosal fundal fibroid can be easily removed early in the operation to provide more operating space and to simplify the operation. If the myomas are centrally located with adequate lateral space for dissection and exposure, enucleation should be postponed until after the ovarian and uterine arteries are secured. However, with broad ligament myomas overlying the uterine arteries and other critically positioned myomas (i.e., lateral, fundal, posterior), a selective myomectomy must be first accomplished before the operation is able to be continued (Figs 12.1 to 12.3).

The technique for myomectomy prior to uterine artery ligation is described below.

The first step of enucleation starts with injection of a dilute solution of vasopressin (10–20 U in 100 mL of saline) into the serosa around the entire circumference of the myoma. Direct intravascular injection should be avoided and the anesthesiologist should be informed when vasopressin is used. The serosal surface is incised with a laparoscopic endoknife or scissors. The incision is carried down until the fibroid is located and the pseudocapsular plane is identified. It is critical to dissect

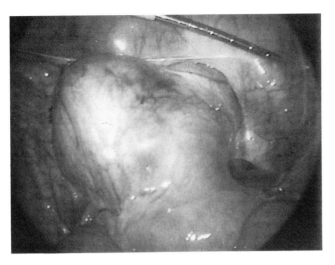

FIGURE 12.1

A large, 10-cm myoma occupying the anterior uterine wall obstructs bladder mobilization.

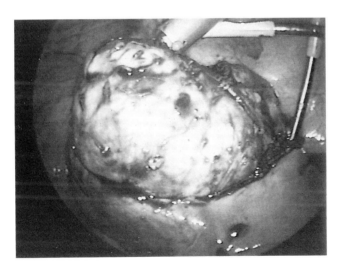

FIGURE 12.2

Enucleation of the obstructing ("key") myoma from the uterus using endocoagulation techniques.

Laparoscopic Hysterectomy for Large Myomatous Uteri   231

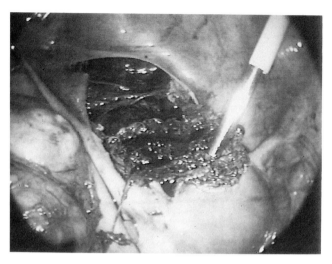

FIGURE 12.3

The "key" myoma removed, with the anterior wall and bladder completely exposed.

within the pseudocapsular plane to minimize bleeding (Fig 12.4). Enucleation of a fibroid from the myometrium can be accomplished with a variety of energy sources. Often, a combination of energy sources will be needed for myoma enucleation. My personal preference is to develop and dissect the pseudocapsular plane with a point tip endocoagulator set at 130°F. The large myoma can be grasped and stabilized with a 10-mm corkscrew instrument or an endoscopic tenaculum. The deeper vascular myoma bed can be carefully dissected with the aid of unipolar or bipolar electrocoagulation. Dissection of the deeper tissue planes must be slowly developed and all vessels precisely secured to prevent excessive bleeding. However, strict adherence to identifying and dissecting within the pseudocapsular plane will result in surprisingly little blood loss (Plate 20). Following complete enucleation, additional hemostasis in the myoma bed can be achieved with endocoagulation, bipolar desiccation, or with an argon beam coagulator. The free myoma can be stored in the upper abdomen and removed through the vagina at the appropriate time. It may be necessary to remove additional myomas, in a similar manner, at various

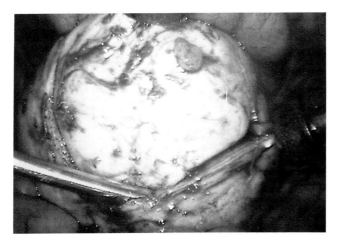

FIGURE 12.4

Dissection within the pseudocapsular plane to minimize bleeding during selective myomectomy *prior to* uterine artery ligation.

stages of the operation to improve exposure and to decrease uterine volume.

At times, management of the adnexal structures may be extremely difficult in the presence of a large myomatous uterus. An ovary may be obscured by the myoma or pulled close to the uterus with a shortened utero-ovarian ligament. A myomectomy must be initially performed to expose and transsect this ligament. Bipolar coagulation is a safe and cost-effective energy source with which to transect the utero-ovarian ligament. Likewise, the infundibulopelvic ligament may be shortened with limited exposure and access. The uterus usually can be displaced to one side and the ureter identified passing over the pelvic brim. The ovarian vasculature can then be grasped, isolated, and secured with bipolar desiccation, endoloops, or an extracorporeal suture ligature. Because of the inherent spatial constraints, it is often difficult to pass a stapling device across the infundibulopelvic ligament. Conserving the ovaries initially and then returning to extirpate them after the uterus has been removed may be a safer and more practical strategy.

With the presence of a large uterus, visual identification of the ureter may be difficult and dissection technically impossible. If the uterus is 12 weeks' gestational size or greater, extends out toward the lateral

Laparoscopic Hysterectomy for Large Myomatous Uteri   233

pelvic side walls, or contains multiple large fibroids, I will place lighted ureteral stents at the beginning of the operation. These illuminated stents permit the surgeon to visually identify the ureters at any level in the pelvis and to follow their course during all stages of the dissection (Plate 21). The stented ureter also provides the surgeon with an additional tactile sensation for identification. This technique is very appreciated when enucleating a broad ligament myoma, ligating the uterine arteries deep in the pelvis, or controlling bleeding from anomalous uterine vessels. A lighted ureteral stent provides the surgeon with a greater comfort level and an increased margin of safety when confronted with challenging pathology or an intraoperative bleeding complication.

Mobilization of the bladder off the cervix can be another problem associated with a large myomatous uterus. This step is often performed prior to ligating the uterine arteries. However, a large fundal or anterior wall fibroid may obscure or distort the anterior bladder peritoneum. In some cases, enucleation of the key anterior fibroid, in the manner described, must first be performed to expose the corpocervical junction. At times, better visualization of the bladder reflection can be achieved by moving the laparoscope to a lower secondary trocar. One must proceed cautiously with this bladder dissection, since this is a new and unfamiliar orientation between camera and instruments.

A third way to approach the problem of bladder identification is to place a sponge under the bladder. At the very beginning of the operation, prior to insertion of the uterine manipulator, the anterior vaginal wall is infiltrated with a small amount of dilute vasopressin. With the anterior cervix grasped and pulled downward, a 2- to 3-cm incision is made along the anterior vagina, just below the bladder border. Using sharp and blunt dissection, the connective tissue plane is carefully developed between the posterior wall of the bladder and the anterior cervix. The dissection is carried upward to the level of the vesicouterine fold, but the anterior peritoneum is not entered. One can often palpate the presence of low uterine myomas after this dissection is completed. A moist sponge is then packed high into this space, creating a bulge at the corpocervical junction. This bulge can be readily seen with the laparoscope and dramatically helps to identify and mobilize the bladder (Plate 22). At the correct time a laparoscopic anterior culdotomy can be made by incising the thin peritoneum overlying the sponge.

With a large uterus, exposure and access to the uterine arteries may be most difficult. A broad uterus, extending out toward the pelvic side walls, will have limited space and thus impose severe technical restrictions. When possible, a key myoma can be carefully enucleated to increase operating space and exposure. A fibroid overlying the uterine vessels or in close proximity to the ureter should be removed by an experienced laparoscopist. With a large myomatous uterus, the uterine vasculature may lie deeper in the pelvis than anticipated and create a formidable effort to ligate. In other situations, the vessels are prominently displayed and can be easily secured. The surgeon must decide whether to ligate the uterine vessels with a laparoscopic technique or to secure the vessels from the vaginal approach. If laparoscopic morselation of the uterus will be required for specimen removal through the vagina, the uterine vessels must be ligated from above. A variety of electrosurgery, clips, stapling, and suturing techniques can be used to ligate the uterine artery and vein (Plate 23). The surgeon must be experienced with all modalities and use the correct one to avoid complications. Due to the variability of the pathology, one operation may require multiple ligation techniques.

After the uterine vessels are completely secured, the large myomas can be enucleated to permit easier vaginal removal (Plate 24). An incision can be made across the corpocervical junction and the large bulky corpus can be totally detached from the cervix. This step will help to improve exposure to the lower pelvis, establish better hemostasis, enable inspection of the ureters, and provide for easier removal of the cervix through the vagina. It should be emphasized, however, that if the uterine pathology does not dictate a laparoscopic ligation of the uterine vessels, the surgeon may be wiser to approach this step through the vagina.

An anterior culdotomy can easily be performed by incising across the anterior bladder peritoneum overlying the sponge. After incision, the sponge is not removed as it prevents loss of the pneumoperitoneum. Following removal of any obstructions into the cul-de-sac, a posterior colpotomy can be accomplished with a variety of laparoscopic techniques. With creation of both culdotomy incisions from above, the vaginal portion of the operation is greatly facilitated. There is less bleeding and easier placement of the vaginal instruments when the cervix remains high. In addition, enucleated myomas and other morcellated tissues can be easily passed through the posterior culdotomy incision before the uterus is removed.

Following complete detachment from all supporting structures, the large uterus can be manipulated through the vagina. However, great care must be exercised if the uterus remains too large for the vaginal tract. The uterus can be morcellated from the vaginal side with a coring technique and selective fibroids enucleated to reduce the uterine volume (Fig 12.5). All laparoscopic tissue specimens should be conveniently positioned for easy identification and removal through the vagina. A vaginal pack or diaphragm, inserted into the vagina, allows for reinflation of the abdominal cavity. This technique permits for retrieval of any elusive myomas and their removal through the vagina. Following closure of the vaginal cuff, it is important to inspect all pedicles for good hemostasis with a laparoscope. While removing a large uterus, a vascular pedicle could be easily traumatized and become the source of postoperative bleeding.

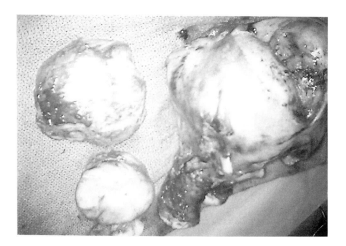

FIGURE 12.5

A 16-week gestational sized uterus after a laparoscopic-assisted vaginal hysterectomy using the techniques as described.

The upper limits of uterine size compatible with laparoscopic hysterectomy technique remains unestablished. Whereas uteri in excess of 20 weeks' gestational size have been removed, most experienced laparoscopists would consider a 14- to 16-week gestational-sized uterus to be a formidable operation. Size alone, however, may not be the limiting factor. Rather, location of crucial fibroids and associated pathology (i.e., adhesions, endometriosis) may have greater significance. In addition, surgeon skill level, a good surgical assistant, availability of instrumentation, and a well-trained operating room team are additional variables that can influence the choice of cases for laparoscopic surgery.

Laparoscopic hysterectomy of a large myomatous uterus is a very complex operation requiring a multidimensional approach that involves both cognitive and technical skills. Proper patient selection is crucial for performing an uncomplicated laparoscopic operation in a timely manner. The surgeon's technical skills must be equal to the challenges presented by the pelvic pathology. The operational plan should be well devised, but subject to reassessment and changes as new challenges are encountered. The surgery must be performed with the option of multiple modalities and techniques. The surgeon, based on good judgment and experience, should always perform the safest operation that is in the patient's best interest. With these concepts in practice, laparoscopic hysterectomy of large myomatous uteri will result in good outcome and afford many additional patients the benefits of laparoscopic surgery.

13

Laparoscopic Supracervical Hysterectomy

Harrith M. Hasson

L aparoscopic hysterectomy has emerged as an alternative to abdominal or vaginal hysterectomy. Three main types have been described: total laparoscopic hysterectomy (TLH), supracervical laparoscopic hysterectomy (SLH), and laparoscopic-assisted vaginal hysterectomy (LAVH). Total laparoscopic hysterectomy and SLH are basically forms of abdominal hysterectomy accomplished by laparoscopic means. Laparoscopic-assisted vaginal hysterectomy is essentially a vaginal hysterectomy preceded by laparoscopic isolation of the adnexa with or without occlusion of the uterine vessels (1). A modified LAVH modeled after the Doderlein vaginal hysterectomy also has been reported (2). When choosing a hysterectomy type, consideration should be given to the concept that removal of the cervix at the time of hysterectomy for benign disease is not warranted (3).

RATIONALE FOR PERFORMING SUPRACERVICAL HYSTERECTOMY

The cervix and the upper third of the vagina serve as the anchor of support within the pelvis. The pelvic organs are supported within the pelvis by the endopelvic fascia, a continuous layer of connective tissue that invests each organ and spreads laterally to the pelvic side walls, where it is attached to the parietal fascia. Approximately two thirds of this supportive structure is attached to the cervix as the cardinal and uterosacral ligaments and one third is attached to the vagina as the upper paracolpium. These ligaments hold the cervix and upper vagina firmly in place within the pelvis. The rest of the uterus is freely mobile. The more attenuated round ligaments that attach the upper part of the uterus to the pelvic wall play a minor role in uterine support and position (4,5). The paracolpium, which is continuous with the cardinal and uterosacral ligaments, maintains the integrity of the vagina (5).

In total hysterectomy the cervical component and a portion of the vaginal component of the supportive structure are severed. This predisposes patients to the development of vaginal vault prolapse and enterocele. Additionally, extended dissection may cause shortening of the vagina and possible sexual dysfunction. Vaginal vault prolapse and enterocele are not uncommon after total abdominal or vaginal hysterectomy (3,6–9).

The cervix and upper vagina also are intimately associated with the Frankenhauser uterovaginal plexus, the major relay station of all autonomic and sensory neurotransmissions from the pelvic organs, upper vagina, and proximal urethra. The bulk of this plexus lies below the broad ligament. It consists of ganglia of various sizes surrounding the cervix and upper vagina, including a large ganglionic plate that is situated on either side of the cervix above the posterior fornix in front of the rectum (10,11).

Surgical removal of the cervix will result in loss of a large segment of ganglia of the Frankenhauser plexus, which is intimately associated with the cervix. The remaining portion of the uterovaginal plexus that is associated with the vagina may not be able to properly handle the information that is travelling to and from the bladder and rectum, which may lead to possible organ dysfunction. Several clinical studies have presented data supporting this concept. (3,12–17).

Recent advances in female sexual response indicate an important role for the cervix and uterus (18–20). Although the existence of internal (vaginal) orgasm has been challenged on the basis that the vagina itself has no nerve endings, this type of orgasm may be triggered by stimulation of the uterovaginal plexus that surrounds the cervix and upper vagina.

Loss of a major portion of the uterovaginal plexus through excision of the cervix probably affects sexual arousal and orgasm in women who previously experienced internal orgasm or in whom sexual arousal is blended. Women who achieve orgasm exclusively through clitoral stimulation would not be affected (3,19). Cervical mucous secretions contribute to vaginal lubrication (21,22). Existing data support these conclusions (3,19,21,23–26).

Other than the force of habit and tradition, the major reason given for removing the cervix routinely at hysterectomy, by any approach, is fear of cancer of the cervix. However, today the risk of undetected cancer development in the cervical stump is overstated. Unlike the 1940s and 1950s, when cancer detection was based on the then "time-honored" cervical biopsy, currently precancerous states, such as squamous intraepithelial lesions (SIL), are diagnosed by cytology, evaluated by colposcopy with a sampling of the endocervix, and treated preferentially with cone biopsy in the form of electroloop excision or CO_2 laser conization (3). Hysterectomy is reserved for patients with persistent or recurrent severe dysplasia or high-grade SIL. Furthermore, it has been shown that prophylactic removal of the cervix does not eliminate the risk of cancer, but rather it shifts the risk to the vaginal epithelium in high-risk patients (27–29). Finally, the question of why leaving the cervix intact after subtotal hysterectomy is any different from leaving it intact after the increasingly popular procedure of endometrial ablation/resection does not have a satisfactory answer. We as physicians do not have a good rationale for prophylactic removal of organs because of fear of cancer, especially when there are good screening tests for the early detection of precancerous lesions, as is the case with the cervix.

The issue of decreased morbidity with subtotal versus total hysterectomy is based on the fact that in supracervical hysterectomy there is no need to dissect the ureter or isolate the main trunk of the uterine artery in the cardinal ligament. There also is less need for bladder mobilization and dissection. This should result in less complications related to urinary tract injury and operative hemorrhage. In a recent report the morbidity from total abdominal hysterectomy was 13.1% and the morbidity from supracervical abdominal hysterectomy was 4.9% (25). For all these reasons, SLH is my preferred method of removing the uterus for benign disease, with or without the adnexa.

INDICATIONS AND CONTRAINDICATIONS

The indications for SLH are identical to those of abdominal hysterectomy for benign disease. The contraindications are listed below.

1. Patient's medical condition and/or degree of obesity (it is inadvisable to keep the patient in Trendelenburg's position with a pneumoperitoneum for a prolonged period of time)
2. Uterine size greater than 18 weeks' of gestation
3. Malignant or premalignant lesions of the cervix, including persistent or recurrent high-grade SIL
4. Malignant or premalignant lesions of the endometrium, including atypical adenomatous hyperplasia
5. Adequate follow-up is not anticipated
6. Patient desires gender reassignment.

Low-grade SIL is not a contraindication to SLH provided that adequate follow-up and treatment are provided. However, most patients with this associated condition will probably prefer to have TLH.

TECHNIQUE

It should be emphasized that with a few exceptions, if the laparoscopic hysterectomy is very easy to perform, it probably was not indicated. Although SLH is in some ways less complicated than TLH, it still requires technically demanding movements that are coordinated between the surgeon and a capable associate surgeon or assistant. The development of a dedicated endoscopy team of physicians and nurses is essential for satisfactory cost-effective outcome of advanced laparoscopic procedures, such as hysterectomy.

Preparation

Preoperative medical therapy is used to reduce the size and vascularity of the uterine mass and conserve menstrual blood loss prior to surgery, as indicated. Prophylactic antibiotics and bowel preparation with Golytely or enema are routine. Following adequate anesthesia, the patient is placed in the lithotomy position. The legs are placed into Allen stirrups (Allen Medical Systems) with the thighs roughly parallel to the floor and the feet resting comfortably in the heel of the boot. The patient's toe, knee, and opposite shoulder are aligned in a straight line. Jelly pads are placed between the boot of the stirrup and the leg of the patient to prevent inappropriate pressure points.

The bladder is emptied and a Foley catheter is left indwelling. An adequate uterine manipulator, such as the Valchetz uterine manipulator (Conkin Surgical Instruments, Toronto, Ontario, Canada), is used to rotate and mobilize the uterus. The patient is placed in a fairly steep Trendelenburg's position to mobilize the bowel out of the pelvic operative field.

Access, Exploration, and Additional Procedures

I use open laparoscopy routinely for primary access, and three secondary access points drawn along the line of an imaginary Pfanensteil incision for operative manipulation. The level of the secondary access points varies with the size of the uterus; the larger the uterus, the higher the level. Five-millimeter stable access cannulas (Marlow Surgical Technologies, Willoughby, OH) are used routinely to facilitate instrument exchanges and to prevent the trocars from slipping in or out of the abdomen during surgery. In difficult cases, I use four access points: two lateral to the inferior epigastric artery (one on each side) and two medial points placed to the right and left of the midline.

Exploration of the pelvis and abdomen is the first step in the operation. This includes systematic exploration of the upper abdomen, the domes of the diaphragm, the liver and gallbladder, the appendix, the omentum, the pelvic organs, and the cul-de-sac. Pelvic peritoneal fluid is aspirated and sent for cytologic evaluation, as indicated. The uterus and adnexa are freed from associated adhesions. Large leiomyomas are

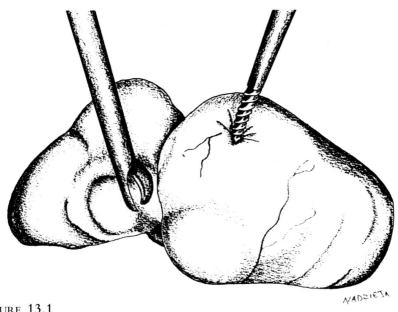

FIGURE 13.1

Debulking the uterine mass by myomectomy prior to initiating hysterectomy. (Reproduced by permission from Hasson HM, Rotman C, Rana N, et al. Experience with laparoscopic hysterectomy. J Am Assoc Gynecol Laparosc 1993;1:1–11.)

excised from the uterus as previously described (1,30) (Fig 13.1) and are stored in the left upper quadrant. Additional procedures that are needed to improve access to the vascular pedicles of the uterus are performed. The laparoscopic procedure is terminated in favor of an open laparotomy if this is warranted by the extent of the lesion and/or the severity of adhesions.

Anterior Dissection and Development of the Bladder Flap

Using the manipulator, an assistant pushes the uterus upward and to one side to place the contralateral round ligament on stretch. The ligament is held in its midportion, coagulated with bipolar forceps, and cut (Fig 13.2). The anterior leaf of each broad ligament is incised parallel to the uterus, and the incisions are curved toward the midline and joined below the white line that represents the vesicouterine fold (Fig

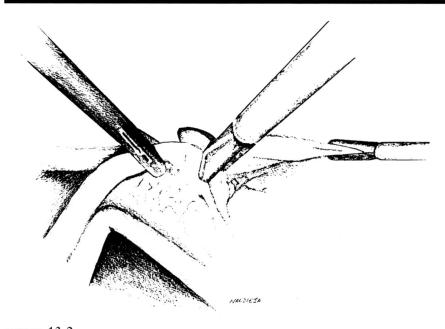

FIGURE 13.2

Cutting the round ligament following coagulation.

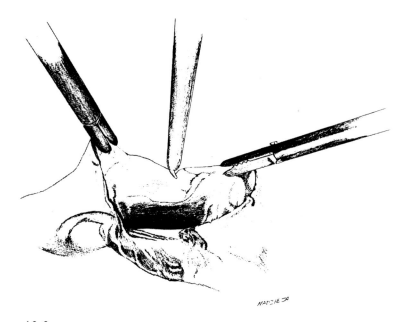

FIGURE 13.3

Incision of the anterior leaf of the broad ligament with unipolar electrode.

244   Laparoscopic Hysterectomy and Pelvic Floor Reconstruction

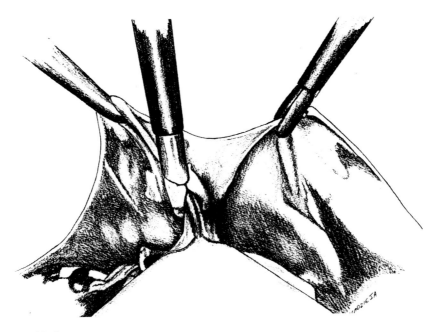

FIGURE **13.4**

Dividing the supravaginal septum to separate the bladder from the cervix (Reproduced by permission from Hasson HM, Rotman C, Rana N, et al. Experience with laparoscopic hysterectomy. J Am Assoc Gynecol Laparosc 1993;1:1–11.)

13.3). Dissection should be carried out superficially, excluding the retroperitoneal areolar tissues to prevent bleeding and staining of the operative field.

The bladder is mobilized out of the operative field by cutting the supravaginal septum (vesicocervical ligament or median raphe), which fuses the bladder to the cervix in the midline (Fig 13.4). The septum is first skeletonized from the sides, then cut in its midportion following coagulation. Subsequent blunt dissection separates the bladder from the cervix and vagina without difficulty. In cases of total hysterectomy, this dissection is easily carried out to the level of the upper vagina. The paracervical fascia is incised in the midline until the glistening pubocervical fascia is seen. Coagulating and cutting the superficial upper portions of the lateral vesicouterine ligaments or bladder pillars completes development of the bladder flap.

Posterior Dissection and Isolation of the Adnexa

Each ovary is held with the three-prong grasper (Linvatec, Clearwater, FL) and the uteroovarian ligament is stretched, coagulated, and cut (Fig 13.5). The posterior leaf of each broad ligament is incised down from this point of dissection to the point of uterosacral ligament insertion into the cervix. A window is made through an avascular area of the broad ligament with gentle blunt dissection (Fig 13.6).

Each fallopian tube, mesosalpinx, and overlying portion of broad ligament is then isolated and detached from the uterus. A suture is passed through the window to encircle and tie off the enclosed tissues with extracorporeal Roeder loop knots or square knots using the newly developed Flamingo sleeve (New Eder, Wood Dale, IL) and the Intercross II knot-pushing forceps (New Eder). The pedicle of tissues on the uterine side is coagulated with bipolar cautery to prevent back

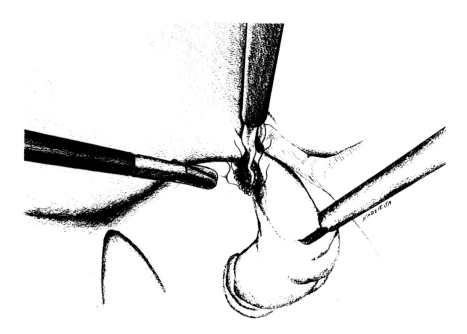

FIGURE **13.5**

Coagulation of the utero-ovarian ligament prior to division. (Reproduced by permission from Hasson HM, Rotman C, Rana N, et al. Experience with laparoscopic hysterectomy. J Am Assoc Gynecol Laparosc 1993;1:1–11.)

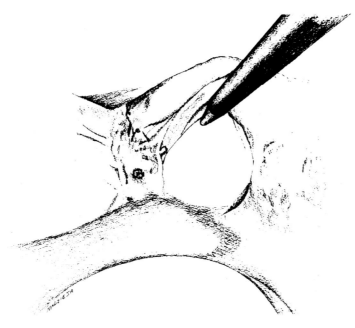

FIGURE 13.6

Creating an opening in the broad ligament. (Reproduced by permission from Hasson HM, Rotman C, Rana N, et al. Experience with laparoscopic hysterectomy. J Am Assoc Gynecol Laparosc 1993;1:1–11.)

bleeding and cut. Alternatively, the isolated tissues are detached from the uterus using bipolar cautery and scissors.

Our group prefers to routinely separate the adnexa from the uterus to simplify the procedure. If indicated, concomitant salpingo-oophorectomy is performed after the uterus has been excised.

Securing the Uterine Vessels

In supracervical hysterectomy, the cervix and surrounding cardinal ligaments are left intact. The main trunk of the uterine artery is not skeletonized and the ureter is not identified. Areolar tissues surrounding the uterine vessels are stripped to expose the vessels as they approach the uterus along the upper confines of the cardinal ligament. However, only the ascending branch of the uterine trunk is skeletonized. Although we have secured the uterine artery and vein with bipolar coagulation and with the application of staples (1), we currently prefer to use a suturing technique.

First, we place tension on the uterine vascular bundle by applying traction through the uterine manipulator as the assistant pushes and rotates the uterus to the contralateral side. Then we apply additional traction and countertraction on the bundle from above with two atraumatic graspers. Subsequently, we use a strong suture on a large straight or ski needle to go under the bundle of artery and vein and tie an extracorporeal knot or square knot. The pedicle of tissues on the uterine side is coagulated with bipolar cautery to prevent back bleeding and cut.

Amputation of the Uterus and Ablation of the Endocervix

The cervix is detached from the uterus a short distance (0.5 to 1 cm) below the uterocervical junction. To separate the uterus, I have used a small surface unipolar electrode, bipolar cautery and scissors, a sharp cold knife, or a combination thereof. To cut the cervix uniformly at the same anteroposterior level, my associates and I have tried several maneuvers, including passing an endoloop suture over the uterine body and tightening the loop around the upper portion of the cervix to provide a landmark for an even circular incision (1).

At this time, our preferred method is to coagulate the cervical tissues further with bipolar cautery, bilaterally, approximately 0.5 cm above the level of occluded vascular bundle. We then carry the coagulation onto the anterior surface of the cervix at the same level to establish a landmark for cervical incision. Subsequently, we cut the cervix from both sides within the coagulated areas with a sharp or electrified scissors, make an incision in the anterior surface of the cervix at the same level with a sharp knife, and quickly carry the incision into the cervix to completely amputate it from the uterus (Fig 13.7).

When the uterus is freed, it is transported to the left upper abdomen for temporary storage. Hemostasis is secured by coagulating bleeding points. The upper portion of the endocervical mucosa is ablated or removed from the stump with a spatula unipolar electrode from above. A loop electric excision procedure may be added from below to remove

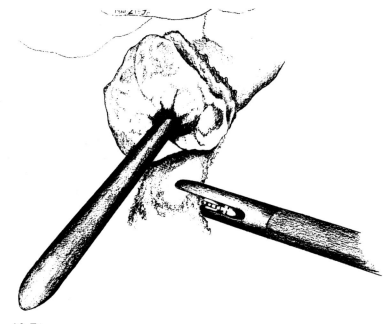

FIGURE 13.7

Detaching the cervix from the uterus.

most, if not all, of the endocervical epithelium. However, I prefer to perform a loop electric excision procedure only if indicated by subsequent cytology and colposcopy.

Initially, the walls of the cervix and the cut peritoneal edges were drawn together with continuous suture. This step was subsequently deleted when it was noted at second look that the pelvic peritoneum heals without adhesions regardless of suture approximation.

Concomitant Adnexectomy

If indicated, salpingo-oophorectomy can be performed as described elsewhere.

Removal of the Specimen

The stored uterus and other pelvic masses are removed through a colpotomy or minilaparotomy incision. Reducing the size of pelvic masses and withdrawing the smaller pieces from the abdominal cavity is the most cumbersome and time-consuming step of the operation. We have tried several methods with varying degrees of success, including morcellation according to Semm, the orange peel technique (30), bisection, posterior colpotomy, and minilaparotomy with externalization or morcellation outside the abdomen (1).

Recently, my associate, Carlos Rotman, MD, devised a simplified laparoscopic abdominal morcellation technique that we have found much easier and faster to perform. Essentially, the specimen is held securely from both sides and sliced longitudinally with a sharp knife. The slices are then removed through a slightly enlarged incision following removal of the laparoscopy cannula. Instruments and methods for this technique will be reported in the near future.

Lavage, Inspection, and Closure

Following complete removal of the specimens, the pelvic cavity is lavaged, the operative sites are inspected, and any small bleeding points are controlled. The secondary access trocars are removed under vision, and the primary access cannula is withdrawn after deflating the abdomen. The skin incisions are infiltrated with a local anesthetic to minimize postoperative discomfort. The open laparoscopy and enlarged removal incisions are closed in layers. The skin of other incisions is approximated. The Foley catheter is removed and the operation is completed.

CLINICAL EXPERIENCE

Our experience with SLH in more than 100 cases during the last 3.5 years confirms the safety and efficacy of the procedure. With increased experience, currently our average estimated blood loss is less than 100 mL. No blood transfusions were given from the beginning of the series. Our usual operative time is currently between 1 and 3 hours, depending on the size of the uterine mass and the extent of adhesions and other associated lesions.

In our series, the estimated blood loss associated with SLH was approximately one third of that associated with LAVH. Similar results were noted by Lyons (31). The estimated blood loss was significantly less with SLH compared with LAVH. The mean length of hospital stay in our series is less than 1 day for SLH compared with 1.8 days for LAVH. In Lyons' series, the length of hospital stay was decreased by approximately one half when SLH replaced LAVH (31). In our experience and that of Lyons, SLH was associated with less morbidity compared with LAVH. Schwartz (32) compared 20 SLH procedures he performed with 232 LAVH procedures from the literature and reported lower morbidity, blood loss, and recovery times with SLH. We have found the SLH and TLH procedures to be associated with low morbidity, short hospital stay, and early return to work. However, SLH was associated with a lower estimated blood loss, shorter operative time, and lower morbidity than TLH.

To date, there have been no instances of febrile morbidity, hemorrhage requiring transfusion, life-threatening events, or unplanned return to surgery in our series of SLH. When this type of complication outcome is compared with complication outcomes reported with abdominal or vaginal hysterectomy, as shown in Table 13.1 (33,34), the advantages of SLH are readily appreciated.

We have noted very few complications in our series. One patient sustained a bladder laceration that was repaired without incident during the laparoscopic procedure, and five patients had cyclic cervical bleeding. Of these five patients, two experienced spontaneous cessation within a few months, two continued to have scanty menses and are not concerned, and one had her cervix removed vaginally at another institution.

Histology revealed endometriosis. Because of these occurrences, patients are currently counselled that they may have scanty menses after the surgery. Most patients do not mind. Another patient had her stump removed when she became concerned about an abnormal Pap smear. Histology revealed chronic cervicitis without dysplasia.

Lyons (31), Schwartz (32), and Pelosi and Pelosi (35) have described other successful techniques for performing SLH. These surgeons remove the specimen through an extended primary umbilical incision. Semm (36) teaches a technique of intracervical enucleation, similar to that described by Lahey (37), who used an exclusive laparotomy

TABLE 13.1

Complication rates in abdominal and vaginal hysterectomy

COMPLICATION	RATE IN TAH[a]	RATE IN TVH[b]	RATE IN COMBINED SERIES[c]
Febrile morbidity	32.3%	15.3%	10%
Hemorrhage requiring transfusion	15.4%	8.3%	4.7%
Unplanned return to surgery	1.7%	5.1%	4.3%
Life-threatening events	0.4%	0	1.2%

Abbreviations: TAH, total abdominal hysterectomy; TVH, total vaginal hysterectomy.
[a] Data obtained from 1283 TAH cases (33). Dicker RC, Greenspan JR, Strauss LT, et al. Complications of abdominal and vaginal hysterectomy among women of reproductive age in the United States. Am J Obstet Gynecol 1982;144:841–848.
[b] Data obtained from 568 TVH cases (33). Dicker RC, Greenspan JR, Strauss LT, et al. Complications of abdominal and vaginal hysterectomy among women of reproductive age in the United States. Am J Obstet Gynecol 1982;144:841–848.
[c] Data obtained from 257 total hysterectomy cases (174 TAH and 83 TVH) (34). Gambone JC, Reiter RC, Lench JB. Quality assurance indicators and short-term outcome of hysterectomy. Obstet Gynecol 1990;76:841–845.

approach. Transabdominal excision of the endocervix at the time of abdominal subtotal hysterectomy has not become popular because of the excessive blood loss associated with it (37,38). The Semm procedure adds several technical refinements by pelviscopy and new instrumentation for coring out the cervical canal, coagulating the remaining endocervix from below, and morcellating the uterine mass from above. A recent study by Vietz and Ahn (39) using the Semm procedure in 102 patients yielded results comparable to other SLH techniques: low morbidity, little blood loss, short recovery time, and no major complications.

CONCLUSION

Supracervical laparoscopic hysterectomy has been shown to be safe and effective. It is preferred to total vaginal, abdominal, or laparoscopic hysterectomy for the treatment of benign gynecologic disease. Patients undergoing supracervical hysterectomy should be followed with periodic pelvic examinations and cytologic screening as if they have endometrial ablation or an intact uterus. The cervix is not a useless organ; it should not be removed without proper indication.

REFERENCES

1. Hasson HM, Rotman C, Rana N, et al. Experience with laparoscopic hysterectomy. J Am Assoc Gynecol Laparosc 1993;1:1–11.
2. Saye WB, Espy GB III, Bishop MR, et al. Laparoscopic Doderlein hysterectomy: a rational alternative to traditional abdominal hysterectomy. Surg Laparosc Endosc 1993;3:88–94.
3. Hasson HM. Cervical removal at hysterectomy for benign disease: risks and benefits. J Reprod Med 1993;38:780–790.
4. Romanes GJ, ed. Cunningham's text book of anatomy. Oxford: Oxford University, 1981:571–572.
5. DeLancey JL. Anatomic aspects of vaginal eversion after hysterectomy. Am J Obstet Gynecol 1992;166:1717–1728.
6. Richardson AC, Williams GA. Treatment of prolapse of the vagina following hysterectomy. Am J Obstet Gynecol 1969;105:90–93.
7. Symmonds RE, Williams TJ, Lee RA, Webb MJ. Posthysterectomy enterocele and vaginal vault prolapse. Am J Obstet Gynecol 1981;140:852–859.
8. Lansman HH. Post hysterectomy vault prolapse. Sacral colpoplexy with dura mater graft. Obstet Gynecol 1983;63:577–582.
9. Kauppila O, Punnonen R, Teisala K. Prolapse of the vagina after hysterectomy. Surg Obstet Gynecol 1985;161:9–11.
10. Mundy AR. An anatomical explanation for bladder dysfunction following rectal and uterine surgery. Br J Urol 1982;54:501–504.
11. Pritchard JA, MacDonald PC. The anatomy of the female reproductive tract. In: Pritchard JA, MacDonald PC, eds. Willams obstetrics. 16th ed. New York: Appleton-Century-Crofts, 1980:11–39.
12. Kilkku P, Hirvonen T, Gronroos M. Supravaginal uterine amputation vs. abdominal hysterectomy: the effects on urinary symptoms with special reference to pollakisuria, nocturia and dysuria. Maturitas 1981;3:197–204.
13. Kilkku P. Supravaginal uterine amputation versus hysterectomy with refer-

ence to subjective bladder symptoms and incontinence. Acta Obstet Gynecol Scand 1985;64:375–379.

14. Hanley HG. The late urological complications of total hysterectomy. Br J Urol 1969;41:682–684.

15. Vervest HA, deJonge MK, Vervest JS, et al. Micturition symptoms and urinary incontinence after non-radical hysterectomy. Acta Obstet Gynecol Scand 1988;67:141–146.

16. Taylor T, Smith AN. Effect of hysterectomy on bowel function. BMJ 1989;299:300–301.

17. Prior A, Stanley K, Smith ARB, Read NW. Effect of hysterectomy on anorectal and urethrovesical physiology. Gut 1992;33:264–267.

18. Clark L. Is there a difference between a clitoral and a vaginal orgasm? J Sex Res 1970;6:27–29.

19. Zussman L, Zussman S, Sunley R, Bjornson E. Sexual response after hysterectomy-oophorectomy: recent studies and reconsideration of psychogenesis. Am J Obstet Gynecol 1981;140:725–729.

20. Williamson ML. Sexual adjustment after hysterectomy. JOGNN 1992;21:42–47.

21. Dennerstein L, Wood C, Burrows GD. Sexual responses following hysterectomy and oophorectomy. Obstet Gynecol 1977;49:92–96.

22. Sloan D. The emotional and psychosexual aspects of hysterectomy. Am J Obstet Gynecol 1978;131:598–605.

23. Kilkku P, Gronroos M, Hirvonen T, Rauramo L. Supravaginal uterine amputation vs. hysterectomy: effects on libido and orgasm. Acta Obstet Gynecol Scand 1983;62:147–152.

24. Schofield MJ, Bennet A, Redman S, et al. Self-reported long-term outcomes of hysterectomy. Br J Obstet Gynaecol 1991;98:1129–1136.

25. Nathorst-Boos, Fuchs T, vonSchoultz B. Consumer's attitude to hysterectomy. The experience of 678 women. Acta Obstet Gynecol Scand 1992;71:230–234.

26. Helstrom L, Lundberg PO, Sorbom D, et al. Sexuality after hysterectomy: a factor analysis of women's sexual lives before and after subtotal hysterectomy. Obstet Gynecol 1993;81:357–362.

27. Jimerson GK, Merrill JA. Cancer and dysplasis of the posthysterectomy vaginal cuff. Gynecol Oncol 1976;4:328–334.

28. Bell J, Sevin BU, Averette H, Nadji M. Vaginal cancer after hysterectomy for benign disease: value of cytologic screening. Obstet Gynecol 1984;64:699–702.

29. Hoffman MS, Roberts WS, LaPolla JP, et al. Neoplasia in vaginal cuff epithelial inclusion cysts after hysterectomy. J Reprod Med 1989;34:412–414.

30. Hasson HM, Rotman C, Rana N, et al. Laparoscopic myomectomy. Obstet Gynecol 1992;80:884–888.

31. Lyons T. Supracervical laparoscopic hysterectomy—a comparison: morbidity and mortality results with LAVH. J Reprod Med 1993;38:763–767.

32. Schwartz RO. Laparoscopic hysterectomy. Supracervical vs assisted vaginal. J Reprod Med 1994;39:625–630.

33. Dicker RC, Greenspan JR, Strauss LT, et al. Complications of abdominal and vaginal hysterectomy among women of reproductive age in the United States. Am J Obstet Gynecol 1982;144:841–848.

34. Gambone JC, Reiter RC, Lench JB. Quality assurance indicators and short-term outcome of hysterectomy. Obstet Gynecol 1990;76:841–845.

35. Pelosi MA, Pelosi MA. Laparoscopic supracervical hysterectomy using a single umbilical puncture. Mini-laparoscopy. J Reprod Med 1992;37:774–784.

36. Semm K. Hysterectomy via laparotomy or pelviscopy. A new CASH method without colpotomy. Geburtshilfe Frauenheilkd 1991;51:996–1003.

37. Lahey FH. A simple method of removing the cervix with the uterus in hysterectomy. Surg Gynecol Obstet 1928;46:257–260.

38. Rauramo M. On excision of the cervical canal in conjunction with uterus amputation. Acta Obstet Gynecol Scand 1949;28:381–387.

39. Vietz PF, Ahn TS. A new approach to hysterectomy without colpotomy: pelviscopic intrafascial hysterectomy. Am J Obstet Gynecol 1994;170:609–613.

14

Laparoscopic Hysterectomy in the Management of Gynecologic Malignancies: Extraperitoneal Laparoscopic Hysterectomy

Nicholas Kadar

S imple and radical laparoscopic hysterectomies play a central role in the laparoscopic surgical treatment of many gynecologic malignancies, just as they do when the operations are carried out via a laparotomy. In most cases, the operations are combined with laparoscopic pelvic and/or aortic lymphadenectomy. Description of the operative techniques for laparoscopic-assisted vaginal radical hysterectomy and for laparoscopic-assisted pelvic and aortic lymphadenectomy is outside the scope of this chapter, and the interested reader is referred to my text, *Atlas of Laparoscopic Pelvic Surgery*, for technical details of these operations (1). The discussion in this chapter will focus on the indications for laparoscopic (simple) hysterectomy and on the technical aspects of my extraperitoneal technique.

INDICATIONS

Malignancies of the uterus provide the most common oncologic indications for simple hysterectomy. These are almost always carcinomas, but will occasionally be a pure sarcoma or a mixed müllerian tumor. Simple hysterectomy is also an integral part of the operative treatment of ovarian carcinoma, and it is used to treat microinvasive carcinoma of the cervix. Occasional oncologic indications for simple hysterectomy include such conditions as chorioadenoma destruens ("invasive mole") (i.e., gestational trophoblastic disease localized to the uterus).

Radical hysterectomy combined with pelvic lymphadenectomy is largely used to treat stage IB & IIA carcinoma of the cervix, but an occasional patient with vaginal carcinoma, or stage IIB carcinoma of the endometrium, may be a candidate for the operation. This operation will not be discussed further here.

CARCINOMA OF THE ENDOMETRIUM

Our approach to the management of endometrial carcinoma is outlined in Figs 14.1 and 14.2. The mainstay of therapy is simple hysterectomy, and the most important management decisions to be made are 1) which patients to subject to a lymphadenectomy, 2) what kind of lymphadenectomy to carry out, and 3) how to use the results of the lymphadenectomy to select subsequent therapy. These questions are considered in detail elsewhere (2) and can only be summarized here.

INDICATIONS FOR LYMPHADENECTOMY

Using data published by the Gynecologic Oncology Group, as well as our own data, we have calculated the number of lymphadenectomies that would need to be performed to identify one patient with pelvic and aortic lymph node metastases for the various combinations of tumor grade and depth of myometrial invasion that could be used as selection criteria for lymphadenectomy. Based on the assumption that 60% of women with positive pelvic nodes and 40% of women with positive aortic nodes could be cured of their disease by the addition of postoperative radiation therapy, we also calculated for each criterion (1) the number of lymphadenectomies required to prevent one death from

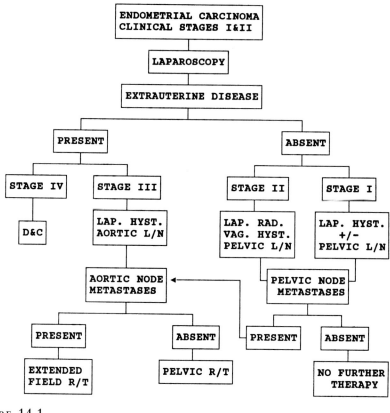

FIGURE 14.1

Laparoscopic management of endometrial carcinoma. (Reproduced by permission from Kadar N. Atlas of laparoscopic pelvic surgery. Boston: Blackwell Science, 1995:198.)

pelvic and aortic lymph node metastasis, and (2) the number of lymphadenectomies required to prevent one additional death from pelvic and aortic lymph node metastases over and above that required to prevent one death for the next less-sensitive criterion.

The results for selected criteria are shown in Tables 14.1 and 14.2. These figures actually exaggerate the therapeutic value of lymphadenectomy in women with disease confined to the corpus and cervix because the analysis was based on data pertaining to women with *clinical* stage I disease, some of whom actually had extrauterine disease, and these patients accounted for 50% of the cases with positive pelvic nodes and 44% of the cases with positive aortic nodes (2). In other

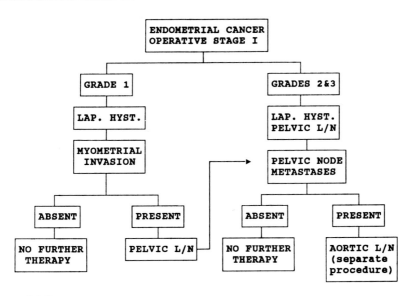

FIGURE 14.2

Laparoscopic management of endometrial carcinoma. (Reproduced by permission from Kadar N. Atlas of laparoscopic pelvic surgery. Boston: Blackwell Science, 1995:199.)

TABLE 14.1

Therapeutic index of selective pelvic lymphadenectomy

CRITERIA	A	B	C	D	E
None	0%	0%	9.3%	—	—
D3	60%	22%	6.0%	6.6	—
G2–3	91%	71%	4.2%	13.9	28
G2–3 and D3	95%	74%	4.0%	13.9	27
G2–3 and D1–3	100%	93%	3.7%	16.6	32

Abbreviations: A, proportion of patients with positive pelvic nodes identified; B, proportion of patients subjected to pelvic lymphadenectomy; C, death rate from pelvic nodal disease; D, number of lymphadenectomies required to prevent one death from pelvic nodal disease; E, number of lymphadenectomies required to prevent one additional death from pelvic nodal disease; G2–3, tumor grade 2–3; D1–3, depth of myometrial invasion to 1 (inner third), 2 (middle third), or 3 (outer third).

TABLE 14.2

Therapeutic index of selective aortic lymphadenectomy

CRITERIA	A	B	C	D	E
None	0%	0%	5.4%	—	—
D3	71%	22%	3.9%	14	—
G3 and D3	76%	37%	3.8%	22	111
G2–3	91%	71%	3.5%	36	108
G2–3 and D2–3	97%	77%	3.3%	36	95
G2–3 and D1–3	100%	93%	3.3%	44	118

Abbreviations: A, proportion of patients with positive aortic nodes identified; B, proportion of patients subjected to aortic lymphadenectomy; C, death rate from aortic nodal disease; D, number of lymphadenectomies required to prevent one death from aortic nodal disease; E, number of lymphadenectomies required to prevent one additional death from aortic nodal disease; G1–3 tumor grade 1–3; D1–3 depth of myometrial invasion to 1 (inner third), 2 (middle third), or 3 (outer third).

words, the criteria would be less sensitive in women who did not have gross extrauterine disease, and more lymphadenectomies would be required to salvage one patient than those tables indicate. Nonetheless, the following conclusions were drawn.

Pelvic Nodes

Table 14.1 indicates that if pelvic lymphadenectomy is carried out in all women with endometrial carcinoma, except those who have grade 1 lesions and no myometrial invasion (line 5), 93% of women would be subjected to pelvic lymphadenectomy, all those with positive pelvic nodes would be identified (column A), 17 pelvic lymphadenectomies would be required to salvage one patient with pelvic lymph node metastasis (column D), mortality would be reduced by almost 6% (column C, line 1 minus line 5), and approximately 30 lymphadenectomies would be required to cure one additional patient with positive pelvic nodes who was not salvaged by adopting a less-sensitive criterion (column E). It seems justifiable to carry out a pelvic lymphadenectomy in these cases because pelvic lymphadenectomy is not associated with a 3% mortality or a 3% serious morbidity rate (3). It also seems worthwhile extending the indications somewhat to simplify therapy and eliminate the need to assess myometrial invasion by intraoperative frozen sections and/or preoperative imaging studies. Thus, we carry out pelvic lymphadenectomy in all women except those with grade 1 lesions and no identifiable tumor in the opened uterus (Figs 14.1 and 14.2).

Aortic Nodes

From the results shown in Table 14.2, we believe it would be difficult to justify aortic lymphadenectomy in the same group of patients who are candidates for pelvic lymphadenectomy. Although the death rate could be reduced by 2% at a "cost" of 44 aortic lymphadenectomies per patient saved (column C, line 1 minus line 6), which could possibly be justified, the more telling statistics appear in column E. This column shows that it takes 100 or more lymphadenectomies to salvage a patient with aortic lymph node metastases who would not be salvaged by using deep myometrial invasion as the indication for aortic lymphadenectomy, and, as we noted at the outset, these are optimistic figures. Thus, in our view, aortic lymphadenectomy cannot be justified in women who have endometrial cancer grossly confined to the uterus unless they have deep (outer third) myometrial invasion.

We took the analysis one step further and compared deep myometrial invasion with pelvic lymph node metastases as a criterion for aortic lymphadenectomy. Obviously, if deep myometrial invasion is used as the criterion, the aortic lymphadenectomy can be carried out at the time of the primary operation, but if pelvic lymph node metastasis is used as the criterion, this must be deferred to a second operation. Approximately 5% to 7% of women with endometrial carcinoma who do not have gross extrauterine or cervical disease can be expected to have pelvic lymph node metastases, and this proportion of women would be subjected to two operations if pelvic lymph node metastases were used as the indication for aortic lymphadenectomy. However, using this criterion, 23% more women with aortic lymph node metastases would be identified and 35% fewer primary aortic lymphadenectomies would need to be performed. In other words, for every 100 aortic lymphadenectomies performed as a second procedure, seven more women would be salvaged and 157 primary aortic lymphadenectomies would be avoided. Aortic lymphadenectomy does not carry a 7% mortality rate (3); therefore, we believe this approach to be preferable even if the complications eliminated by avoiding 157 primary aortic lymphadenectomies are ignored. Moreover, the disadvantages of a two-stage approach are minimized if the operations are performed laparoscopically.

Thus, although it has been inferred from the 1988 FIGO staging for endometrial carcinoma and the surgical protocols of collaborative groups such as the Gynecologic Oncology Group that aortic lymphadenectomy should be performed whenever pelvic lymphadenectomy is carried out, this cannot be justified in clinical practice in our view. Many women require only pelvic lymphadenectomy or only aortic lymphadenectomy (e.g., those who have gross extrauterine or cervical disease), not both.

Rigid adherence to the unsupported view that lymphadenectomy in endometrial cancer necessarily means both pelvic and aortic lymphadenectomy has also needlessly disqualified obese women, precisely the ones most likely to benefit from avoidance of a laparotomy incision, from laparoscopic lymphadenectomy. Laparoscopic aortic lymphadenectomy has proved to be difficult to perform in women weighing more than 180 pounds (4), but the same restrictions do not apply to pelvic lymphadenectomy, and I have successfully performed pelvic lymphadenectomy in women weighing as much as 300 pounds (5). Therefore, if aortic lymphadenectomy were restricted to women who had pelvic lymph node metastases, most women, especially obese women who tend to have more favorable tumors, could be satisfactorily managed laparoscopically because most do not need an aortic lymphadenectomy.

LYMPH NODE SAMPLING VERSUS LYMPHADENECTOMY

Lymph node sampling means different things to different people. When applied to the selective removal of clinically enlarged lymph nodes, as practiced by Wertheim, for example, the term was both accurate and descriptive. However, we now know that at least 50% to 70% of lymph node metastases are clinically silent and cannot be detected by simply inspecting the lymph nodes at surgery. It follows a priori, therefore, that lymph node sampling will be insensitive at identifying nodal disease. It is accepted that a lymphadenectomy is never complete in the sense that every lymph node in the targeted area will be removed, but clearly this is a weak argument for purposefully not attempting a complete excision.

Arguments favoring the use of lymph node sampling, however defined, seem to rely on the proposition that there should be a difference between a staging and a therapeutic operation, but this is a proposition we do not accept. Patients with lymph node metastases may not benefit from adjunctive radiation or chemotherapy, but even if they do, that does not mean that the lymphadenectomy contributed nothing to their survival. Even if by identifying the presence of nodal metastases, lymphadenectomy served only to signal the need for additional therapy to achieve cure; a complete procedure would still be indicated because a selective operation might miss nodal metastases in some patients, who would thereby be denied potentially curative therapy. It is for this reason that Donohue (6), commenting on retroperitoneal lymphadenectomy in testicular tumors, stated, "our position is that the more thorough the lymphadenectomy, the more accurate the staging," a view that we would endorse. Breast cancer is the classic example of a malignancy that disseminates early in its natural history and in the treatment of which, therefore, lymphadenectomy is not curative. Nonetheless, to my knowledge no one has argued for selective removal of the primary lymph nodes in breast cancer just because an axillary dissection is not therapeutic and serves only to direct further therapy.

Thus, we manage the pelvic lymph nodes in endometrial cancer in exactly the same way as we do in cervical cancer. That is, we carry out the same kind of lymphadenectomy, and we irradiate the pelvis if the nodes are positive unless only minimal microscopic lymph node metastases are present.

OVARIAN CARCINOMA

The role of laparoscopy in the management of ovarian carcinoma is controversial. There is no question that huge, fixed pelvic masses, which require extensive retroperitoneal dissection and often proctocolectomy and retrograde hysterectomy to remove them, cannot be removed laparoscopically. However, one can usually identify women who have this type of lesion before surgery, or if not, certainly after assessing the pelvis laparoscopically. Moreover, the value of neoadjuvant chemotherapy in this setting is currently being investigated (7). Final answers are not available as yet, but it is entirely possible that neoadjuvant therapy, by shrinking the malignancy, may allow us to circumvent this type of surgery altogether in many patients. Even if the disease cannot be treated laparoscopically after neoadjuvant chemotherapy has done its work, the laparoscope will still have spared the patient one laparotomy, which, given what these patients usually have to go through, is not a respite that should be dismissed lightly.

At the other extreme are cases of advanced ovarian cancer with normal-sized ovaries, a situation also referred to as primary peritoneal carcinomatosis. "Debulking" plays no part in the management of these tumors, and, although these women do usually undergo laparotomy, hysterectomy, oophorectomy, and omentectomy, it is legitimate to question what is actually being achieved by this. We would argue that surgery achieves nothing besides a diagnosis and that these women are ideal candidates for laparoscopic management.

The majority of women with advanced ovarian cancer (probably 60% to 80%) have lesions in between these extremes. A proportion of these patients will have a large omental cake, or large plaques of tumor involving small bowel, that also will not be suitable for laparoscopic resection. In many other cases, however, the term "debulking" is simply a way of saying total abdominal hysterectomy, bilateral salpingo-oophorectomy, and omentectomy. Although these women often are also subjected to pelvic and aortic lymphadenectomy, there is no evidence that this will actually benefit the patient or alter her treatment, even if it changes her stage.

Experience with laparoscopic hysterectomy in women with benign pelvic masses suggests that many of these patients could almost certainly be "debulked" laparoscopically (i.e., undergo hysterectomy, oophorectomy, and omentectomy). Although this would obviously need to be demonstrated by actual experience, it is clearly far from self-evident that the laparoscopic management of advanced ovarian cancer is either misplaced or doomed to failure in most cases, as has been suggested. Tumor seeding of the abdominal wall along the trocar tract is a real and legitimate concern (8,9), but given that this is never seen in the laparotomy scars of women who have had advanced disease and ascites, prompt chemotherapy, closure of the peritoneum below the trocar insertion sites, or coagulation of the trocar tracts alone or in combination should avert this problem.

TUMOR DISSEMINATION DURING LAPAROSCOPY

Although laparoscopic cystectomy usually involves cyst rupture, oophorectomy does not, and it is not immediately obvious that laparoscopic oophorectomy carries a greater risk of cyst rupture than open oophorectomy. The greatest risk of rupture with laparoscopic oophorectomy is during removal of the specimen, but removal without rupture has been facilitated by the availability of an impermeable bag in which the ovary can be housed during removal, as well as by better techniques for colpotomy. Moreover, even if the cyst does rupture, seeding of the peritoneal cavity is much less likely with the techniques of extraction currently being used than with laparotomy. In fact, the available data suggest that most adnexal masses that are removed by laparoscopic oophorectomy or salpingo-oophorectomy are not ruptured in the process (10–13). Common sense suggests that the likelihood of rupture during removal increases with the size of the cyst. But the larger the cyst, the more likely the tumor is to have already disseminated, in which case the issue of rupture becomes irrelevant. Most ovarian carcinomas occur in postmenopausal women, and postmenopausal women with adnexal masses are not candidates for ovarian cystectomy.

Therefore, it is unclear to this author by what line of reasoning one arrives at a proscription of laparoscopic oophorectomy in post-menopausal women with suspicious adnexal masses.

TECHNIQUE OF EXTRAPERITONEAL LAPAROSCOPIC HYSTERECTOMY

Operations that can be successfully approached laparoscopically in the same way as at laparotomy have generally presented few problems to surgeons adept at laparoscopic techniques. The most obvious examples are cholecystectomy, and pelvic and aortic lymphadenectomy. Hysterectomy, by contrast, cannot be approached successfully in the same way as an abdominal hysterectomy, and the operation has become mired in controversy. Technical problems encountered during laparoscopic hysterectomy do not simply reflect a surgeon's lack of anatomical knowledge, surgical experience, or adequate laparoscopic training, or indeed even the inherent difficulty of laparoscopic surgery. This may be deduced from the fact that ureteric injuries, for example, have occurred during laparoscopic hysterectomy in the hands of the most experienced laparoscopic surgeons (14) as well as gynecologic oncologists proficient at performing more difficult radical operations laparoscopically and whose knowledge of pelvic anatomy is beyond dispute (15–17).

LAPAROSCOPIC VERSUS ABDOMINAL HYSTERECTOMY: IMPORTANT DIFFERENCES

The Ureter Must Be Identified

Dissection of the retroperitoneum and identification of the ureters are seldom necessary during abdominal hysterectomy for benign pathology. A clamp can be placed safely on the infundibulopelvic ligament without visualizing the ureter if the ureter is first identified in the broad ligament by palpation. The technique for placing clamps on the uterine arteries, parametria, and cardinal and uterosacral ligaments also ensures that only tissue directly adjacent to the cervix, and therefore medial to the ureter, will be included in the clamps, and identification of the ureter is again not required to ensure its safety. These techniques are obviously not available to the laparoscopic surgeon, and unless the laparoscopic part of the operation is restricted to adhesiolysis, excision of endometriosis, and oophorectomy, the ureters must be identified to make the operation safe. The numerous recorded, and doubtless many more unrecorded, ureteric injuries during laparoscopic hysterectomy attest to this fact.

Open Techniques for Ureteric Identification Cannot Be Used

The ureter is easily identified during abdominal hysterectomy by blunt dissection medial to the hypogastric artery, which is, in turn, easily identified by palpation after the broad ligament is opened. As discussed in Chapter 1, the ureter cannot be identified laparoscopically by simply opening the broad ligament, for it is covered by the infundibulopelvic ligament. The hypogastric arteries also cannot be seen except in the thinnest of patients, for they are covered by fatty areolar tissue. The precise level at which to open the pararectal space is therefore not obvious at first, and it is all too easy to start dissecting either too proximally or too distally. Annoying bleeding then occurs, which, although rarely sufficient to be of concern in itself, stains the surrounding tissues, making it very difficult to identify the underlying ureter and hypogastric artery.

Sequence of the Operation Must Be Altered

Abdominal hysterectomy begins with division of the round and then the infundibulopelvic ligaments, and many gynecologists start laparoscopic hysterectomy in the same way. If this is done, however, the parametrial tissues become increasingly floppy and difficult to place on tension, and blunt dissection of the extraperitoneal tissue planes will be extremely difficult, if not impossible. This is of no consequence as long as there are no plans to divide the uterosacral or cardinal ligaments. However, if a true laparoscopic hysterectomy is to be performed, the ureters must be identified, as we have noted, and if the hysterectomy is started in the same way as an abdominal hysterectomy, most of the time it will not be possible to identify the ureter where it matters, in the depths of the pelvis by the cardinal ligament.

Bladder Dissection and Anterior Colpotomy Illogical

Laparoscopic dissection of the bladder off the cervix has become part of a laparoscopic hysterectomy for no apparent reason other than that this is what is done during an abdominal hysterectomy. However, it is a step that makes little sense and reveals better than any other the extent to which our approach to laparoscopic hysterectomy has been influenced by the technique of abdominal hysterectomy. During abdominal hysterectomy, the vagina is entered anteriorly simply because, when viewed through an abdominal incision, it is the anterior rather than the posterior vaginal wall that presents itself *en face* to the surgeon. There are no deeper reasons for entering the vagina by this route. Indeed, in a vaginal hysterectomy, in which anterior colpotomy carries no such advantages over a posterior colpotomy, many vaginal surgeons start the operation by incising the posterior vaginal wall rather than with a circumferential incision around the cervix.

Unless total laparoscopic hysterectomy is to be performed, and the vaginal cuff sutured laparoscopically, laparoscopic bladder dissection makes no sense at all. First, unless the uterus is greatly enlarged, it is easier to make a posterior colpotomy laparoscopically than an anterior one, provided that a suitable vaginal manipulator is used that allows anteversion of the uterus. Second, if the vaginal cuff is to be closed transvaginally, laparoscopic dissection of the bladder will only serve to bring the bladder and distal ureter down into harm's way and make closure of the cuff more difficult.

Steps of the Operation Undefined

Hysterectomy entails a limited number of operative steps regardless of the route by which they are carried out. For abdominal and vaginal hysterectomy, these steps are clearly defined and the sequence in which they are performed is reversed. In a laparoscopic hysterectomy it is unclear which steps must or should be carried out laparoscopically and which ones vaginally. The number of permutations is rather large and the scope for disagreement is wide. There is a danger, therefore, that questions of technique will become embroiled with the rather different question of which steps to perform laparoscopically. To the extent that what is to be done affects how it can be done, the two questions are related, but it is helpful to keep them separate. The difficulties of laparoscopic hysterectomy do not stem from disagreements over what to do laparoscopically, but from how to approach what is to be done laparoscopically, and this approach, as we have tried to show, cannot be the same as that used in an abdominal hysterectomy.

LAPAROSCOPIC HYSTERECTOMY: OVERALL STRATEGY

Our extraperitoneal approach to laparoscopic hysterectomy evolved out of the technical difficulties encountered when laparoscopic hysterectomy was approached in the same way as an abdominal hysterectomy. It incorporates two strategies that have no real parallel in an abdominal hysterectomy.

First, the sequence of the steps is altered, and the uterine artery divided before the upper blood supply and supports of the uterus to preserve the natural tension in the tissues and to facilitate dissection of the retroperitoneum.

Second, the obliterated hypogastric arteries are isolated and traced retrogradely to the origin of the uterine vessels. This seemingly circuitous step allows the uterine arteries not only to be identified, but to be completely freed; the pararectal spaces to be accurately located and opened; and the ureter identified.

Once this preparatory dissection has been completed, laparoscopic hysterectomy becomes a simple matter of dividing a few structures by whatever means the surgeon wishes, although we strongly encourage traditional techniques of scissor dissection.

The Retroperitoneal Dissection (Steps 1–5)

The first stage of the hysterectomy consists of a retroperitoneal dissection, in the course of which the paravesical and pararectal spaces are developed, and the ureter and uterine arteries are identified and dissected free. These steps have been described in detail in Chapter 8 and will only be summarized here.

Step 1: The pelvic side wall triangles are opened (Fig 2.8A).

Step 2: The ureter is identified at the pelvic brim (Plate 25).

Step 3: The obliterated hypogastric arteries are identified extraperitoneally (Plate 25).

Step 4: The paravesical spaces are developed (Figs 2.9 and 14.3).

Step 5: The pararectal spaces are developed and the ureters freed from the distal part of the broad ligament (Fig 2.10).

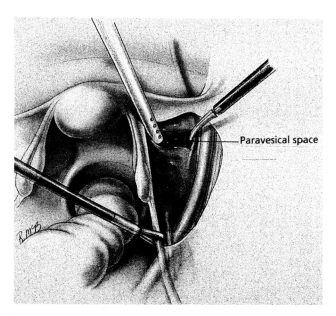

FIGURE 14.3

The medial paravesical space is opened. (Reproduced by permission from Kadar N. Atlas of laparoscopic pelvic surgery. Boston: Blackwell Science, 1995:108.)

The Hysterectomy

Step 6: The uterine arteries, round ligaments, and infundibulopelvic ligaments are divided.

Areolar tissue that still covers the anterior aspect of the uterine artery and cardinal ligament is dissected off bluntly by pushing the uterine artery backward and medially and the areolar covering forward and laterally. A vertical band of areolar tissue will separate from the anterior surface of the uterine artery and cardinal ligament if it did not already do so when the medial paravesical space was developed. The superior vesical artery will be seen lying in this areolar tissue as the tissue is placed on tension by pushing the umbilical ligament laterally (Fig 2.10). The uterine arteries are next desiccated with bipolar forceps or clipped with Laproclips and divided (Fig 14.4). Our preferred method is to clip the uterine arteries (and infundibulopelvic ligaments) with

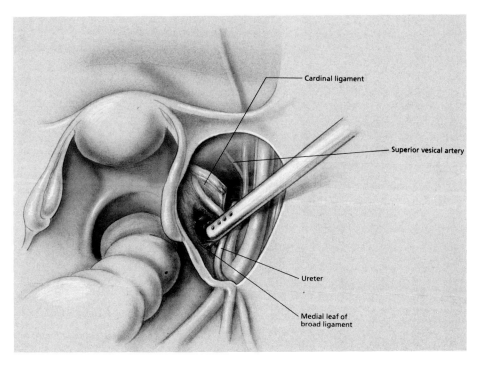

FIGURE 14.4

The uterine arteries are divided. (Reproduced by permission from Kadar N. Atlas of laparoscopic pelvic surgery. Boston: Blackwell Science, 1995:110.)

LH in the Management of Gynecologic Malignancies   271

Laproclips (Davis & Geck, Danbury, CT) because this is quicker and more reliable hemostasis is obtained. The round ligament is divided next, and the incision is continued along the anterior leaf of the broad ligament and the bladder peritoneum to the contralateral side, but the bladder is not dissected off the vagina. Finally, the infundibulopelvic ligaments are desiccated, ligated with silk, or doubly clipped with Laproclips and divided, and the incision continued along the medial leaf

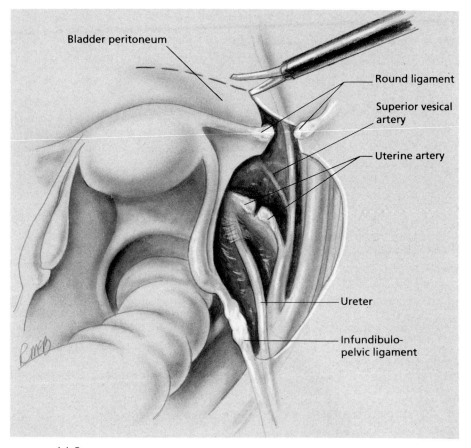

FIGURE 14.5

The infundibulopelvic ligament has been desiccated, the round ligament divided, and the incision extended along the anterior broad ligament and bladder peritoneum (step 6). (Reproduced by permission from Kadar N. Atlas of laparoscopic pelvic surgery. Boston: Blackwell Science, 1995:111.)

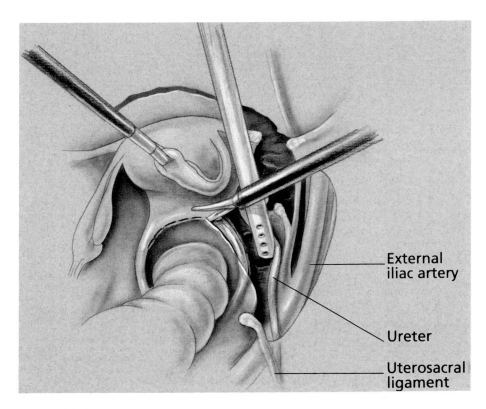

External
iliac artery

Ureter

Uterosacral
ligament

FIGURE 14.6

The infundibulopelvic ligament has been divided and the incision extended along the broad ligament to the uterosacral ligament. The ureter is retracted laterally as the uterosacral ligament is divided. (Reproduced by permission from Kadar N. Atlas of laparoscopic pelvic surgery. Boston: Blackwell Science, 1995:111.)

of the broad ligament toward the uterus to where the ureters have been reflected laterally (Fig 14.5). If bipolar coagulation is used, it is important to use the forceps efficiently. Rather than repeatedly taking it in and out of the peritoneal cavity, we generally coagulate the uterine artery and the round, and infundibulopelvic ligaments in sequence before dividing them. The smoke generated must be continuously suctioned during desiccation.

Step 7: The posterior dissection. The uterosacral ligaments are divided and the posterior vaginal wall is incised.

A plane is developed between the peritoneum and the uterosacral ligaments. The peritoneum is incised, and the incision extended to the pouch of Douglas, which is opened. The incision is continued across the midline to meet a similar incision in the peritoneum of the opposite broad ligament. The ureters are retracted laterally, and the uterosacral ligaments are divided with the closed tips of the dissecting scissors using a monopolar current (Fig 14.6).

The uterus is sharply anteflexed with the uterine mobilizer to an almost vertical position, whereupon a bulge resembling the cervix will appear at its lower end, which is in fact the hub of the instrument against the posterior vaginal wall. The posterior vaginal wall is incised against

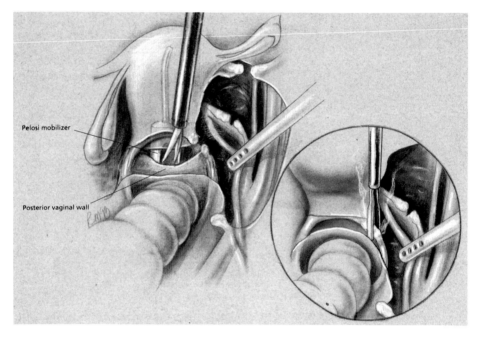

FIGURE 14.7

The posterior vaginal wall is opened against the hub of the Pelosi uterine mobilizer (Apple Medical, Bolton, MA) . (Reproduced by permission from Kadar N. Atlas of laparoscopic pelvic surgery. Boston: Blackwell Science, 1995:112.)

this bulge with the points of the dissecting scissors closed using a monopolar current (Fig 14.7). The incision should not be too close to the cervical attachment of the posterior vaginal wall, otherwise the incision will be too proximal to facilitate the vaginal part of the procedure. Contact between the dissecting scissors and the hub of the mobilizer is of no consequence because the surface area is large and any current that flows down the instrument will be dissipated along low current density pathways (see Chapter 3).

Step 8: The hysterectomy is completed vaginally.

The cervix is grasped with two single-toothed tenacula and elevated to expose the incision in the posterior vaginal wall; a long, self-weighted speculum is placed in the peritoneal cavity. The incision is then continued across the front of the cervix with a scalpel, the bladder dissected sharply off the cervix, the anterior cul-de-sac entered, and the bladder retracted with a deaver. A Zeppelin clamp (Zannutti, Torrance, CA) is placed on each cardinal ligament, the ligaments are divided and sutured, and the specimen is removed. The vagina is closed horizontally with a running, nonlocking stitch. The pneumoperitoneum is re-established, and the pelvis is irrigated copiously and checked for hemostasis.

REFERENCES

1. Kadar N. Atlas of laparoscopic pelvic surgery. Boston: Blackwell Science, Boston, 1995:205–247.
2. Kadar N, Homesley HD, Malfetano J. Some new perspectives on the indications for pelvic and para-aortic lymphadenectomy in the management of endometrial carcinoma. Gynaecol Endosc 1995;4:109–118.
3. Homesley HD, Kadar N, Lentz S, Barrett R. Selective pelvic and periaortic lymphadenectomy does not increase morbidity in surgical staging of endometrial carcinoma. Am J Obstet Gynecol 1992;167:1225–1230.
4. Childers JA, Hatch KD, Tran AN, Surwit EA. Laparoscopic para-aortic lymphadenectomy in gynecologic malignancies. Obstet Gynecol 1993;82:741–747.
5. Kadar N, Pelosi MA. Laparoscopically assisted hysterectomy in women weighing 200 pounds or more. Gynaecol Endosc 1994;3:159–162.

6. Donohue JP. Retroperitoneal lymphadenectomy. Urol Clin North Am 1977;4:509–521.

7. Jacob JH, Gershenson DM, Morris M, et al. Neoadjuvant chemotherapy and interval debulking for advanced epithelial ovarian cancer. Gynecol Oncol 1991;42:146–150.

8. Hsiu J, Given FT, Kemp GM. Tumor implantation after diagnostic laparoscopic biopsy of serous ovarian tumors of low malignant potential. Obstet Gynecol 1986;68:90–93s.

9. Gleeson NC, Nicosia SV, Mark JE, et al. Abdominal wall metastases from ovarian cancer after laparoscopy. Am J Obstet Gynecol 1993;169:522–523.

10. Bratschi HU, Heiz B. Video laparoscopic in total removal of ovarian tumors of uncertain origin in a bag through posterior colpotomy. Presented at the Second European Congress in Gynecological Endoscopy and New Surgical Techniques, Heidelberg, Germany October 21–23, 1993, p 13. Abstract.

11. Hettenbach A, Possover M, Morawski A. Laparoscopic surgery of ovarian tumors in post menopausal women. Presented at the Second European Congress in Gynecological Endoscopy and New Surgical Techniques, Heidelberg, Germany, October 21–23, 1993, p 60. Abstract.

12. Ottersen T. Laparoscopic (plastic bag) surgery; what are the benefits? Presented at the Second European Congress in Gynecological Endoscopy and New Surgical Techniques, Heidelberg, Germany, October 21–23, 1993, p 93. Abstract.

13. Ulrich U. The use of endobags in operative laparoscopy. Presented at the Second European Congress in Gynecological Endoscopy and New Surgical Techniques, Heidelberg, Germany, October 21–23, 1993, p 158. Abstract.

14. Hourcabie JA, Bruhat M-A. One hundred and three cases of laparoscopic hysterectomy using endo-GIA staples and a device for presenting the vaginal fornices. Gynaecol Endosc 1993;2:65–72.

15. Hunter RW, McCartney AJ. Can laparoscopic assisted hysterectomy safely replace abdominal hysterectomy? Br J Obstet Gynaecol 1993;100:932–934.

16. Childers JA, Brzechffa PR, Hatch KD, Surwit EA. Laparoscopically assisted surgical staging (LASS) of endometrial cancer. Gynecol Oncol 1993;51:33–38.

17. Kadar N, Lemmerling L. Urinary tract injuries during laparoscopically assisted hysterectomy: causes and prevention. Am J Obstet Gynecol 1994;170:253–254.

15

Complications of Laparoscopic Hysterectomy: Prevention, Recognition, and Management

C.Y. Liu

The first laparoscopic hysterectomy performed in the United States was in January 1988. Published literature regarding this procedure is still limited. The reported surgeries were performed by experienced laparoscopic surgeons, but nonetheless were associated with some serious complications. Laparoscopic hysterectomy is not an inocuous procedure; it carries the combined risks of both operative laparoscopy and hysterectomy.

In our (Liu and Reich, see Chapter 10) series of 518 cases of laparoscopic hysterectomy and total laparoscopic hysterectomy, the complication rate was 5.7%. These complications included febrile morbidity (2.1%), injury to the urinary tract system (1.3%), injury to the bowel (1.1%), delayed postoperative vaginal cuff bleedings (0.5%), unanticipated blood transfusions (0.3%), and pulmonary embolism (0.2%) (Table 10.3). As a rule, the more complex the pelvic pathology and the more technically difficult the procedure, the more likely that serious complications will occur. This chapter will systematically address the possible sites of complications, precautionary measures for avoiding intraoperative complications, and, should they occur, management of the complications.

VESSEL INJURY

Perforation of Abdominal Wall Vessels

The likelihood exists that if he or she performs enough laparoscopic procedures, every gynecologist will perforate one or more of the major abdominal wall vessels. Of primary concern are the deep and superficial epigastric vessels of the abdominal wall when secondary trocars are placed in the lower abdomen. The deep inferior epigastric artery arises from the external iliac artery right before the latter enters into the femoral canal. Shortly after coming out of the external iliac artery, the deep inferior epigastric artery branches out into the rectus abdomini muscle, where it usually has a tributary running along the lateral border of the rectus muscle. The superficial epigastric artery arises from the femoral artery near the inguinal ring and courses medially over the rectus muscle toward the midline. Since the deep inferior epigastric vessels traverse beneath the rectus muscle and immediately above the parietal peritoneum, they usually can be readily seen through the laparoscope. The superficial epigastric vessels usually also can be seen through the transillumination of the abdominal wall when the tip of the laparoscope is placed near or against the abdominal wall. However, in obese patients and in patients with surgical scars in the lower abdomen, especially a scar resulting from Pfannenstiel's incision, these vessels may be obscured. When these vessels are not visible, the risk of vessel injury will be increased; however, injury may be minimized by placing the trocars *medial* to the obliterated umbilical artery or *lateral* to the site where the round ligament inserts into the inguinal canal.

The obliterated umbilical artery and the round ligament always can be identified even in very obese patients. When the secondary trocar is placed near the level of the umbilicus, the inferior epigastric vessels are much more difficult to identify; however, because the rectus muscle is more obvious, the trocar should be placed lateral to the rectus muscle to avoid puncturing the tributary of the inferior epigastric vessels. The secondary trocars always should be inserted under direct visualization, never placed blindly, and they should be placed perpendicular to the fascia to avoid lacerating the vessels close to the trocar insertion sites.

If vessel injury is noted at the time of trocar insertion, it is important to remember that the trocar sleeve should be left in place. *Do not remove the sleeve.* Because the sleeve is the only marker for the location of that injured vessel, removal would result in difficulty in finding the bleeding vessel within a large hematoma. Furthermore, the sleeve acts as a drain for the blood to escape into the peritoneal cavity, thus preventing large hematoma formation.

The deep inferior epigastric vessels lie just above the parietal peritoneum. Unless the artery is completely severed and retracted, bipolar forceps inserted from the other side of the abdomen compress and desiccate the vessel and the tissues adjacent to the sleeve usually allowing the bleeding to be controlled. It is important to remember that the deep inferior epigastric vessels have significant anastomosis with internal mammary vessels and deep circumflex iliac vessels. Both ends of the injured vessel must be desiccated to achieve adequate hemostasis. When bipolar coagulations around the trocar sleeve fall to control the bleeding and the hematoma is rapidly increasing in size, the blood vessel is most likely completely severed and retracted, in which case the skin incision around the trocar sleeve should be enlarged longitudinally and dissection carried down, following the sleeve. The bleeding vessel on both ends should be secured and ligated.

The popular method of using an inflated Foley catheter tip to compress the bleeding site may not work if the artery is completely severed and retracted. Large trocars (>10 mm) are more likely to completely sever the vessel compared with small trocars (≤5 mm). Therefore, whenever possible, a small trocar (≤5 mm) with a conical tip, rather than a pyramidal tip with three sharpened edges, should be used to avoid lacerating or completely severing the vessel. Instruments designed for closing the fascial layer of the large trocar puncture site are available (Fig 15.1). These instruments also can be used to control bleeding from a lacerated epigastric vessel.

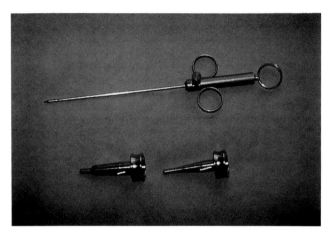

FIGURE 15.1

Instruments designed for the purpose of closing the fascial layer of the large trocar puncture site. These instruments can also be used to control bleeding from a lacerated epigastric vessel.

Intraoperative Hemorrhage

Massive and troublesome intraoperative hemorrhage can occur with a slipped ligature tie or hemoclips, large ovarian or uterine artery injury, or premature division before the vessels are completely desiccated. The principles to follow in dealing with massive bleeding laparoscopically are the same as those in open laparotomy: *compression, suction and irrigation of the bleeding site*, and *clear identification of the bleeder*. After the bleeder is clearly identified, it can be controlled either by suture ligation, electrodesiccation, or hemoclip application. The majority of bleedings can be controlled by bipolar desiccation alone; however, the surrounding anatomy needs to be checked prior to initiation of electrodesiccation to avoid thermal injury to vital structures, such as the ureter, bladder, or bowels. Suture ligation or application of the hemoclips is more appropriate when the bleeder is close to the vital structures.

The key to preventing premature division before the large vessels are completely desiccated is to have the assistant or circulating nurse carefully observe the ammeter on the generator of the electrosurgery unit to make sure that the flow of the electrical current has completely ceased between the prongs of the bipolar forceps. If the vessels are not completely desiccated and occluded, the electrical current will continue to flow between the tips of the forceps and the needle of the ammeter will not return to the 0 position. If a large vessel is still unable to be desiccated after 8 to 10 seconds of application of the bipolar forceps, the two prongs of the forceps must not have completely grasped it, in which case the forceps must be reapplied. Injury to the external iliac vessels, aorta, or vena cava requires immediate laparotomy and intraoperative consultation with a vascular surgeon.

URINARY TRACT SYSTEM INJURY

Bladder Injury

Bladder injury occurs in approximately 0.5% to 1% of all major pelvic surgery cases. Laparoscopic hysterectomy should have approximately the same rate of injuries as other major pelvic surgical procedures. However, in our series of 518 laparoscopic hysterectomies, six (1.5%) bladder injuries occurred, which is slightly higher than reported in abdominal hysterectomy.

There are basically two types of bladder injuries that may occur during laparoscopic hysterectomy: intraperitoneal and extraperitoneal bladder injuries. Intraperitoneal bladder injury involves perforation of the bladder and its covering peritoneum, resulting in urine leakage into the peritoneal cavity. In extraperitoneal bladder injury, the peritoneum remains intact and the urine leaks into Retzius' space. Bladder injury during laparoscopic hysterectomy is always caused either mechanically by instruments, such as improperly placed trocar and scissors, or thermally from electrosurgery and/or laser.

Recognition of Bladder Injury

Intraoperatively: Intraperitoneal bladder injury can be easily recognized by leakage of indigo carmine dye. However, in rare occasions with small trocar injury, there may not be any leakage of dye. A strong suspicion of injury is needed to make the proper diagnosis. If the trocar tip appears to be pushing through the muscular organ, bladder injury should be ruled out by performing cystoscopic examination. Cystoscopic examination also is necessary in cases in which excessive electrosurgery has been performed around the bladder.

Postoperatively: Unexplained hematuria found during postoperative catheterization, decreased urine output, anuria, suprapubic swelling and pain, and abdominal distention with an elevated blood urea nitrogen level may be indicative of bladder injury. A cystogram and a cystoscopic examination should be performed to make the proper diagnosis. Thermal injury to the bladder wall usually does not manifest itself immediately after surgery. Sudden hematuria or a vesicovaginal fistula 7 to 14 days postoperatively may be the first sign of thermal injury to the bladder. Cystoscopic examination should be performed to confirm the diagnosis.

Prevention of Bladder Injury: The following steps are very helpful in preventing injury to the bladder during laparoscopic hysterectomy.

Step 1: The bladder should be emptied prior to surgery. We routinely instill 15 to 20 mL of concentrated indigo carmine dye into the bladder after it is emptied. This facilitates the early recognition of bladder injury during surgery. It is not necessary to leave the Foley catheter in the bladder during prolonged complicated laparoscopic procedures, which usually require extensive uterine or vaginal manipulation from below by the assistant. The catheter may inadvertently be pulled and tucked by the assistant while manipulating the uterus or vagina, thereby bruising the trigon area of the bladder with the balloon tip of the catheter. If the bladder becomes distended during surgery, it can be emptied using a straight catheter.

Step 2: Insert all secondary trocars under direct visualization. This is especially important when the anatomy is distorted due to infection, extensive endometriosis, or previous surgery.

Step 3: Separate the bladder from the low uterine segment by using sharp dissection. *Never dissect the bladder bluntly.* This is especially important when the patient has had a previous cesarean section, infection, or endometriosis.

Step 4: If an automatic multifire stapling device is to be used during the hysterectomy, make sure the bladder is not inside the jaws of the laparoscopic stapling device before firing it.

Step 5: Avoid using electrosurgery extensively around the bladder, especially with monopolar electrosurgery in a coagulation mode. Brisk bleeding from around the bladder usually indicates injury to the muscular layer of the bladder wall. Hemostatic suture, rather than electrocoagulation, will reduce the possibility of bladder injury.

Management of Bladder Injury: Any bladder injury must be evaluated cystoscopically; the integrity of both ureters needs to be confirmed. For a small extraperitoneal bladder injury, catheterization with Foley catheter for 10 to 14 days should be adequate. However, for a larger injury, a mini-laparotomy with standard two-layer repair using absorbable sutures should be done, followed by 10 to 14 days of catheterization. For intraperitoneal bladder lacerations less than 1 cm in length, a two-layer pursestring suture with 2-0 absorbable sutures can be used. The first pursestring suture includes the muscular and mucosal portions, and the second pursestring suture includes the serosa and muscular layers. If the laceration of the bladder is longer than 1 cm, the bladder is mobilized to ensure the suture site is free from tension. A standard two-layer closure should then be done. We recommend using a 3-0 delayed absorbable suture with an SH needle for the first-layer closure, which includes the muscular and mucosal portions of the bladder, using continuous nonlocking running stitches. Two hundred fifty to 300 mL of indigo carmine dye or sterile infant formula should be instilled into the bladder after the first layer is closed to ensure the repair is water tight. If any leakage is observed from the suture line, the bladder is deflated and a figure-of-eight suture is placed at the leaking site. The bladder is reinflated with 250 to 300 mL of dye or infant formula and checked for leakage. If there is no leakage from the suture line, the bladder is then deflated and a second layer of stitches, which includes the serosa and muscular portions of the bladder, is placed with 2-0 delayed absorbable sutures using either interrupted or continuous stitches. The bladder is then drained with a Foley catheter for 10 to 14 days.

A cystoscopic examination is performed after every case of bladder repair to ensure that the entire injury is repaired and that the integrity of the ureters is not compromised. Laparoscopic repair of intraperitoneal bladder injury can be easily performed if the surgeon is proficient in laparoscopic suturing technique. If the injury is caused by through-and-through thermal burn, the devitalized tissue of the thermal injury of the bladder wall needs to be excised and the defect repaired with the two-layer technique described above.

Ureteral Injury

The incidence of ureteral injury in laparoscopic hysterectomy is unknown, although in our (Liu and Reich, see Chapter 10) series of 518 laparoscopic hysterectomies there was only one ureteral injury. However, our private correspondence with gynecologic laparoscopists from around the world leads us to believe that the incidence of ureteral injury in laparoscopic-assisted hysterectomy is higher than in traditional abdominal or vaginal hysterectomy, which is reported to vary between 0.4% and 1.5%. Most ureteral injuries during laparoscopic hysterectomy occur in the area between the ureteric canal and the bladder base. The patients at risk for ureteral injury should be identified prior to surgery. Patients with a history of extensive pelvic inflammatory disease or endometriosis, preoperative pelvic findings of a large pelvic mass, intraligamentary leiomyomata, obliterated cul-de-sac, and induration in the paracervical area should arouse suspicion of ureteral involvement. Preoperative evaluation with an intravenous pyelogram is helpful in patients with these conditions.

Prevention of Ureteral Injury: The best way to prevent ureteral injury during laparoscopic hysterectomy is to be certain of its location at all times during the procedure. With laparoscopic surgery, one loses the ability to palpate the pelvic organs, but one gains a much improved visibility of the pelvic structures; this is the reason we are not in favor of using preoperative ureteral catheterization in high-risk patients. One may argue that transillumination of the ureter through the recently developed lighted ureteral catheter makes the course of the ureter obvious during laparoscopy. However, because the presently available lighted ureteral catheters are all rather rigid and are larger in caliber, the mucosa of the ureter can be easily damaged by the heat emited from the lighted catheter and from intraoperative manipulation of the catheter against the ureter.

The ureteral injury can be especially severe in cases of preexisting periureteral fibrosis and scarring, which may be secondary to previous infection or endometriosis. We recommend routine identification and dissection of the pelvic ureters at the beginning of the hysterectomy; by doing so, the ureteral locations are clear throughout the entire surgical procedure. We have not had any ureteral injury since we began the practice of ureteral identification and dissection as the first step of any laparoscopic hysterectomy. The anatomy of the pelvic ureter and the technique of identification and dissection of the ureter are described in detail in Chapter 8.

Recognition of Ureteral Injury

Intraoperatively: Ureteral injuries have the best prognosis when they are recognized and repaired intraoperatively. A delay in diagnosis can lead to the development of progressively deteriorated renal function. As many as 25% of unrecognized ureteral injuries result in eventual loss of the affected kidney. Any complicated laparoscopic pelvic surgery should prompt the surgeon to look for possible ureteral injury, even though no obvious damage has been recognized. The steps for detection of intraoperative ureteral injury have been described in detail in Chapter 8.

Postoperatively: Patients with undetected ureteral injuries will present various signs and symptoms, such as flank pain, costovertebral angle tenderness, unexplained fever and chills, abdominal distention, and ileus. A strong suspicion of ureteral injury and prompt investigation with an intravenous pyelogram is crucial for diagnosis of the postoperative ureteral injury. Cystoscopy and retrograde pyelography often are needed to determine the exact location of the lesion or obstruction.

Treatment of Ureteral Injury: As soon as intraoperative ureteral injury is detected, immediate laparotomy with ureteral repair is recommended. Although there are a few gynecologists who can effectively repair ureteral injury laparoscopically, one must consider one's own experience and skills and maintain caution about one's own limits, especially when laparoscopic repair of ureteral injury is intended. Consultation with colleagues experienced in ureteral repair is highly recommended. The timing of repair of postoperatively recognized ureteral injuries is more complicated; the patient's general condition, the degree of edema, and the associated local inflammation should be carefully evaluated, since the surgical procedure for this type of ureteral reconstruction usually is more difficult and lengthy, although some physicians feel that early intervention, as soon as diagnosis of ureteral injury is made, does not increase the postoperative complications or sequelae. However, we recommend that in the presence of edema, local inflammation, and poor general condition of the patient, ureteral reconstruction should be postponed 4 to 6 weeks, unless a percutaneous nephrostomy cannot be done or there is evidence of progressively deteriorating renal function in spite of intensive conservative treatment.

Surgical Considerations: Regardless of whether the injury is recognized intraoperatively or postoperatively, the surgery for ureteral reconstruction should adhere to the following principles:

1. Have adequate debridement and use only the healthy part of the ureter for reanastomosis.
2. Avoid using too many sutures.
3. Avoid any tension at the anastomotic site.
4. Obtain complete hemostasis if possible.
5. Insert an indwelling ureteral catheter and place retroperitoneal drainage.

There are essentially three options for ureteral repair: end-to-end reanastomosis, ureteroneocystostomy, and transureteroureterostomy.

End-to-End Reanastomosis: If the site of ureteral injury is above the midpelvis and the injury is not very extensive, then end-to-end anastomosis of the ureter can be performed easily, first by debriding the injured portion and then mobilizing the ureter to avoid undue tension on the anastomotic site. A double J ureteral catheter is inserted and some type of extraperitoneal suction drainage, such as a Jackson-Pratt drain, is placed close to the anastomotic site. The bladder is drained with a urethral or suprapubic catheter.

Ureteroneocystostomy: Most ureteral injuries in laparoscopic hysterectomies occur around the area of either the ureteric canal or along the site of the cardinal ligament between the ureteric canal and the base of the bladder, which is located deep in the pelvis. After resection of the damaged section of the ureter, the continuity of the urinary tract can best be restored by performing a ureteroneocystostomy rather than an end-to-end ureteroureterostomy. To avoid any tension in the anastomotic site, the bladder must be mobilized from the back of the pubis. An anterior cystostomy is performed and the ureter is brought through the wall of the bladder by means of a submucosal tunnel; an end-to-side, mucosa-to-mucosa anastomosis between the end of the ureter and the sidewall of the bladder is then performed. A double J ureteral catheter is inserted and a Jackson-Pratt drain is inserted retroperitoneally close to the anastomotic site but not touching it. If adequate mobilization of the bladder is difficult, a bladder hitch can be done by simply displacing the bladder upward and attaching it to the fascia of the iliopsoas muscle. Similarly, the upper segment of the ureter can be further mobilized to reduce the tension on the anastomotic site.

Transureteroureterostomy: If a large segment of the ureter has been damaged and a ureteroneocystostomy is not possible, a transureteroureterostomy by an experienced urologist is advised.

BOWEL INJURY

Bowel injury during laparoscopic hysterectomy is uncommon; when it occurs, it usually is associated with trocar insertion, extensive intraperitoneal adhesions, or endometriosis. In our series of 518 cases of laparoscopic hysterectomies, we had two small bowel injuries occur during enterolysis due to extensive adhesions. One superficial thermal injury of the anterior wall of the sigmoid colon occurred. Two intentional anterior rectal wall resections for full-thickness endometriosis were performed. Two patients developed Richter's hernia in the 12-mm trocar sites postoperatively. Early recognition of bowel injury is crucial; it is preferable to detect it during surgery so that immediate implementation of appropriate treatment can reduce morbidity.

Small Bowel Injury

Most of the small bowel injuries during laparoscopic hysterectomies are caused by trocar insertion and enterolysis secondary to extensive adhesions. Patients with a history of multiple laparotomies, prior ruptured appendix, inflammatory bowel disease, previous pelvic inflammatory disease, and extensive endometriosis are particularly at risk for the presence of bowel adhesions. Trocar injury of the small bowel usually occurs when there are bowel adhesions to the anterior abdominal wall, especially around the umbilical area.

Recognition of Small Bowel Injury: There are basically three different causes for small bowel injuries during laparoscopic hysterectomy: trocar injury, injury secondary to enterolysis or electrosurgery, and Richter's hernia.

Trocar Injury: If the umbilical trocar has made a large laceration in the small bowel, the surgeon may be able to laparoscopically view the mucosal surface of the small bowel. In addition, contents of the small bowel may be seen leaking from the laceration or a hematoma may be present on the small bowel surface. If adhesions are detected around the umbilical area, even though there is no evidence of bowel injury, inspection of the umbilical trocar in its entirety with a 5-mm laparoscope through a secondary trocar sleeve must be performed to ensure that there is no occult or through-and-through small bowel laceration. If a trocar or laparoscope is detected inside the small bowel lumen, *do not remove it* before the laparotomy or laparoscopic repair of the injury, for it will seal the puncture and serve to identify the site of laceration.

Injury Secondary to Enterolysis or Electrosurgery: When dense adhesions exist and require extensive enterolysis and electrosurgery for hemostasis, small bowel injury usually is obvious. Monopolar electrosurgical energy should not be used around the small bowel unless the surgeon possesses the highest level of expertise. Another drawback to the wide use of electrosurgery is that discharge of static electric energy from the trocar sleeve or instruments can produce bowel injury. In such cases, electrical burns can be difficult to detect and evaluate because the injury usually is outside the laparoscopic viewing field. Furthermore, monopolar electrical injury of the small bowel often appears smaller than it actually is. The mechanism and prevention of injuries caused by electrosurgery are detailed in Chapter 4.

Richter's Hernia: Due to the manipulation of the trocar sleeve during the operative laparoscopy, fascia and peritoneal defects can easily become enlarged, often allowing a loop of small intestine to herniate into this defect and become incarcerated. Therefore, any fascia defect of the puncture site for any trocar larger than 10 mm should be closed to prevent the formation of Richter's hernia. There are various instruments available for this purpose. Richter's hernia usually manifests signs and symptoms of small bowel obstruction within 48 hours of surgery.

Avoiding Small Bowel Injury: Most small bowel injuries occur during the insertion of the Verres needle for pneumoperitoneum or initial trocar insertion. Unintentional preperitoneal insufflation can complicate the initial trocar insertion; this occurrence is more common in obese patients. *Do not attempt to reinsert the trocar in cases of preperitoneal insufflation.* The risk of injuring the intra-abdominal organs is much higher since the ballooned-out peritoneum is now in much closer proximity to the abdominal organs, and small bowel injury can occur easily with the tip of the trocar. Preperitoneal gas should be emptied through the trocar sleeve, after which pneumoperitoneum can be re-established.

Factors that may cause the surgeon to perform an uncontrolled sudden trocar entry into the abdominal cavity include an inadequate umbilical incision, scar tissue from a prior laparoscopy or laparotomy, and a dull trocar. These are in the absence of intra-abdominal adhesions or other predisposing pelvic pathology.

Trocar insertions in patients at risk for small bowel adhesions to the anterior abdominal wall should follow the techniques illustrated in Chapter 7.

Treatment of Small Bowel Injury: The small bowel injury caused by the Verres needle usually is inocuous as long as no leakage of bowel contents is observed and the laceration does not involve the mesenteric vessels. Superficial bowel injury caused by the trocar seals readily and requires no further treatment. When the lacerations involve the muscularis or mucosa, repair with sutures is needed. When the lacerations are small, they can be repaired either laparoscopically or through laparotomy. However, if the laceration exceeds one half the diameter of the lumen, or if the mesenteric blood supply is interrupted or damaged, a segmental resection and anastomosis should be performed through laparotomy. For small lacerations that do not compromise the mesenteric blood supply, we recommend using a two-layer closure. The first layer, which includes the muscularis and mucosa, uses 3-0 absorbable sutures, either with interrupted or continuously running nonlocking stitches. The second layer of reinforcing sutures of 3-0 silk Lembert stitches is used to approximate the muscularis and serosal edges. All lacerations should be closed transversely to prevent the possibility of narrowing the bowel lumen.

Thorough lavage of the entire abdomen and pelvis with copious amounts of Ringer's lactate solution after the bowel repair is completed is essential to eliminate the possibility of peritonitis. A nasogastric tube should be placed and postoperatively removed when the patient starts to pass flatus. Our experience shows that the postoperative recovery for patients who had laparoscopic small bowel repair is short. Their bowel function resumes rather quickly, and all patients are able to have the nasogastric tube removed within 24 hours of surgery.

When the patient presents signs and symptoms of possible small bowel obstruction or peritonitis after discharge from the hospital, an *immediate* second-look laparoscopy or laparotomy should be done as soon as the patient is stabilized. This is to rule out unrecognized intestinal perforation or Richter's hernia. The prognosis is usually favorable if the intervention is made before the incarcerated bowel is damaged or before extensive peritonitis has developed in the case of undetected bowel perforation. For Richter's hernia, the trapped loop of the small bowel usually can be pulled out of the previous trocar puncture site and the abdominal wall defect sutured, either laparoscopically or through laparotomy.

Wheeless presented a seven-point plan for the management of patients with peritonitis secondary to unrecognized bowel perforation:

1. Preoperative stabilization with fluids, electrolytes, and nasogastric suction.
2. Exploratory laparotomy with repair or resection of the injured bowel.
3. Resection of all necrotic tissue.
4. Copious and repeated lavage with saline of the abdomen.
5. Pelvic drainage through the vagina using a closed drainage system.
6. Aggressive antibiotic therapy.
7. Starting a mini-dose of heparin (5000 U every 8 hours) for embolus prophylaxis.

LARGE INTESTINE INJURY

Injury to the colon during laparoscopic surgery is uncommon. The actual incidence is unknown at present. In our (Liu and Reich, Chapter 10) series of 518 cases of laparoscopic hysterectomies, we had one case of superficial thermal injury of the sigmoid colon and two cases of intentional resection of the anterior rectal wall due to full-thickness bowel wall infiltration of endometriosis. We do not consider these two cases of intentional resection of the rectal wall in our series as complications, but rather as part of the therapeutic process.

Recognition and Prevention of Injuries to the Large Intestine

Colon Injury Due to Trocar Insertion: Most injuries to the large intestine occur during trocar insertion. The incidence of trocar injury to the large intestine is estimated to be approximately 0.1%. The transverse colon and sigmoid colon are most commonly traumatized by the trocar insertion. This usually happens during blind insertion of the umbilical trocar. This fact can be explained by consideration of the anatomy of the large intestines. Because the ascending and descending colon are on the lateral sides of the abdominal cavity and are retroperitoneally located, there is no medial displacement by intraperitoneal adhesions. In contrast, the transverse colon is the most mobile portion of the colon and the entire length is attached to the greater curvature of the stomach by the gastrocolonic ligament. The upper end of the omentum apron is attached to the anterior aspect of the transverse colon. Therefore, the transverse colon can be easily displaced inferiorly to the middle of the abdominal cavity when there is omental adhesion to the anterior abdominal wall or when there is gastric distention secondary to mask ventilation prior to a difficult intubation during the initial stage of anesthesia. The sigmoid colon also is at risk because of its midline location in the path of the uncontrolled advancing trocar.

The diagnosis of colon injury is obvious if fecal material is noted on the tip of the trocar or in the abdomen during the procedure. However, if the injury to the bowel is not a full-thickness perforation or if the colon is empty, the only sign may be a rent and bleeding from the site of injury. Therefore, it is important to conduct a systematic and thorough inspection of the abdominal organs during the initial viewing through the laparoscope to rule out any injury that might have been sustained during the trocar insertion. A distended stomach and anterior omental adhesions should draw special attention to the possibility of colon injury.

To prevent trocar injury to the large intestine during laparoscopic hysterectomy, careful review of the patient's history usually can identify those patients at risk. The risk of bowel injury is increased in patients with previous abdominal surgery, including bowel resection, colostomy, appendectomy for ruptured appendix, or a history of intestinal obstruction or inflammatory bowel disease. Trocar insertions in high-risk patients should follow the guidelines described in Chapter 7. A nasogastric tube should always be used in patients known to have difficulty with endotracheal intubation at the initial stage of anesthesia; better yet, it should be used in all cases to prevent the gastric distention and subsequent inferior displacement of the transverse colon. The importance of having an adequate umbilical incision and sharp trocar to prevent injury to the bowel has already been emphasized in this chapter in the section on avoiding small bowel injury.

Colon Injury Secondary to Electrosurgery and Laser: Laparoscopic hysterectomy requires extensive use of electrosurgical devices for hemostasis and tissue division, which can produce thermal injury to the bowel. The rectosigmoid colon is especially vulnerable because of its close proximity to the uterus and ovaries. The inherent risk of burn injury to the bowel, ureter, and skin necessitates the use of bipolar rather than unipolar electrosurgical devices. Burn injury to the rectosigmoid colon from bipolar forceps is almost always caused by poor exposure; that is, the surgeon did not see the prong tips of the forceps touching the rectosigmoid colon when he or she stepped on the pedal. Therefore, the surgeon must first make sure that both prongs are in clear view and away from the bowel before stepping on the pedal. Viewing the magnified operative field on the video monitor is not only less fatiguing for the surgeon, but also is valuable in reducing the incidence of bowel injury. Colon injury caused by bipolar electrocoagulation can be readily identified by viewing the blanched area on the surface of the bowel.

Colon injury caused by unipolar electrosurgery can be difficult to detect and evaluate. This injury usually is due to direct burn or discharge of static electricity built up in the trocar sleeve. The mechanisms of the capacitating coupling and the faulty electrosurgical equipment are detailed in Chapter 4. According to Thompson and Wheeless, signs and symptoms of electric bowel burns appear between 3 and 7 days postoperatively. Wheeless also reported that only two of 33 known bowel burn patients developed perforation. With the exception of cecum, the wall of the colon is much thicker than the wall of the small bowels. This accounts for the fact that the large intestines are more resistant to thermal injury than the small bowel.

Although there is theoretical risk of colon injury by laser energy, in reality the risk is extremely low, especially in the hand of a surgeon well trained in the use of a laser. The only laser that may potentially inflict significant trauma to the colon is the Nd-YAG laser delivered through the bare fiber tip. Fortunately, as far as we know, all gynecologists using the Nd-YAG laser to perform laparoscopic hysterectomies are using it with sapphire tips, which practically eliminate the risk of colon injury by laser if used judiciously.

Colon Injury Related to the Obliterated Cul-de-sac: Cul-de-sac obliteration, caused either by endometriosis or by previous pelvic inflammatory disease, presents a difficult challenge for the gynecologic surgeon. The sigmoid colon and rectum are at risk with obliterated cul-de-sac. Accidental entry into the rectum or sigmoid colon during their separation from the posterior wall of the uterus and cervix, or during excision of infiltrating endometriosis on the rectal wall, can cause a serious major complication if the bowel is unrepaired or improperly repaired. Intentional bowel entry for adequate excision of full-thickness infiltrating endometriosis of the bowel wall seldom results in any complication, which probably reflects the expertise of a surgeon who has experience and skill in performing this difficult procedure.

After extensive dissection of the cul-de-sac, a careful inspection for complete hemostasis and evidence of possible bowel injury should be done. It also is prudent to perform a thorough rectovaginal examination to ensure that all the infiltrating endometriosis has been excised and to be certain that no rectal injury has occurred during the dissection.

Management of Colon Injury

Early recognition of large bowel injury, preferably before the patient leaves the operating room, is crucial to avoid catastrophic consequences. Patients at risk for large bowel injury are those who have had previous bowel surgery, such as bowel resections and colostomies. Also at risk are patients who have the following conditions: a history of bowel obstruction and extensive intra-abdominal adhesions, a history of bowel inflammatory disease, or a history of or presence of obliterated cul-de-sac with rectal nodules. These at-risk patients should be identified preoperatively, and standard bowel preparation should be implemented prior to surgery. Our standard bowel preparations include 1) neomycin 1 gm every 4 hours and erythromycin 500 mg every 6 hours by mouth starting 48 hours before surgery, 2) a clear liquid diet starting 36 hours before surgery, and 3) Golytely (Braintree Laboratories, Braintree, MA) 4 liters by mouth beginning the afternoon before surgery. This bowel preparation regimen has worked well for us both in open laparotomy and in laparoscopic surgery.

SUGGESTED READINGS

Ball TL, Platt MA. Urological complications of endometriosis. Am J Obstet Gynecol 1962;84:1516–1518.

Bradford JA, Ireland EW, Warwick BG. Ureteric endometriosis: 3 case reports and a review of the literature. Aust N Z J Gynecol 1989;29:421–424.

Case AS. Diagnostic studies in bladder rupture. Urol Clin North Am 1989;16:267–273.

Corriere JN Jr, Sandler CM. Management of the extraperitoneal bladder rupture. Urol Clin North Am 1989;16:275–277.

Corson SL. Major vessel injury during laparoscopy. Am J Obstet Gynecol 1980;138:589.

Fry DE, Milholen L, Harbrecht PJ. Iatrogenic ureteral injury. Options in management. Arch Surg 1983;118:454–457.

Gomel V, James C. Intraoperative management of ureteral injury during operative laparoscopy. Fertil Steril 1991;55:416–419.

Grainger DA, Soderstrom RM, Schiff SF, et al. ureteral injury at laparoscopy: insights into diagnosis, management, and prevention. Obstet Gynecol 1990;75:839–843.

Harrow BR. A neglected maneuver for ureterovesical implantation following injury at gynecological operations. J Urol 1968;100:280–287.

Hoch WH, Kursh ED, Persky L. Early aggressive management of intraoperative ureteral injuries. J Urol 1975;114:530–532.

Hulka JF. Major vessel injury during laparoscopy. Am J Obstet Gynecol 1980;138:590.

Hurd WW, Pear ML, DeLancey JOL. Laparoscopic injury of abdominal wall blood vessels: a report of three cases. Obstet Gynecol 1993;82:673–676.

Mann WJ, Arato M, Pastiner B, et al. Ureteral injuries in an obstetric and gynecology training program: etiology and management. Obstet Gynecol 1988;72:82–85.

Neto WA, Lopes RN, Cury M, et al. Vesical endometriosis. Urology 1984;24:271–274.

Penfield AJ. Trocar and needle injury. In: Phillips JM, ed. Laparoscopy. Baltimore: Williams & Wilkins, 1977:236–241.

Peters PC. Intraperitoneal rupture of the bladder. Urol Clin North Am 1989;16:279–282.

Phillips JM, Julka JF, Peterson HB. American Association of Gynecologic Laparoscopist's 1982 membership survey. J Reprod Med 1984;29:592–594.

Reich H, McGlynn F. Laparoscopic repair of bladder injury. Obstet Gynecol 1990;76:909–910.

Shah PM, Kim K, Ramirez-Schon G, et al. Elevated blood urea nitrogen: an aid to the diagnosis of intraperitoneal rupture of the bladder. J Urol 1979;122:741–743.

Shin CS. Vascular injury secondary to laparoscopy. NY State J Med 1982;82:935–936.

Symmonds RE. Ureteral injuries associated with gynecologic surgery: prevention and management. Clin Obstet Gynecol 1976;19:623–644.

Tarkington MA, Dejter SW Jr, Bresette JF. Early surgical management of extensive gynecologic ureteral injuries. Surgery 1991;173:17–21.

Thompson BH, Wheeless CR Jr. Gastrointestinal complications of laparoscopic sterilization. Obstet Gynecol 1973;41:669–676.

Wheeless CR Jr. Gastrointestinal injuries associated with laparoscopy. In: Phillips JM, ed. Endoscopy in gynecology. Downey, CA: American Association of Gynecological Laparoscopists, 1978:317–324.

Yuzpe AA. Pneumoperitoneum needle and trocar injuries in laparoscopy. A survey on possible contributing factors and prevention. J Reprod Med 1990;35:485–490.

Zinman LM, Libertino JA, Roth RA. Management of operative ureteral injury. Urology 1978;12:290–303.

PART THREE

Pelvic Floor Reconstruction

16

Anatomy and Clinical Evaluation of Pelvic Floor Defects

C.Y. Liu

T he goal of laparoscopic repair of pelvic floor defects is to restore normal functioning by correcting or even sometimes intentionally overcorrecting the defects. The supporting system in the pelvic floor is dynamic rather than static, with the pelvic striated muscles, primarily the levator ani muscles, playing the most important role in this dynamic support. The endopelvic fascia and ligaments that attach the pelvic viscera to the pelvic side walls become important in supporting the pelvic organs only when the levator ani muscles have been damaged and can no longer function normally.

For example, the majority of cases of stress urinary incontinence are caused by loss of posterior support of the proximal urethra and bladder neck. Anatomically, the proximal parts of the urethra and bladder neck are not normally fixed in a static position; rather, they are dynamically supported by the resting tone of the levator ani muscle (Fig 16.1). Contraction of the levator ani muscles during, or in anticipation of, increase in intra-abdominal pressure can elevate the bladder neck, while relaxation of the same muscles during urination can drop the bladder neck and obliterate the posterior urethrovesical angle. When the levator

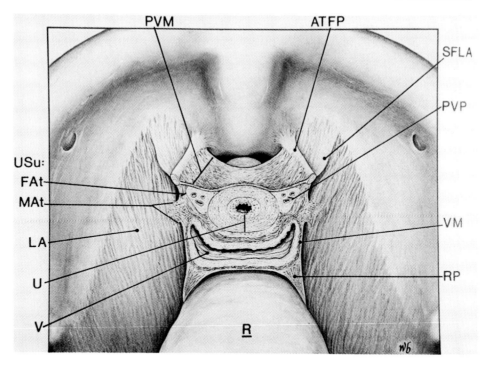

FIGURE 16.1

Cross-section of the urethra (U), vagina (V), arcus tendineus fascia pelvis (ATFP), and superior fascia of levator ani (SFLA) just below the vesical neck (drawn from cadaver dissection). The pubovesical muscles lie anterior to the urethra and anterior and superior to the paraurethral vascular plexus (PVP). The urethral supports (USu) attach the vagina and vaginal surface of the urethra to the levator ani muscles (MAt, muscular attachment) and to the superior fascia of the levator ani (FAt, fascial attachment). R, rectum; RP, rectal pillar; VM, vaginal wall muscularis. (From DeLancey JOL. Pubovesical ligament: A separate structure from the urethral supports. Neurourol Urodynam 1989;8:57. Copyright © 1989. Reprinted by permission of Wiley-Liss, Inc, a subsidiary of John Wiley & Sons, Inc.)

ani muscles are damaged due to childbirth or to a constant increase in intra-abdominal pressure, as in chronic pulmonary diseases, constipation, or constant heavy lifting and straining activities, the levator muscles are no longer able to close the pelvic floor and support the pelvic organs. In such cases, the endopelvic fascia and ligaments must assume primary support of the pelvic organs. Unfortunately, the endopelvic fascia, being a fibromuscular tissue consisting of collagen, elastin, and smooth muscle fiber, is poorly suited to support the pelvic organs, which are under constant gravitational pull and increased intra-abdominal pressures. Exposed to prolonged pressure and tension, the endopelvic fascia will stretch and eventually break, resulting in loss of support to the pelvic organs and eventual clinical manifestations of vaginal prolapse and urinary and/or fecal incontinence. Because the defect in the pelvic floor usually is multiple and not limited just to the obvious component, the entire pelvic floor supporting system must be thoroughly evaluated before and during surgery, and all defects must be reconstructed concurrently.

Unfortunately, the current surgical practice for the repair of pelvic floor defects, primarily relies on the strength of the endopelvic fascia, which clearly is not ideal for providing the kind of dynamic support necessary for the pelvic floor. Due to recent advances in the knowledge and understanding of neuroanatomy and neurophysiology, it is hoped that the prevention and management of pelvic floor defects will be better understood and effective in the near future.

When evaluating patients with pelvic floor defects for surgery, the surgeon must have a clear knowledge of the anatomic alterations that will result from each individual repair. Restorative surgery for stress urinary incontinence, for example, will change the direction of force vectors to the posterior cul-de-sac of the pelvis, so that any existing deficiency in that area, however slight, may well become a marked deficiency postoperatively, necessitating further surgery. Up to 28% of patients undergoing a Burch-type colposuspension develop middle and/ or posterior compartment deficiency and subsequently manifest enterocele, rectocele, and vaginal vault prolapse, requiring additional surgery. Obliteration of the cul-de-sac and repair of coexisting mid and posterior compartment defects concurrently with retropubic colposuspension may eliminate the need for further reparative surgery.

Laparoscopic surgery provides unique advantages in identifying and confirming the existing pelvic floor defects. With general anesthesia and more than 15 mm Hg of intra-abdominal pressure provided by positive pneumoperitoneum, the pelvic floor defects can be easily identified and confirmed both before and after surgery. Positive intra–abdominal pressure helps the surgeon ensure that all defects have been repaired. This can be confirmed visually (by viewing the pelvic floor through the laparoscope) and digitally (by palpating the pelvic floor through the vagina).

ANATOMY OF THE PELVIC FLOOR SUPPORT

Every surgeon interested in performing pelvic floor reconstruction needs to be familiar with the structures discussed below.

Pelvic Sidewall

The pelvic sidewall comprises the vertical walls of the pelvis to which the pelvic floor attaches. The ultimate support of all the pelvic organs and soft tissues, the anterior pelvic sidewall consists of the symphysis pubis and the pubic bone; the obturator interna muscle and the arcus tendineus fascia, which stretches between the pubic bone and ischial spine, form the anterolateral part of the pelvic side wall; the pyriformis muscle, which occupies the greater sciatic foramen with the coccygeus muscle connecting to its lower border, becomes the posterolateral wall; and the sacrum occupies the posterior wall. All the pelvic viscera are connected to the pelvic side walls by the endopelvic fascia. The direction of the force vector of the increased intra–abdominal pressure is dispersed by the curvature of the lumbosacral spine and the angle of inclination of the pelvis onto the lower abdominal wall and pubic bone. The remaining forces are directed posteriorly against the levator plate and sacrum.

Endopelvic Fascia

The endopelvic fascia is one continuous body of connective tissue that contains a considerable quantity of smooth muscle. The uppermost portion of the endopelvic fascia is composed of cardinouterosacral ligaments that are incorporated into pubocervical fascia and bladder pillars caudally. These portions of endopelvic fascia suspend the upper part of the vagina and cervix to the pelvic sidewalls through their attachment to

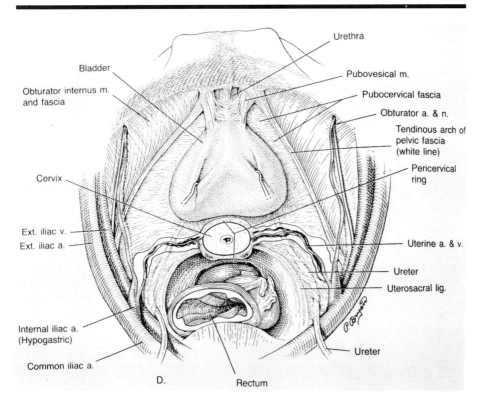

Bladder

Urethra

Obturator internus m. and fascia

Pubovesical m.

Pubocervical fascia

Obturator a. & n.

Tendinous arch of pelvic fascia (white line)

Pericervical ring

Cervix

Ext. iliac v.

Ext. iliac a.

Uterine a. & v.

Ureter

Uterosacral lig.

Internal iliac a. (Hypogastric)

Common iliac a.

Ureter

D.

Rectum

FIGURE 16.2

Attachment of the cardinal and uterosacral ligaments to the pericervical ring of connective tissue that supports the cervix. Also note the attachment of the pubocervical fascia at the tendinous arch of the pelvic fascia. (Reproduced by permission from Skandalakis JE, et al, eds. Hernia: surgical anatomy and technique. New York: McGraw-Hill, 1989:244.)

the pericervical ring. The midportion of the vagina attaches to the arcus tendineus fascia of the pelvis (white line) on both sides through the pubocervical fascia in the front and through the rectovaginal septum in the back. This comes in closer contact with the pelvic walls than does the upper portion of the vagina, which is suspended by the cardinouterosacral ligaments. The rectovaginal septum contains an abundance of fibromuscular tissue, which lies ventral to the rectovaginal space. Superiorly it blends with the cardinouterosacral ligaments, inferiorly it fuses with the perineal body, and laterally it attaches to the superior fascia of the pelvic diaphragm (Fig 16.2).

Anatomy and Clinical Evaluation of Pelvic Floor Defects   303

Levator Ani Muscle

Often referred to as the levator plate or pelvic diaphragm, the levator ani muscle consists of both pubococcygeus and iliococcygeus muscles. The pubococcygeus muscle is a thick, U-shaped muscular band that begins at the inner portion of the pubic bone and passes downward into the anus between the internal and external sphincters. Although some of the muscle fibers in this region go back to attach to the coccyx, the bulk of the muscle circles around the dorsal parts of the anorectal junction and then returns to the other side of the pubic bone. This muscle functions as a sling to compress and close the lumen of the vagina, rectum, and urethra by pulling them anteriorly toward the pubic bones. The iliococcygeus muscle is a thin sheet of muscle that comes out from the arcus tendineus fascia of the levator ani of the fascia of the obturator internus muscle. The two sheets of the iliococcygeus muscles from either side are joined in a midline raphe just above the anococcygeal raphe. The levator ani muscle forms the shelf on which the pelvic viscera rests. It also pulls these organs anteriorly toward the pubic bones.

Urogenital Diaphragm

Frequently referred to as the perineal membrane, the urogenital diaphragm spans the anterior portion of the pelvic outlet and connects the perineal body to the ischiopubic rami. The bulbocavernous, ischiocavernous, superficial transverse perineal, and anal sphincter muscles form the floor that seals off the lower aspect of the pelvic cavity. The urogenital diaphragm does not provide much support for the pelvic organs; its main role is to attach the lateral wall of the vagina and the perineal body to the ischial pubic rami.

Vagina

The vaginal wall consists of the pubocervical fascia anteriorly and rectovaginal septum posteriorly. The vaginal lumen is lined by mucosal epithelium that attaches to the vaginal wall. The upper anterior wall of the vagina and its attachment to the pelvic side walls and levator ani muscles support the urethra, the base of the bladder, including the trigone, and the uterus. Since the anterior wall of the vagina rests on the posterior wall of the vagina, these organs also are supported to some degree by the posterior vaginal wall. The rectovaginal septum is a dense layer of fibromuscular tissue between the vagina and rectum. Superiorly it merges with the base of the cardinouterosacral ligament and cul-de-sac peritoneum (Fig 16.2), on each side laterally it attaches to the pelvic side walls at the fascia of the levator ani muscle, and distally it fuses with the perineal body. The rectovaginal septum, when intact with all its attachments, supports the cul-de-sac and posterior wall of the vagina and prevents the formation of enterocele, rectocele, and vaginal prolapse. The support of the vagina will be discussed further in Chapter 20.

PREOPERATIVE EVALUATION OF THE PELVIC FLOOR SUPPORT

There are many and varied clinical classification systems used by surgeons to describe the severity of pelvic floor defects, with each system delineating the criteria for grading the degree of defects and for comparing preoperative findings with postoperative results. The same grading criteria are used to compare therapeutic results in different series of patients. However, there is still no consensus among gynecologists as to which system best serves the purpose. While it is important to standardize a grading system for comparing therapeutic results, the grading system per se does not necessarily indicate the underlying anatomic defects, it only denotes the degree of prolapse.

There are several different anatomic defects that can result in clinically manifested prolapse. For example, a clinically manifested cystocele can be the result of a break in the paravaginal area between the pubocervical fascia and the arcus tendineus fascia of the pelvis or it can be caused by a vertical or transverse break in the middle or upper part of the pubocervical fascia. Therefore, it is crucial to accurately identify the defect(s) that cause the prolapse, and only then can an appropriate operative procedure be planned that will either repair the defect with restoration of normal anatomy or create a compensatory overcorrection of the defect. A cystourethrocele caused by paravaginal defect can be repaired with either a paravaginal suspension to restore the normal anatomy or with a paravaginal repair combined with a Burch type of colposuspension to create a compenstory overcorrection of the defect.

For convenience, in clinical practice we divide the pelvic floor defects into three compartment categories; each compartment connects with and supports the others. The urethrocele and cystocele belong to the anterior compartment defect; the uterovaginal prolapse belongs to the middle compartment defect; and the enterocele and rectocele belong to the posterior compartment defect.

Detailed digital palpation of the pelvic floor is combined with careful visual inspection of the defect(s) while the patient is at rest and during strain. A posterior half of a bivalve vaginal speculum (Fig 16.3) is most useful to retract the anterior and posterior vaginal wall during examination. Evaluation of pelvic floor defect(s) is best accomplished with the patient in the semireclining position since the true extent of relaxation usually cannot be achieved in the supine position. In our practice, we have our patients recline 45 to 60 degrees on the examining table with both legs bent and resting on the footings of the examination table in a semisquatting position (Fig 16.4). The examination table (preferably electrically powered) is raised to avoid straining the examin-

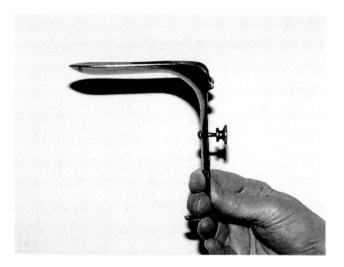

FIGURE 16.3

The posterior half of a Grave's bivalve vaginal speculum is most helpful in assaying the various degrees of pelvic floor defects.

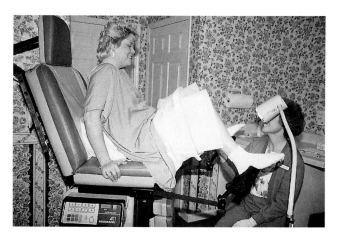

FIGURE 16.4

The patient's position on the examination table for assaying pelvic floor defects.

er's neck and back. Using the hymenal ring as the O point, the degree of prolapse with the patient at rest and at maximum strain is observed and described; for instance, the cervix is 1 cm above the hymenal ring at rest and 2 cm below the hymenal ring with maximum strain. Next, the posterior half of a vaginal speculum is inserted deep into the vagina, retracting the posterior wall of the vagina to evaluate the anterior compartment defect (Fig 16.5). The location of the urethrovaginal crease and the pattern of the vaginal rugale are especially important. The anterior compartment defect(s) is then carefully noted. There are three different defects in the anterior vaginal wall that can result in cystocele formation: the central defect, lateral defect, and transverse defect.

Central Defect

The central defect is caused by a tear or break in the midportion of the pubocervical fascial hammock, resulting in herniation of the bladder through this layer of tissue. The cystocele caused by the central defect also is called distention cystocele; the vaginal mucosal rugae usually are lost in this type of cystocele. When a distention cystourethrocele is suspected, insert a disposable straight plastic catheter into the bladder and palpate the base of the bladder and urethra. One can note on palpation

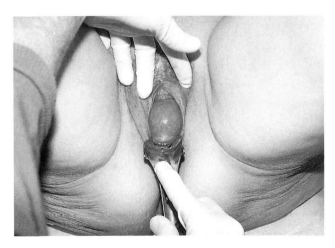

FIGURE 16.5

Visual evaluation of an anterior compartment defect. A urethrocystocele is examined by placing the posterior half of a bivalve speculum into the vagina and pressing the posterior vaginal wall downward while patient is at rest and at maximum strain.

that there is only vaginal mucosa and bladder wall or urethral mucosa between the examining finger and the catheter.

Lateral Defect

The lateral defect is a result of separation of the paravaginal attachment of the pubocervical fascia from the pelvic side walls. The cystocele caused by paravaginal defect(s) also is called displacement cystocele and is by far the most common type of cystocele. The paravaginal defect can be unilateral or bilateral. Careful palpation of the anterior vaginal wall to establish the degree of lateral mobility of the urethra usually can determine the existence of paravaginal defects. Paravaginal defects also can be detected by placing the index finger along the lateral sulci of the vagina, at which time the patient is then asked to squeeze her vagina and rectum. In the absence of a paravaginal defect, the anterior vaginal wall is pulled upward and laterally. A defect in the paravaginal area is evidenced by little or no upward movement of the anterior vaginal wall.

A sponge ring forceps also can be used for the clinical evaluation of paravaginal defects. The forceps are opened with the ring tips placed at each lateral side of the anterior vaginal wall, elevating and supporting the vagina to its lateral sidewalls. In patients with a paravaginal defect(s), this maneuver will elevate and support the vagina to its normal position.

Transverse Defect

The transverse defect is due to the separation of the pubocervical fascia from the pericervical ring. The vesical neck usually remains well supported. When the fascia separates from the cervix, the base of the bladder herniates down in between the bladder and the cervix, obliterating the anterior vaginal fornix. The transverse defect, when it occurs alone, does not alter the mobility of the vesical neck. The clinical symptoms of the transverse defect is not stress urinary incontinence, but incomplete voiding.

Differentiation among these three defects is important when planning reparative surgery. For example, traditional anterior colporrhaphy works well for correcting distention cystoceles (central defects), but it is ineffective for repairing displacement cystoceles (paravaginal defects).

For examination of posterior compartment defects, the physician must turn the half speculum 180 degrees to retract the anterior vaginal wall upward so that the posterior vaginal wall defect can be evaluated (Fig 16.6). The posterior vaginal wall is maintained and supported by the rectovaginal septum (Denonvilliers' fascia) and its peripheral attachments. Defects in this area generally occur at its peripheral margins. When defects are in the central end under the cul-de-sac, an enterocele results, and when defects occur further down, where the vagina and rectum are in apposition, a rectocele occurs. The defects in this compartment are sometimes difficult to assess, especially between the enterocele and high rectocele, which coexist in most cases. When the posterior vaginal wall is observed to be descending below the hymenal ring, significant posterior compartment defects exist. This may be caused by a rectocele, an enterocele, or both. Enteroceles usually can be diagnosed by rectovaginal examination. They usually appear as a distinct bulging sac above the rectocele. This is especially clear when the patient is performing Valsalva's maneuver during the rectovaginal examination. However, its diagnosis can be difficult. Using a tenaculum to elevate the cervix and

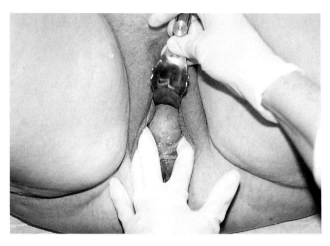

FIGURE 16.6

Visual evaluation of a posterior compartment defect. A rectocele is evaluated by placing the posterior half of a bivalve speculum into the vagina and retracting the anterior wall of the vagina upward while patient is at rest and at maximum strain.

depress part of the posterior vaginal wall and perineum, the examiner can observe the cul-de-sac while the patient strains; an enterocele will bulge in this area and often, but not always, will obliterate the posterior fornix. To evaluate the posterior vaginal wall in patients with vaginal prolapse, it is important to push the cervix or vaginal cuff up to its normal position while performing the rectal examination. A small rectocele may not be apparent unless a rectal examination with careful palpation is done while the posterior vaginal wall is being held upward under slight tension. Examination of the perineal body is important to rule out pseudorectocele, which is caused by a deficiency in the perineal body and allows the normal rectum to bulge into the vagina.

The degree of the middle compartment defect is determined by the location of the cervix or of the apex of the vagina in patients who have had a previous hysterectomy. When the uterus is in place, the position of the cervix serves as a marker for poor support of the upper vagina (Fig 16.7). However, descent of the vaginal apex often is missed in cases of posthysterectomy vaginal prolapse when a large cystocele and/or rectocele is present. In these cases, if the vaginal vault is not suspended,

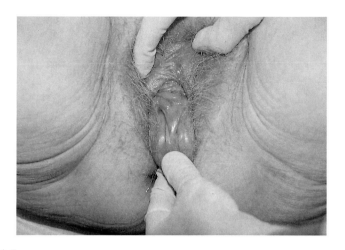

FIGURE 16.7

Complete genital procidentia.

or if only the anterior and posterior compartment defects are repaired, the operation will be unsuccessful and the prolapse will recur.

Because multiple defects in the pelvic support frequently occur in more than one compartment, careful assessment of the defects preoperatively followed by intraoperative confirmation is critical. Performing several individualized restorative operative techniques concurrently is often needed to achieve the best results. Although the following few chapters will describe the technique of repairing individual defects, the reader is reminded that in the majority of cases, repair of multiple pelvic supporting defects is the rule, not the exception.

SUGGESTED READINGS

Baden WF, Walker TA. Physical diagnosis in the evaluation of vaginal relaxation. Clin Obstet Gynecol 1972;15:1055.

DeLancey JOL. Anatomy and physiology of urinary continence. Clin Obstet Gynecol 1990;33:298.

DeLancey JOL, Richardson AC. Anatomy of genital support. In: Benson TJ, ed. Female pelvic floor disorders: investigation and management. New York: WW Norton, 1992:19–26.

Anatomy and Clinical Evaluation of Pelvic Floor Defects   311

Koelbl H, Strassegger H, Riss PA, Gruber H. Morphologic and functional aspect of pelvic floor muscles in patients with pelvic relaxation and genuine stress incontinence. Obstet Gynecol 1989;74:789–793.

Nichols DH, Milley PS. Surgical significance of the rectovaginal septum. Am J Obstet Gynecol 1970;108:215–220.

Oelrich TM. The striated urogenital sphincter muscle in the female. Anat Rec 1983:205:233–232.

Richardson AC. Anatomic evaluation of pelvic floor defects by physical examination. Presented at the Fifth International Vaginal Surgery Conference. St Louis, March 17, 1994.

TeLinde RW. Prolapse of the uterus and allied conditions. Am J Obstet Gynecol 1966;94:444–463.

Wiskind AK, Creighton SM, Stanton SL. The incidence of prolapse after the Burch colposuspension. Am J Obstet Gynecol 1992;167:399–405.

17

Laparoscopic Retropubic Colposuspension

C.Y. Liu

T The birth of modern gynecology witnessed a beginning of the recognition of and efforts to repair urinary fistulae. In 1852, Marion Sims, credited as being the father of modern gynecology, reported the cure of 252 fistulae out of 320 attempts. Like Sims, Howard Kelly, the first professor of gynecology at Johns Hopkins Medical School, believed that the fields of urology and gynecology were closely related and should not be separated. In 1914, Kelly and Dumm described the condition of urinary incontinence not related to fistulae and pioneered surgical treatment for this problem (1). For the rest of his life, Dr Kelly was a champion for women's rights in seeking alleviation for miseries caused by urinary incontinence as he continued to pursue the cure for this condition. More than 200 different types of operations have been described for the treatment of stress urinary incontinence in women since Kelly first suggested plication as a component of anterior colporrhaphy. Furthermore, these procedures have many modifications, indicating the complexity of problems involved in stress urinary incontinence. Recent remarkable advances in our knowledge of the histology, biochemistry, and neurophysiology of the female urinary system give us a somewhat better understanding of the pathophysiology of female urinary incontinence.

It is now recognized that there are two basic types of stress urinary incontinence: hypermobility stress urinary incontinence, which is due to poor fibromuscular support of the proximal urethra and vesical neck, and intrinsic sphincteric insufficiency, which is caused by poor closure of the internal sphincteric mechanism of the urethra. It is important to point out that most patients with genuine stress urinary incontinence have the intrinsic sphincteric mechanism intact, but it is functioning poorly due to the displacement of the urethrovesical junction and the proximal part of the urethra due to loss of fibromuscular support.

Mild to moderate stress urinary incontinence usually can be managed nonsurgically with medications, therapeutic devices, or pelvic floor training. However, more severe stress urinary incontinence that requires the constant use of perineal pads or diapers may benefit from surgery. Because the severity of stress urinary incontinence is purely subjective, the decision to have surgery should come from the patient, *not* from the physician. Surgery should not be undertaken until the stress incontinence is to the degree that causes the patient to request it. The objectives of surgery should be outlined and clearly articulated to the patient prior to surgery, and any unrealistic expectations of surgical outcomes should be corrected. The patient must understand that surgery will only relieve stress incontinence; it will not cure detrusor instability, nocturia, urinary urgency, or other problems unrelated to stress incontinence. Never promise that the patient will become completely dry after surgery. The purpose of surgery is defeated in a dry patient who requires constant self-catheterization, which creates a new problem. The objective of surgery is satisfaction with a restored normal functioning bladder by a patient who once again can enjoy normal activities free of incontinence.

When the decision for surgery has been made, choosing the procedure most appropriate for the given patient's condition is crucial. The operation should be tailored to the type of incontinence. For those patients who have hypermobility stress urinary incontinence, the ultimate goal of surgery, is to restore the normal anatomic position of the urethrovesical junction and the proximal part of the urethra for the proper functioning of the urethral sphincter. Thus, the objectives of anti-incontinent surgery are as follows:

1. To elevate and stabilize the suburethral fascia (pubocervical fascia) to prevent excessive displacement of the urethra during periods of increased intra–abdominal pressure.
2. To allow for the posterior rotational descent of the bladder base.
3. To preserve the pliability and compressibility of the urethra.
4. To avoid compromising the urethral sphincteric mechanism (2,3).

There currently are three procedures available for patients with hypermobility stress incontinence:

1. Retropubic urethropexy, such as the Marshall-Marchetti-Krantz procedure (4), Burch's colposuspension procedure (5,6), and paravaginal suspension (7–9).
2. The needle bladder neck suspension procedure, such as the Raz, (10), Stamey (11), modified Pereyra (12), and Gittes (13) procedures.
3. The suburethral sling procedure (14,15).

Choosing an appropriate surgical procedure involves consideration of the following: 1) the status of the operation (whether it is a primary or recurrent procedure), 2) the degree of concomitant pelvic relaxation, 3) the long-term cure rate, and 4) the incidence of complications.

The needle bladder neck suspension provides a simple and quick way to suspend the urethrovesical junction. However, recent evidence suggests that long-term results with needle suspension procedures are not as effective as with retropubic urethropexy (16,17). Furthermore, the high incidence of postoperative urinary retention secondary to the suburethral sling procedure makes it a poor choice if the patient is unwilling, or unable, to perform intermittent self-catheterization. Both operations also have an increased incidence of postoperative uterovaginal prolapse and enterocele formation. Recently there seems to be a consensus, especially among gynecologists, that retropubic colposuspension (Burch's procedure) is the surgical treatment of choice for patients with genuine stress urinary incontinence who have intact urethral sphincters but whose urethrovesical junction is displaced. For those patients with a poor urethral sphincteric mechanism, suburethral sling procedures, periurethral injections (such as GAX collagen [18] and Teflon past [19]), or an artificial urinary sphincter (20) will be more appropriate.

This chapter will address only the laparoscopic treatment of urinary stress incontinence with Burch's colposuspension procedure.

EVOLUTION OF THE PROCEDURE

In 1949, Marshall et al reported their results of vesicourethral suspension on 50 patients (five men and 45 women) with stress urinary incontinence. In these cases, the periurethral fascia was sutured to the back of the symphysis pubis. These investigators reported a success rate of 82%; in the remaining patients, 7% had improvement and 11% failed (4). This retropubic suspension of the bladder neck has been modified by many surgeons since its publication. In 1961, Burch reported his modification of the Marshall-Marchetti-Krantz procedure by using Cooper's ligament instead of the periosteum of the pubic bone to avoid the occasional complication of osteitis pubis and to obtain more secure points of urethrovaginal fixation. All 53 patients in his initial series were relieved of their incontinence (21). In 1968, his subsequent series of 143 patients had an overall success rate of 93% with rare recurrences even beyond 20 months of follow-up (5). Because his most frequent complication was the development of enterocele (7.6%), Burch emphasized the need for obliteration of the cul-de-sac.

In 1976, Tanagho reported modification of Burch's procedure by advocating no dissection within 2 cm of the urethra or vesical neck and removing the fatty tissue lateral to this area to stimulate fibrosis and fixation to the retropubis (6). In this modified procedure, the sutures must be tied without undue tension to avoid necrosis and breakdown at the suture placement site and to avoid compressing or kinking the proximal part of the urethra. It is not necessary to bring the anterior vaginal wall all the way to meet Cooper's ligaments. Instead of using no. 1 chromic catgut, as in Burch's original procedure, Tanagho used two delayed absorbable sutures (no. 1 Dexon), one placed at the midurethral level and the other at the urethrovesical junction on both sides of the urethra.

In 1979, Cardozo et al reported that 18% of patients who underwent retropubic urethropexy developed detrusor instability (22). Potential etiologic factors include sutures through the bladder, vesical neck obstruction, and extensive surgical dissection around the urethrovesical junction, further supporting the important surgical principles outlined by Tanagho. The Tanagho modification of Burch's colposuspension procedure is widely accepted and has become the standard for performing Burch's procedure today.

With advanced technologic developments in laparoscopic and video equipment and improved skill in performing operative laparoscopy, we have no difficulty in applying the important surgical principles for retropubic colposuspension in laparoscopy. In some cases we can even exceed traditional surgery in meeting the stringent surgical criteria of Burch's procedure: adequate exposure with good visibility of the operative field, accurate dissection of the retropubic space, perfect hemostasis, precise placement of the paraurethral sutures, and approximation of tissue without undue tension.

PREOPERATIVE WORK-UP

Prior to surgery, the diagnosis of genuine stress urinary incontinence must be confirmed and differentiated from other causes of incontinence, such as detrusor instability and overflow incontinence. The preoperative evaluation includes a complete history and physical examination with particular emphasis on neurologic history and current medication. Urinary incontinence questionnaires and the patient's voiding diary (urolog) can provide invaluable information. The lower neurologic examination, with emphasis on the sensory and motor dermatone pattern of S_2, S_3, and S_4, are important. Pelvic examination to assess the concomitant pelvic floor defects as previously described is crucial for avoiding additional surgeries.

Other office tests include urinalysis and urine culture, a stress test, and a Q-Tip test, as well as a simple office cystometry and measurement

TABLE 17.1

Patients requiring multichannel urodynamic studies

Age > 60

Previous unsuccessful anti-incontinent surgery

Any deviation in the office tests

Continuous or unpredictable leakage

of the residual urine. If there is any deviation in the results of these tests, if the patient is frail and old (>60 years), or if the patient has had previous unsuccessful anti-incontinent surgery, more sophisticated multichannel urodynamic studies should be performed before any treatment is rendered (Table 17.1).

OPERATIVE TECHNIQUE IN LAPAROSCOPIC RETROPUBIC COLPOSUSPENSION

Under general anethesia with endotrachael intubation, the patient is placed in a low dorsolithotomic position with both legs supported in Allen's universal stirrups (Edgewater Medical System, Cleveland, OH) (Fig 17.1). An 18 or 20 Fr Foley catheter with a 30-mL balloon tip is then inserted into the bladder. After the bladder is emptied, 50 mL of concentrated indigo carmine dye is instilled into the bladder. The Foley catheter is then clamped. Accidental penetration of the bladder during the procedure will be recognized immediately by the escape of blue dye. A 10-mm laparoscope is inserted through a vertical intraumbilical incision, and four 5-mm puncture sites are made in the lower abdomen. The lower pair of puncture sites is made lateral to the deep inferior epigastric vessels and the upper pair is placed lateral to the abdominal rectus muscle at about the umbilical level (Fig 10.2). Careful inspection is made of the internal viscus. The patient is then placed in a 20-degree Trendelenburg's position, and the pelvic organs are then meticulously examined. All visible pathologies, such as adhesions and endometriosis, are excised by using various types of laparoscopic instruments. Additional

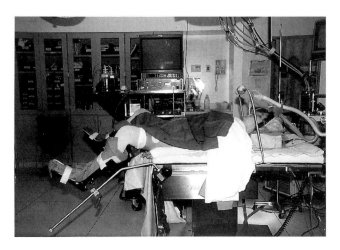

FIGURE 17.1

Patient's position for laparoscopic retropubic colposuspension.

procedures, such as adnexectomy and hysterectomy, vaginal vault suspension, and repair of the enterocele and rectocele, are performed if
indicated. The cul-de-sac is obliterated using 2-0 permanent sutures
with the modified Moschcowitz technique (23) through the laparoscope.
More than one pursestring suture may need to be used to obliterate
the cul-de-sac. It is important also to obliterate the channels on both
sides of the sigmoid colon to prevent future enterocele formation
(Plate 26A–B).

A transverse incision is made with laparoscopic scissors on the
parietal peritoneum about 1 in above the symphysis pubis in between
two umbilical ligaments. The anterior peritoneum is dissected away from
the anterior abdominal wall toward the pubic bone, and the retropubic
space is entered and dissected with scissors. However, no dissection is
carried out within 2 to 2.5 cm of the urethra.

Anatomic landmarks, such as the symphysis pubis, Cooper's ligaments, obturator canal, aberrant obturator vein, obturator neurovascular
bundle, arcus tendineus fascia of pelvis, and arcus tendineus fascia of
levator ani, are identified (Plate 27). As much paravaginal fat as possible
is removed to promote fibrosis and scar formation in the paravaginal
area. The bladder is mobilized medially and the pearly white, glistening
appearance of the pubocervical fascia should be identified on both sides

Laparoscopic Retropubic Colposuspension   319

of the urethra (Plate 28). During retropubic dissection and bladder mobilization, the paraurethral vascular plexus can sometimes be injured, causing troublesome bleeding. However, hemostasis can always be achieved by bipolar electrocoagulation and/or sutures. Four sutures of nonabsorbable material, such as no. 2 Gortex (W.L. Gore & Associates, Phoenix, AZ), are used to raise and pull the anterior vaginal wall forward and up toward the Cooper's ligaments. A pair of sutures is placed at the level of the midurethral and urethrovesical junction, inserted at least 2 cm from the urethra and the urethrovesical junction. A double bite of the whole thickness of the anterior vaginal wall, avoiding the vaginal canal, is taken and is then passed through the Cooper's ligament of the ipsilateral side at a level immediately above the location of the anterior vaginal wall suture (Plate 29 and Fig 17.2). During the placement of sutures, the assistant, or preferably the operating surgeon, places his or her middle and index fingers at the level of the urethrovesical junction with the tips of the fingers at the junction of the

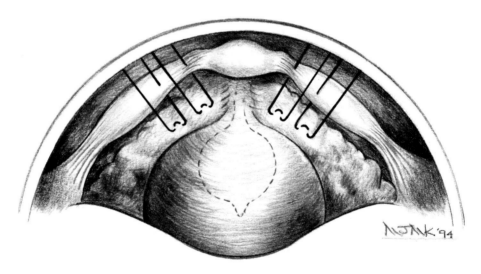

FIGURE 17.2

Two sutures are placed on each side of the urethra, one at the midurethral level and the other at the level of the urethrovesical junction. Both sutures are placed through the ipsilateral side of the Cooper's ligament. Both sutures are double looped and placed deep into the anterior vaginal wall, avoiding the vaginal mucosa.

Foley catheter balloon and the drainage tube. The assistant should wear protective devices on the finger tips to prevent accidental needle pricks. Tenting of the anterior vaginal wall in this manner facilitates the correct placement of the sutures. Once the sutures are correctly placed, they can be tied using the extracorporal knot-tying technique with the Clark-Reich knot pusher. Tying is facilitated by the assistant pushing the finger in the vagina up toward the Cooper's ligament. The procedure is then repeated on the contralateral side. Particular care must be taken to avoid tying knots too tightly. It is not necessary to have the vaginal wall in direct contact with the Cooper's ligament. Adequate support will be obtained if the sutures are tied without undue tension; excessive tension will compress or kink the urethra, and may produce necrosis at the suture sites, possibly resulting in suture release and surgical failure. The retropubic space is then irrigated with copious amounts of Ringer's lactate solution. Any bleeders are coagulated with bipolar forceps and, occasionally, sutures. A suprapubic catheter is inserted into the bladder under direct visualization (Plate 30) and the peritoneal defect is closed with 2-0 absorbable sutures. No drain is necessary in the retropubic space since adequate hemostasis can always be obtained laparoscopically. Cystoscopic examination is then performed to ensure that no suture material has penetrated through or onto the bladder wall. Five milliliters of indigo carmine dye and 10 mg of furosemide (Lasix) may then be injected intravenously to confirm the integrity of the ureters. The peristalsis and ejection of dye from ureteral orifices can be clearly observed cystoscopically (24,25) (Fig 8.9).

POSTOPERATIVE CARE

The postoperative care is similar to that of any major laparoscopic surgery. The majority of patients can be discharged from the hospital within 24 hours of the surgery with mild analgesic medication. Some patients, however, will be discharged with an indwelling suprapubic catheter that can be removed when their residual urine amounts are less than 50 mL in three consecutive voidings.

All patients are allowed to drive and return to work within 2 weeks of the surgery, providing their jobs do not require much physical exertion. Detailed instructions regarding their postoperative physical activities are given. Patients are instructed to limit activities for at least 3 months following surgery to promote strong fibrosis and scar tissue formation in the retropubic area, which will ensure a better long-term result from the surgery. Therefore, no heavy lifting, pushing, stooping, bending, or reaching should be undertaken during this time.

COMPLICATIONS

The complications of traditional abdominal retropubic colposuspension include intraoperative urethral and bladder injury, ureteral kinking and obstruction, retropubic hematoma and abscess, urinary tract infection, urinary retention, postoperative detrusor instability, enterocele, genital prolapse, and sexual dysfunction. In our series of 186 laparoscopic retropubic colposuspension (as of June 1994), the overall complication rate was 7.3% (Table 17.2). There was no conversion to laparotomy in our series. Four of our patients had intraoperative bladder injuries, all of which occurred on the dome of the bladder during the initial entry into the retropubic space; one of the patients had undergone a previous Marshall-Marchetti-Krantz procedure. The bladder injuries were recog-

TABLE 17.2

Complications in 186 laparoscopic retropubic colposuspensions

COMPLICATION	NO. OF PATIENTS	RATE[a]
Bladder injury	4	2.1
Urinary retention	4	2.1
Ureteral obstruction	1	0.5
Detrusor instability	4	2.1
Gross hematuria[b]	1	0.5
Total	14	7.3

[a] Rate per 100 women undergoing laparoscopic Burch's procedures.
[b] Gross hematuria was secondary to the insertion of the suprapubic catheter.

nized and repaired laparoscopically. Four patients developed postoperative voiding difficulty with urinary retention that required prolonged catheterization for more than 10 days. Four patients developed de novo detrusor instability; all improved with the administration of oxybutynin (Ditropan) and bladder retraining. One patient developed a right ureteral obstruction after a combined paravaginal suspension and Burch's colposuspension procedure; a second-look laparoscopy and cystoscopy performed 10 days after the initial surgery revealed a kinked right ureter, which was relieved laparoscopically by releasing the retropubic colposuspension sutures on the right side. Another patient had gross hematuria from the suprapubic catheter site, which also required a second cystoscopic examination. The suprapubic catheter was removed and the bleeder was coagulated cystoscopically. No other complications, such as retropubic hematoma, abscess, or urinary fistula, occurred in our series (26,27).

RESULTS

Between April 1991 and June 1994, 186 patients in our center underwent laparoscopic retropubic colposuspensions for the treatment of genuine stress urinary incontinence. The length of follow-up is shown on Table 17.3. Thirty-nine of the patients (30%) were from out of state and received follow-up care from their own gynecologists. A follow-up

TABLE 17.3

Length of follow-up (as of June 1994)

FOLLOW-UP	NO. OF PATIENTS
>6 mo	30
6 mo–1 yr	24
1–2yr	71
>2 yr	61
Total	186

survey was sent to 132 patients whose surgeries had been performed more than 1 year previously. They were asked to respond to one of the following questions:

1. I have definitely improved and am glad that I had surgery.
2. Occasionally I still notice leakage when I cough, sneeze, or laugh, but I am glad that I had surgery.
3. I have not noticed any improvement since surgery.

One hundred twenty-six patients responded to the survey, of whom 82 (65.1%) agreed with the first statement, 31 (24.6%) agreed with the second statement, and 13 (10.3%) agreed with the third statement.

ALTERNATIVE TECHNIQUES

Some investigators currently are using synthetic mesh, stapling one end of the mesh to the anterior vaginal wall and the other end to the Cooper's ligament, to suspend the anterior vaginal wall and elevate the urethrovesical junction (28) (Fig 17.3). Others are using a combined laparoscopic and vaginal approach (29). The retropubic space is approached extraperitoneally and under laparoscopic guidance, the Pereyra needle with the suture on it is used to puncture through the Cooper's ligament and to go through the anterior vaginal wall. The needle is then reversed through the anterior vaginal wall and Cooper's ligament again. The sutures are then tied on the Cooper's ligament laparoscopically. The shortcomings of the extraperitoneal retropubic colposuspension include inability to inspect and detect any unsuspected abdominal and pelvic pathology, and inability to repair the concomitant middle and posterior compartment defects simultaneously. The results of these alternative techniques remain unknown.

SUMMARY

There are two distinctive types of stress urinary incontinence: one has an intact intrinsic sphincteric mechanism of the urethra but with poor

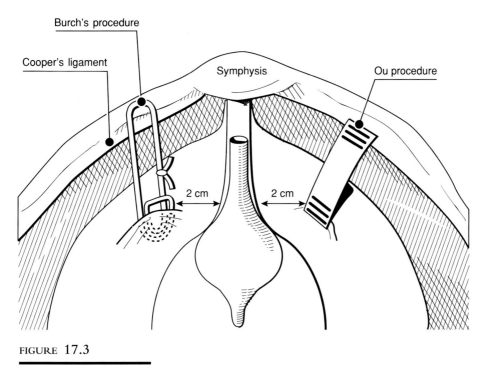

Cooper's ligament

Burch's procedure

Symphysis

Ou procedure

2 cm

2 cm

FIGURE 17.3

The anterior vaginal wall is suspended to the Cooper's ligament by prolene mesh, which is stapled to the anterior vaginal wall on one end and to the Cooper's ligament on the other.

fibromuscular support of the proximal urethra and the urethrovesical junction, and the other has urethral sphincter dysfunction. Burch's procedure can only elevate the anterior vaginal wall that supports the bladder neck and restores its normal anatomic position, but cannot correct the urethral sphincteric dysfunction. A displaced and hypermobile bladder neck and proximal urethra are results of the defect in the pelvic floor supporting system. When such a defect is of such magnitude that surgery is required, the defect in the pelvic floor is usually not limited to the presenting symptom. Therefore, reparative surgery for any pelvic floor defect, be it for the repair of cystourethrocele, enterocele, rectocele, or uterovaginal prolapse, must not be thought of as an isolated procedure; the pelvic floor must be treated as a whole instead of piecemeal. Furthermore, the surgeon who performs the pelvic floor defect surgery must have a clear picture of the anatomic alteration created by the operation. Patients who undergo Burch's colposuspension procedure, for example, will have altered vaginal axis after the operation. When the anterior wall of the vagina is being pulled up to a high retropubic position, as in Burch's procedure, the posterior wall of the vagina will also be tented up, resulting in a wide-open cul-de-sac. This will change the force vectors in the middle and posterior compartments of the pelvic floor, so that any deficiency in these compartments, however slight, is likely to increase in severity postoperatively, thereby requiring further surgery. Wiskind et al reported that up to 28% of patients who had undergone Burch's colposuspension procedure developed middle and posterior compartment deficiencies and subsequent enterocele, rectocele, or vaginal vault prolapse (29). Therefore, the entire pelvic floor support must be thoroughly investigated and considered before and during any reconstructive surgery.

Patients with urethral sphincteric dysfunction may exhibit low urethral closure pressures on their urethral pressure studies. Recent evidence suggests that the failure rate of patients with low urethral closure pressure who undergo Burch's procedure is high. McGuire noted a high incidence of unsuccessful anti-incontinence surgery among such patients (30). Sand et al found that the failure rate of retropubic colposuspension among patients with low urethral closure pressure was 54% (31). Bowen et al came to the same conclusion (32). Therefore, it is important to recognize this risk factor and to properly screen and counsel patients before surgery. A suburethral sling procedure or periurethral GAX collagen injection might be preferable for these patients.

With increased intra-abdominal pressure during laparoscopy, the pelvic floor defects are more easily identified, and repair of these defects either laparoscopically or vaginally must be carried out concomitantly with laparoscopic retropubic colposuspension.

Although the majority of failures of anti-incontinence surgery occur within the first 2 years after the procedure, the failure rate increases with time. The main cause of immediate surgical failure usually is due to not placing the paraurethral anchoring sutures deep enough and not incorporating a sufficient amount of the anterior vaginal wall. Placing the sutures in a figure-of-eight fashion is helpful. The outcome of the repair depends on anchoring this suture securely into the pubocervical fascia around the bladder neck, and the strength of this suture should be tested by pulling on it forcefully to make sure it is anchored into the tissue before attaching it to the Cooper's ligament.

The laparoscopic approach to retropubic colposuspension provides better visualization of Retzius's space than the traditional laparotomy. This facilitates dissection of the retropubic space and mobilization of the bladder. With greater magnification from the video display system, the important anatomic landmarks and the vessels are more easily visualized, thus contributing to greater accuracy in the placement of sutures, a decrease in blood loss, and an easily achieved complete hemostasis. No drain is necessary in the retropubic space.

I have been performing laparoscopic retropubic colposuspension for the past 5 years and although my series of patients is still small and the follow-up time is short (Table 17.3), I remain encouraged by the results. Patients who had a laparoscopic retropubic colposuspension had less discomfort, much shorter hospital stays, and quicker recoveries than patients who underwent a similar procedure through an abdominal incision. I believe laparoscopic retropubic colposuspension can be a satisfactory alternative to abdominal retropubic colposuspension in well-selected patients.

REFERENCES

1. Kelly HA, Dumm WM. Urinary incontinence in women without manifest injury to the bladder. Surg Gynecol Obstet 1914;18:444.
2. Hertogs K, Stanton SL. Lateral bead-chain urethrocystography after sucessful and unsuccessful colposuspension. Br J Obstet Gynecol 1985; 92:1179–1183.
3. Hertogs K, Stanton SL. Mechanism of urinary continence after colposuspension: barrier studies. Br J Obstet Gynecol 1985;92:1184–1188.
4. Marshall VF, Marchetti AA, Krantz KE. The correction of stress incontinence by simple vesicourethral suspension. Surg Gynecol Obstet 1949; 88:509–518.
5. Burch JC. Cooper's ligament urethrovesical suspension for stress incontinence. Am J Obstet Gynecol 1968;100:764–774.

6. Tanagho EA. Colpocystourethropexy: the way we do it. J Urol 1976;116: 751–753.

7. Richardson AC, Lyon JB, Williams NL. Treatment of stress urinary incontinence due to paravaginal fascial defect. Obstet Gynecol 1981;57:357–362.

8. Shull BL, Baden WF. A six-year experience with paravaginal defect repair for stress urinary incontinence. Am J Obstet Gynecol 1989;160:1432–1440.

9. White GR. An anatomic operation for the cure of cystocele. Am J Obstet Dis Wom Child 1912;56:286–290.

10. Raz S, Klutke CG, Colomb J. Four-corner bladder and urethra suspension for moderate cystocele. J Urol 1989;142:712–715.

11. Stamey TA. Endoscopic suspension of the vesical neck for urinary incontinence in females. Ann Surg 1980;192:465–471.

12. Pereyra AJ, Lebherz TB, Frowdon WA, Poers JA. Pubourethral support in perspective: modified Pereyra procedure for urinary incontinence. Obstet Gynecol 1981;59:643–648.

13. Gittes RF, Loughlin KR. No-incision pubovaginal suspension for stress incontinence. J Urol 1987;138:568–570.

14. Beck RP, McCormick S, Nordstrom L. The fascia lata sling procedure for treating recurrent genuine stress incontinence. Obstet Gynecol 1988;72: 699–703.

15. Horbach NS, Blanco JS, Ostergard DR, et al. A suburethral sling procedure with polytetrafluoroethylene for the treatment of genuine stress incontinence in patients with low urethral closure pressure. Obstet Gynecol 1988;71:648–657.

16. Bergman A, Ballard CA, Koonings PP. Comparison of three different surgical procedures for genuine stress incontinence: prospective randomized study. Am J Obstet Gynecol 1989;160:1102–1106.

17. Bergman A, Ballard CA, Koonings PP. Primary stress urinary incontinence and pelvic relaxation: prospective randomized comparison of three different operations. Am J Obstet Gynecol 1989;161:97–101.

18. Kieswetter H, Fischer M, Wober L, Flamm J. Endoscopic implantation of collagen (GAX) for the treatment of urinary incontinence. Br J Urol 1992;69:22–25.

19. Beckingham IJ, Wemyss-Holden G, Lawrence WT. Longterm follow-up of women treated with periurethral Teflon injections for stress incontinence. Br J Urol 1992;69:580–583.

20. Webster GD, Perez LM, Khoury JM, Timmons SL. Management of type III stress urinary incontinence using artificial urinary sphincter. Urology 1992;39:499–503.
21. Burch JC. Urethrovaginal fixation to Cooper's ligament for correction of stress incontinence, cystocele and prolapse. Am J Obstet Gynecol 1961;81:281–290.
22. Cardozo LD, Stanton SL, Williams JE. Detrusor instability following surgery for genuine stress incontinence. Br J Urol 1979;51:204–207.
23. Moschcowitz AV. The pathogenesis, anatomy, and cure of prolapse of the rectum. Surg Gynecol Obstet 1912;15:7–21.
24. St Lezin MA, Stoller ML. Surgical ureteral injuries. Urology 1991;38:497–506.
25. Symmonds RE. Ureteral injuries associated with gynecological surgery: prevention and management. Clin Obstet Gynecol 1976;19:623.
26. Liu CY. Laparoscopic retropubic colposuspension: a review of 58 cases. J Reprod Med 1993;38:526–530.
27. Liu CY, Paek WS. Laparoscopic retropubic colposuspension (Burch procedure). J Am Assoc Gynecol Laparoscopists 1993;1:31–35.
28. Ou CS, Presthus J, Beadle E. Laparoscopic bladder neck suspension using hernia mesh and surgical staples. J Laparoendoscopic Surg 1993;3:563–566.
29. Wiskind AK, Creighton SM, Stanton SL, The incidence of prolapse after the Burch colposuspension. Am J Obstet Gynecol 1992;167:399–405.
30. McGuire EJ. Urodynamic findings in patients after failure of stress incontinence operation. Prog Clin Biol Res 1981;78:351–360.
31. Sand PK, Bowen LW, Panganiban R, et al. The low pressure urethra as a factor in failed retropubic urethropexy. Obstet Gynecol 1987;69:399–402.
32. Bowen LW, Sand PK, Ostergard DR, et al. Unsuccessful Burch retropubic urethropexy: a case-controlled urodynamic study. Am J Obstet Gynecol 1989;160:452–458.

18

Laparoscopic Cystocele Repair: Paravaginal Suspension

C.Y. Liu

I n the early 1900s, George R. White described transvaginal reattachment of the anterior vaginal fornix to the arcus tendineus fascia of the pelvis as a form of treatment for cystocele (1,2). In 1948, K.M. Figurnov described vaginal surgery for urinary incontinence that was very similar to White's procedure (3). Then, in 1959, Durfee published a modification of the Marshall–Marchetti–Krantz procedure, putting an additional stitch from the "musculofascial dome of the vagina to the lateral pelvic sidewall in the obturator membrane" (4). In the early 1970s, Richardson et al (5,6) and Baden and Walker (7) rediscovered the sound anatomic principle of repairing the paravaginal defects for the treatment of cystocele. Richardson et al emphasized that the cystocele is not caused by the stretching or attenuation of the pubocervical fascia, but that it is a result of a "break" of the pubocervical fascia from its peripheral attachments or a "break" inside itself.

Support for the bladder and urethra is provided by the pubocervical fascia of the anterior vaginal wall. The pubocervical fascia is a layer of fibromuscular tissue that overlies the vaginal mucosa. (Fig 18.1). Superiorly it connects to the base of broad ligament and extends into the pericervical ring, laterally it attaches on each side to the arcus tendineus

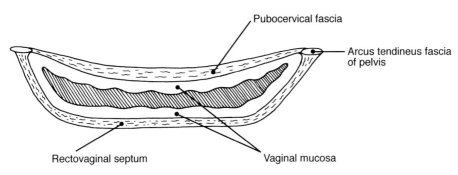

Pubocervical fascia

Arcus tendineus fascia of pelvis

Rectovaginal septum   Vaginal mucosa

FIGURE 18.1

Cross-section of the vagina. The anterior vaginal wall consists of the pubocervical fascia, which lies above the vaginal mucosa. The posterior vaginal wall consists of the rectovaginal septum, which lies below the vaginal mucosa. Support of the middle section of the vagina is provided by its lateral attachments to the pelvic sidewalls.

fascia of the pelvis on the pelvic side walls, and distally it merges with the urogenital diaphragm (Fig 18.2). The pubocervical fascia supports the bladder and urethra by forming a shelf, allowing the bladder neck and proximal urethra to be compressed in an anterioposterior fashion during periods of stress. When this supportive mechanism becomes loosened due to the trauma of childbirth, or for other reasons, the stability of this supportive layer of fascia diminishes and may ultimately fail, leading to the formation of cystocele and the development of stress urinary incontinence (SUI) if the fascial defect involves the support of the bladder neck and the proximal part of the urethra. After careful study of cadaver dissections and clinical cases, Richardson pointed out that there are four different pubocervical fascial defects that can cause cystocele (8,9): the paravaginal defect, transverse defect, midline defect, and distal defect.

Paravaginal Defect

The paravaginal defect is a result of detachment of the pubocervical fascia from its lateral attachment to the fascia of the obturator interna muscle at the level of the arcus tendineus fascia of the pelvis (white line)

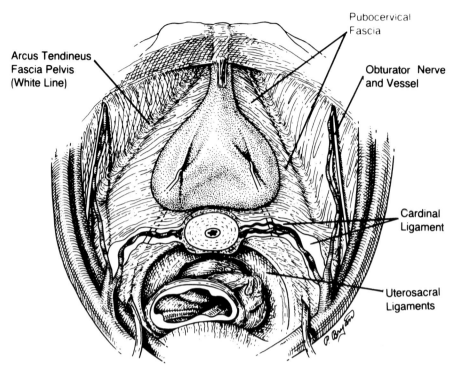

FIGURE 18.2

Pubocervical fascia viewed from above. (Reproduced by permission from Richardson AC. How to correct prolapse paravaginally. Contemp Obstet Gynecol 1990;35(9):100–109.)

(Fig 18.3). It can be unilateral or bilateral. This is by far the most common cause of urethrocystocele, accounting for approximately 80% of all urethrocystoceles. The paravaginal repair operation re-establishes the lateral pelvic side wall attachments of the pubocervical fascia and restores the stability of this hammock by correcting the fundamental anatomic defect of this type of urethrocystocele. Ninety-five percent of patients with paravaginal defects also will have SUI. However, the paravaginal repair is not an operation to repair SUI, but rather a procedure designed to correct a cystocele or urethrocystocele due to a paravaginal defect that may or may not be accompanied by the clinical symptoms of SUI. Yet, according to Richardson, 99% of patients with

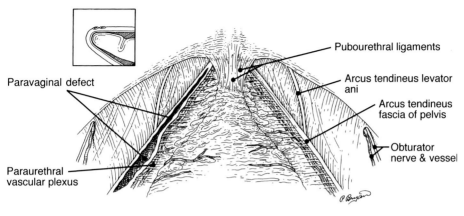

Paravaginal defect

Pubourethral ligaments

Arcus tendineus levator ani

Arcus tendineus fascia of pelvis

Obturator nerve & vessel

Paraurethral vascular plexus

FIGURE 18.3

Paravaginal defect. The pubocervical fascia has detached from the arcus tendineus fascia of the pelvic side wall on the left side.

genuine SUI involving a paravaginal defect are cured if the normal anatomy is restored (9).

Transverse Defect

The transverse defect is the next most common type of defect, resulting from transverse separation of the pubocervical fascia from the pericervical ring into which the cardinal and uterosacral ligaments insert. The base of the bladder herniates into the anterior vaginal fornix and forms a pure cystocele without displacing the urethra or urethrovesical junction. Patients with this type of cystocele do not have clinical manifestations of SUI, but may have problems of completely emptying the bladder. However, in patients with total vaginal procidentia, the transverse defect can occur in combination with paravaginal defect(s).

Midline Defect

The midline defect is caused by a break in the central portion of the hammock-like sling of the pubocervical fascia on which the bladder rests. This may or may not be manifested with SUI, depending on whether the area under the bladder neck is involved in the break. Traditional anterior colporrhaphy works well for this defect. However, one must identify the edges of the fascial defects during the repair by

Laparoscopic Cystocele Repair: Paravaginal Suspension   333

dissecting the vaginal mucosa off the underlying pubocervical fascia and reapproximating the defects.

Distal Defect

The distal defect is the result of an avulsion of the urethral attachment to the urogenital diaphragm as it passes under the symphysis pubis. Occurring rarely, this type of defect often is seen in patients who have had surgical amputation of the distal urethra as part of a radical vulvectomy. However, patients with this defect usually have SUI.

TECHNIQUE OF LAPAROSCOPIC PARAVAGINAL SUSPENSION

Under general anesthesia with endotracheal intubation, the patient is placed in a low dorsolithotomic position with both legs supported in Allen's universal stirrups (Fig 17.1). An 18 or 20 Fr Foley catheter with a 30 mL balloon tip is then inserted into the bladder. After the bladder is emptied, 30 mL of concentrated indigo carmine dye is instilled into the bladder. The Foley catheter is then clamped. Accidental penetration of the bladder during the procedure will be immediately recognized by the escape of blue dye. A 10-mm laparoscope is inserted through a vertical intraumbilical incision, and four 5-mm puncture sites are made in the abdomen. The lower pair of puncture sites is made lateral to the deep inferior epigastric vesssels, and the upper pair is placed lateral to the abdominal rectus muscle at about the umbilical level (Fig 10.2). Careful inspection is made of the internal viscus, after which the patient is then placed in a 15- to 20-degree Trendelenburg's position and the pelvic organs are meticulously examined. All visible pathologies, such as endometriosis or adhesions, are excised, and a hysterectomy and/or salpingo-oophorectomy is also performed if indicated using various types of laparoscopic instruments. Prior to the initiation of the paravaginal suspension, the entire pelvic floor is carefully surveyed both by viewing the pelvis through the laparoscope and by performing digital vaginal examinations simultaneously. All pelvic floor defects detected in the preoperative assessment are now confirmed. Posterior and middle compartmental defects, such as enterocele, and vaginal vault prolapse are first repaired laparoscopically, and a low rectocele and perineorrhaphy are performed vaginally.

A transverse incision is then made on the parietal peritoneum approximately 1 in above the symphysis pubis in between two umbilical ligaments with laparoscopic scissors. The parietal peritoneum is dissected away from the anterior abdominal wall toward the pubic bone, and the retropubic space is entered and dissected with scissors. Anatomic landmarks, such as the symphysis pubis, the obturator foramen, and the obturator neurovascular bundle are identified. The paravaginal defect, i.e., the lateral vaginal sulci, can be seen detaching from the arcus tendineus fascia of the pelvis. As much paravaginal fat as possible is removed to promote fibrosis and scar formation in the paravaginal area. The prominent paraurethral vascular plexus usually can be seen after the fat has been excised.

The bladder is then mobilized medially and the pubocervical fascia exposed. The ischial spine can be located digitally by placing the operator's fingers inside the vagina while viewing through the laparoscope. During the mobilization of the bladder, the assistant places his or her fingers in the vagina and lifts the lateral superior sulcus of the vagina to facilitate the dissection.

The separation of the lateral sulcus from the pelvic side wall can be easily appreciated laparoscopically. Permanent sutures, such as 2-0 prolene, are used to suture the superior lateral sulcus of the vagina to the arcus tendineus fascia of the pelvis (white line). The superior lateral sulcus of the vagina is elevated by the assistant's fingers in the vagina; a full-thickness stitch is placed through the lateral sulcus of the vagina, going beneath the prominent paraurethral vascular plexus if possible, and is then sutured to the white line of the pelvic side wall.

Troublesome bleeding can occur when the paraurethral vascular plexus, which runs longitudinally along the axis of the vagina, is penetrated by the needle. This bleeding invariably will stop when the suspension sutures are tied. To avoid the contamination of the operative field by the blood, the first paravaginal suspension stitch should be placed as close to the ischial spine as possible. Figure-of-eight sutures are used on all the suspension stitches to obtain a better hemostasis and suspension

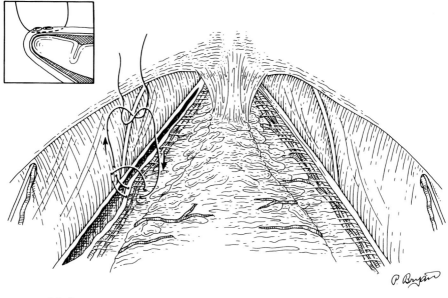

FIGURE 18.4

A figure-of-eight paravaginal suspension suture is placed to obtain a better suspension and hemostasis. Penetration of the paraurethral vascular plexus is common and can cause troublesome bleeding.

(Fig 18.4). Following the placement of this first stitch, additional sutures are placed through the vaginal sulcus with its overlying fascia and the arcus tendineus fascia ventrally toward the symphysis pubis. The last stitch should be as close as possible to the pubic ramus ventrally.

It is important not to injure the pudendal vessels and nerve while putting in the first stitch. Before placing this first stitch, the surgeon should clearly identify the ischial spine by vaginal palpation and by viewing through the laparoscope. The first stitch usually is placed through the white line approximately 1 to 1.5 cm ventral to the ischial spine. Frequent vaginal examination to evaluate the status of suspension during and at the completion of the surgery is important to ensure that good suspension has been achieved with properly placed stitches (Plate 31A–B). If the urethrovesical junction is not well supported and the patient does have SUI, additional Burch stitches should be placed to elevate the urethrovesical junction (Plate 32).

The entire retropubic space is then thoroughly irrigated with copious amounts of Ringer's lactate solution and hemostasis is controlled by either electrosurgery or sutures. No drains are necessary, for complete hemostasis can always be achieved. A suprapubic catheter is not needed unless Burch's procedure is performed concomitantly. A suprapubic catheter is inserted into the bladder under direct visualization. The peritoneal defect is closed with a 2-0 absorbable suture. Cystoscopic examination is then performed to ensure that no suture is inside the bladder or on the bladder wall, and to ascertain the integrity of both ureters by observing the effusion of indigo carmine dye through both ureteral orifices (Fig 8.9).

DISCUSSION

Richardson et al reported more than 95% patient satisfaction with paravaginal repair for their cystoceles and urethrocystoceles (5,6). The criteria they used to define satisfactory results were as follows:

1. Correction of the cystocele and urethrocele.
2. Relief of SUI.
3. Preservation of normal voiding function.
4. No persistent postoperative bladder dysfunction.

Richardson also noticed that the incidence of postoperative voiding difficulty and postoperative de novo detrusor instability is much lower when compared with other types of retropubic colposuspension procedures, such as the Marshall-Marchetti-Krantz procedure or Burch's procedure (10). Shull et al also reported an approximately 95% success rate of restoration of normal anatomy and functions with vaginal paravaginal suspension (11). Both of these investigators emphasize the importance of simultaneous repair of all the coexisting pelvic floor defects.

We have been performing laparoscopic paravaginal suspensions for the past 4 years with satisfactory results. The vast majority of our paravaginal repairs were performed concomitantly with pelvic floor reconstructions (Table 18.1). More than 90% of our patients with marked genital procidentia also underwent paravaginal repair in addition

TABLE 18.1

Concomitant surgeries in 46 laparoscopic paravaginal repairs

PROCEDURES	NO. OF PATIENTS
Vaginal vault suspensions (n = 32)	
Sacrospinous suspensions	15
High McCall vault suspensions	17
Enterocele repairs	38
Occlusion of cul-de-sacs (Moschcowitz technique)	8
Rectocele repairs and perineorrhaphy*	22
Burch's colposuspension procedures	28

* Twelve of 22 patients had low rectoceles, required vaginal rectocele repair and perineorrhaphy.

to vaginal vault suspension. Preoperatively, we routinely map out all the pelvic floor defects by performing detailed pelvic examinations, as described in Chapter 16. Intraoperatively, we confim and substantiate our preoperative findings by digital vaginal examinations under laparoscopic view before initiating the operation. Under positive intra-abdominal pressure, which is created by pneumoperitoneum, pelvic floor defects become much more apparent when viewed through the laparoscope. Digital vaginal examinations afford the surgeon tactile assessment of pelvic floor defects. Therefore, intraoperative findings of the pelvic floor defects not only confirm the preoperative findings, they dictate the ultimate procedures to be performed. At the end of the reconstructive surgery, repeat digital vaginal examination under direct laparoscopic view allows the surgeon to be confident that all the pelvic defects have been repaired.

As of August 1994, we have performed 46 laparoscopic paravaginal repairs with satisfactory results. We define our satisfactory results in terms of both anatomic and functional restorations of the cystoceles and urethroceles (Table 18.2). We have had four recurrences of cystoceles, three of which occurred during the first year of our experience with this procedure. The vaginal wall sutures to the pelvic sidewalls were not placed high enough in the early stage of our experience. However, one

TABLE 18.2

Pelvic floor defects detected during postoperative follow-ups in 46 paravaginal repairs

Defect Sites	No. of Patients (%)
Urethra	0 (0)
Bladder	4 (8.6)
Vaginal vault	0 (0)
Cul-de-sac	2 (4.3)
Rectum	2 (4.3)

cystocele recently recurred within 6 weeks of surgery, in spite of correcting this problem by placing the sutures close to the ischial spine. There have been no voiding disorders, with the exception of two patients who developed postoperative detrusor instability. Both of these patients also had concomitant Burch's colposuspension procedures. No injuries to the bowel, bladder, or ureter occurred, nor were there any retropubic hematoma or abscess formations. The average hospital stay was less than 2 days.

The laparoscopic approach to the paravaginal defect is not a solitary procedure; rather, it is part of a larger operation in which the whole pelvic floor is reconstructed. Laparoscopy provides better visualization of pelvic floor defects, as well as greater precision in placing strategically important stitches in the repair of paravaginal defects. We have followed the sound anatomic and surgical principles of paravaginal repair with the anticipation that the long-term results of this procedure will at least be comparable to the traditional open or vaginal approaches.

REFERENCES

1. White GR. An anatomic operation for the cure of cystocele. Am J Obstet Dis Women Child 1912;65:286–290.
2. White GR. Cystocele, a radical cure by suturing lateral sulci of vagina to white line of pelvic fascia. JAMA 1909;53:1707–1711.

3. Figurnov KM. Surgical treatment of urinary incontinence in women. Akush Ginekol (Mosk) 1948;5:6–11.

4. Durfee RB. The anterior vaginal suspension operation. Am J Obstet Gynecol 1965;92:615–619.

5. Richardson AC, Lyon JB, Williams NL. A new look at pelvic relaxation. Am J Obstet Gynecol 1976;126:568–573.

6. Richardson AC, Lyon JB, William NL. Treatment of stress urinary incontinence due to paravaginal fascial defect. Obstet Gynecol 1981;57:357–362.

7. Baden WF, Walker TA. Urinary stress incontinence: evolution of paravaginal repair. Female Patient 1987;12:89–94.

8. Richardson AC. How to correct prolapse paravaginally. Contemp Obstet Gynecol 1990;35:100–114.

9. Richardson AC. Repair of paravaginal defects. Presented at the 5th International Vaginal Surgery Conference. St Louis, March 1994.

10. Richardson AC. Cystocele. Paravaginal repair. In: Benson JT ed., Female pelvic floor disorders. Chapter 12. New York: WW Norton, 1992:280–287.

11. Shull BL, Capen CV, Riggs MW. Bilateral attachment of the vaginal cuff to ilcoccygeus fascia: an effective method of cuff suspension. Am J Obstet Gynecol 1993;168:1669–1677.

CHAPTER

19

Laparoscopic Enterocele Repair

Thierry G. Vancaillie

An enterocele is defined as the presence of a herniation of the vaginal wall that contains small bowel (1). Theoretically, this herniation can present anywhere along the vaginal axis; however, it is evident that the most likely site for this anatomic defect is the upper half of the posterior vaginal wall. The clinical presentation of an enterocele constitutes a diagnostic challenge. Bulging of the vaginal wall is evident, but it may be difficult to identify the contents of the hernia. A combined rectovaginal examination by an experienced physician leads to the diagnosis in most cases. More sophisticated investigations are helpful to some extent. Ultrasonography with the vaginal probe allows the clinician to study the entire pelvic anatomy, including the bladder neck and vaginal vault support. Moreover, the clinician can perform the testing in rest and stress conditions. This offers a great advantage provided that the examination is performed by the clinician. Other tests, such as magnetic resonance imaging, are of academic importance at this time. Their use in the routine study of pelvic floor relaxation is not warranted.

The etiology of enterocele formation is obscure. The clinical entity, known as enterocele, most likely is the end stage of different pathophysiologic processes (2), involving endogenous and environmental factors. The strength of the pelvic floor tissues is mainly determined by the genetic code and the amount of stress imposed on the pelvic floor resulting from environmental abuse.

The clinical presentation of an enterocele is often obscured by the presence of a more obvious rectocele. Frankly, the occurrence of an isolated enterocele is quite unusual; it is more common in patients who have undergone previous hysterectomy or pelvic floor repair surgery. It is debatable whether the distinction between enterocele and rectocele is that important, considering surgical treatment. Both entities are the result of a weakness at the level of the posterior compartment of the pelvic floor support structures. An argument can be made that during surgical repair of the rectocele, the surgeon should address the possibility of a concomitant enterocele, and vice versa.

Another difficult question is "What are the symptoms of an enterocele?" Patients' complaints are vague and variable. One of the more consistent symptoms is a "feeling of fullness" within the vaginal area. This sensation is reported by patients in the most diversified way. The symptom that is often intentionally omitted by the patient is the inability to have normal sexual intercourse.

The presence of an enterocele in itself is rarely the primary indication for surgery. More commonly, cure of an enterocele is part of a larger intervention. Another indication for the surgical technique, detailed further below, is the prevention of an enterocele in patients undergoing other procedures, such as hysterectomy and bladder neck suspension. The ability to cure an enterocele adds value to the transperitoneal approach for bladder neck suspension.

TECHNIQUE

Independent of the etiology that caused the enterocele, there are specific anatomic findings in patients with pelvic floor relaxation. These findings are attenuation or breakage of the fascial structures (Denonvilliers' fascia, endopelvic fascia) and separation of the crux levatores. The crux levatores consist of the hiatus between the levator muscles and the fascial tissues around the muscle.

In view of these anatomic findings, I propose that the surgery consist of 1) approximating the levator muscles to reduce the levator hiatus and 2) enforcing the attenuated tissues by the use of skin grafts and surgical mesh. My personal preference is Vicryl mesh, which is absorbable, remaining in the body long enough to cause scarring. In addition, complications, such as erosion of foreign material into the rectum or bladder, are less likely to occur.

The structure of the pelvis is narrow and elongated, much like an inverted cone. Technically, this peculiar shape makes unilateral access difficult. It seems logical that combined abdominal and vaginal access would provide the surgeon with the best conditions for reconstructive surgery, and this is where laparoscopy can play a role. Laparoscopy provides abdominal access without the morbidity of a large incision. There is the additional benefit that the optical system of the laparoscope provides excellent viewing of the anatomy, which cannot be obtained with the naked eye.

The vaginal part of the procedure consists mainly of a classical posterior repair, as originally described by Hegar. Several modifications have been incorporated over the last years, resulting from the influence of many physicians. Two surgeons have left a great impression: E.H. Schmidt (Bremen, Germany) and R. Zacharin (Melbourne, Australia); Schmidt for his insistence on identifying the anatomic structures carefully, extending the dissection into painstaking detail, and Zacharin for the idea of using the redundant vaginal skin as a graft to enforce the rectovaginal septum (3). The following is a detailed description of the surgical procedure as currently performed. I am hopeful that the technique will continue to evolve to become even better.

The patient is positioned in the modified lithotomy or "frog" position. The legs are in abduction and the knees bent to allow space for the surgeon and one assistant to fit between the legs so that the procedure can be performed comfortably. The legs are only slightly elevated, in anticipation of the abdominal part of the procedure. A medium-curved deaver is placed into the vagina so as to force the vault in its anatomic position. This deaver will remain in place for the entire procedure. An Ellis clamp is placed on each side of the posterior fourchette at the level of the upper edge of the perineoplasty, which will follow the posterior repair. A transverse incision is made along the vaginal mucosa. It is optional to inject a local anesthetic submucosally to reduce postoperative pain. The vaginal mucosa is grasped in the middle with one or two Ellis clamps, and the vaginal mucosa is separated from the underlying fascia and rectum. Two parallel incisions are made into the vaginal mucosa, thereby isolating a longitudinal strip of vaginal mucosa. This dissection is carried along until the apex or posterior fornix of the vagina is reached. The strip of vaginal tissue is then cut off and maintained in a bath of physiologic solution until ready to be used.

The edges of the vaginal wall are grasped with Ellis clamps and put on tension. The vaginal wall is dissected off the underlying loose connective tissue using a scalpel and Metzenbaum scissors. The attachments of the endopelvic fascia, also called "rectal pillars," are left intact if possible. These rectal pillars contain branches of the pudendal vessels and nerve. Hemorrhage during this dissection is not uncommon. The rectovaginal fossa is opened on both sides. The dissection of the fossa is continued until the levator muscle is clearly identifiable, at least in its anterior course.

Four to six sutures are used to approximate the levator muscles. The middle suture is placed first, followed by the sutures that involve the distal part of the repair and, finally, the sutures that are placed closest to the perineum. The line of sutures is placed in such a way that a curvature is formed in the sagittal direction, similar to the natural curvature of the vagina. The sutures are loosely tied, which goes against traditional doctrine. Tightly fastened sutures are more likely to erode through the tissue. The objective of these sutures is to reduce the gap between the muscles; total occlusion of the hiatus is not necessary. The length of the suture line is more likely to be the determining factor for success rather than the tightness of the individual sutures. In addition, it is important to pay attention to the course imposed on the vagina by the posterior repair.

The next phase consists of insertion of the vaginal skin graft. The graft is sutured with the mucosal aspect down, on top of the levator muscle suture line. The lower edge is fixed with sutures to the perineal body and the lateral edges are fastened to the levator muscles. The distal edge is, for now, left alone. It will later be attached to the sacrouterine ligaments, thereby completing the reinforcement of Denonvilliers' fascia.

The vaginal mucosa is closed using interrupted stitches of absorbable material. At the level of the perineum, two to three sutures are used to approximate the perineal bodies. These sutures are situated in front of the skin graft, underneath the vaginal mucosa suture line. The vaginal part of the procedure is then finished by closing the perineum.

The abdominal part of the procedure starts as any other laparoscopy. I favor the use of a Veress needle prior to inserting the trocar. In case of previous pelvic surgery (except for cesarean section), access is gained through the left subcostal area. After insufflation, a 5-mm endoscope is inserted through a small trocar to view the lower abdominal wall. Adhesiolysis is performed as deemed necessary. Once the 10-mm laparoscope is inserted through the umbilical trocar sheath, attention is turned to the pelvic cavity. The patient is placed in a steep Trendelenburg's position. If necessary, the sigmoid colon is detached from the side wall to increase visualization of the pelvis. Anatomic landmarks are noted: the rectosigmoid, ureters, sacrouterine ligaments, vagina, and bladder.

It is debatable whether the uterus should be removed at the same time. As a general rule, I suggest leaving the uterus if it is not involved in the relaxation process. Obviously, in cases of true uterine prolapse with a pulsion enterocele, a hysterectomy is desirable to restore the anatomy adequately. Leaving the uterus in place, however, facilitates recognition of the anatomic landmarks, especially the cardinal and sacrouterine ligament complex. It also may be postulated that the uterine artery participates in the vascularization of the pelvic support structures and that maintaining this vessel improves the healing and strength of these structures. This is open to further debate.

The following description will ignore the presence or absence of the uterus. Once the anatomic landmarks are identified, the actual surgical procedure starts. The procedure is slightly different, depending on whether a posterior repair has preceded the laparoscopy. In cases without clinically obvious enterocele or rectoenterocele in which laparoscopy is used for bladder neck suspension, the surgeon may opt to obliterate the cul-de-sac to prevent the occurrence or worsening of an enterocele at a later date. The two techniques are slightly different and will be described separately.

Combined Vaginal and Abdominal Approach

The initial incision is made between the sacrouterine ligaments and the rectum, on the outside of the hernia sac, in the form of an inverted horseshoe. The incision is extended down toward the pararectal gutters. The rectovaginal space is bluntly opened. This dissection is simplified because a posterior repair has been performed prior to laparoscopy. It is possible to reach the sacrospinous ligament by dissecting this space toward the side wall. Up to this point, the dissection has been performed in an effort to isolate the structures that will be involved in the surgical repair, namely, the vagina, sacrouterine, and cardinal ligaments. The sutures that were placed on the levator muscles can be seen once the rectovaginal space is opened. The excess peritoneum is cut loose from the anterior wall of the rectum and removed.

The next step consists of anchoring the vaginal skin graft to the sacrouterine ligament complex on both sides (Plate 33). An effort is made to place the sutures as low as possible to continue the curvature given to the posterior repair. These sutures complete the reinforcement of Denonvilliers' fascia. A double sheet of Vicryl mesh is then placed over the skin graft, reaching from one pararectal space to the other, at the level of the levator muscles (Plate 34). The vaginal vault is then attached to the ligament complex with several nonabsorbable sutures that do not pierce through the mucosa, but anchor into the fascial layers (Plate 35).

A pursestring suture is placed to approximate the sacrouterine ligaments in front of the rectum. The peritoneum is then closed with interrupted sutures. Some medial displacement of the ureter is unavoidable. It is important to check on this. A cystoscopy is advisable in all cases in which the surgeon is not certain that there is no damage to the ureters.

Abdominal Approach Only

In patients without clinically evident rectocele or enterocele who undergo a laparoscopy for surgical correction of genuine stress urinary incontinence, the surgeon may consider occluding the cul-de-sac, either to cure a small enterocele that is clinically not evident or to prevent an enterocele from developing as the result of the urethropexy. In these cases, the initial step is the same: the peritoneum is incised on the inside along the sacrouterine ligaments and the posterior aspect of the vagina. The rectovaginal septum is then entered and bluntly dissected. The anatomic structures are well identified, particularly the rectum, vagina, sacrouterine ligaments, ureters, and bladder. It may be necessary to dissect the bladder free from the vaginal vault to optimize identification of the anatomic landmarks. Vicryl mesh may be used to reinforce the upper rectovaginal septum. The first suture approximates the posterior aspect of the sacrouterine ligaments in front of the rectum. Next, the vaginal vault is attached to the sacrouterine ligament at a level that can be reached without tension. The vagina is attached in such a fashion that the vault points downward, again to re-establish a correct axis. Closure of the enterocele follows by additional sutures placed on the sacrouterine ligaments and peritoneum.

RESULTS

The initial attempts to cure an enterocele using laparoscopic techniques were performed in early 1992. The technique has evolved over the years and is still evolving. A study of the first 18 patients has been reported (4). Sixteen of the 18 patients have been successfully treated using the technique described above. The vaginal skin graft, a technique I introduced after a visit to Dr Zacharin during the summer of 1993, has been applied in 11 patients with good success. There were no life-threatening complications. One patient was taken back to the operating room to revise a hematoma of the posterior repair. In three cases, one suture was released and replaced, because it was estimated that one ureter was excessively displaced medially and even incorporated into the suture in one case. There were no cases of permanent ureteral or bladder injury. During the postoperative period, patients, were able to return to a normal diet within 24 hours, except for one patient, who presented with an idiopathic ileus that lasted less than 3 days. Parenteral pain medication was given for the first 24 hours only. The hospital stay was 5 days or less in all cases and was less than 3 days in over 90% of cases. The length of stay directly correlated with the extent of surgery. Additional supportive measures consisted of sitz baths, stool softeners, and prophylactic antibiotics.

CONCLUSION

Laparoscopy is a useful technique that provides abdominal access to the pelvic floor, either as a primary mode of access or as a complement to vaginal surgery. In addition, it offers the surgeon the advantage of improved visualization. The increased taxation of the surgeon's skills is offset by the reduced morbidity for the patient.

REFERENCES

1. Nichols DH. Types of enterocele and principles underlying choice of operation for repair. Obstet Gynecol 1972;40:257–262.
2. Waters EG. Enterocele; cause, diagnosis and treatment. Clin Obstet Gynecol 1961;4:186–198.
3. Zacharin RF. Use of vaginal skin graft in posterior colporrhaphia. Aust N Z J Obstet Gynaecol 1992;32:146.
4. Vancaillie TG, Butler DJ. Laparoscopic enterocele repair—description of a new technique. Gynecol Endosc 1993;2:211–216.

20

Laparoscopic Vaginal Vault Suspension

C.Y. Liu

Genital procidentia is one of the most frustrating and embarrassing disorders confronting the modern woman, who, with increased life expectancy, is interested in maintaining her femininity and capacity for sexual activity. Massive eversion of the vagina (Fig 20.1) is a result of defective pelvic floor support and nearly always coexists with other pelvic floor defects. Therefore, vaginal vault suspension is just a part of the total reconstruction of the pelvic floor, which is necessary for restoration of the normal anatomy and function. This chapter will discuss the laparoscopic approach to complete vaginal eversion.

ANATOMY OF THE VAGINAL SUPPORT

The vagina, a fibromuscular tubular structure, extends from the vestibule to the cervix. In the resting state, the anterior and posterior walls of the vagina are in apposition to one another and appears as an H-shaped lumen, with the principal dimension being transverse. The anterior vaginal wall consists of the pubocervical fascia and vaginal mucosa, while the posterior wall of the vagina consists of the rectovaginal septum and

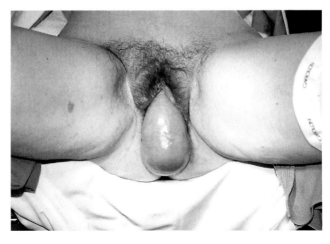

FIGURE **20.1**

Complete uterovaginal procidentia. Small area of mucosal erosion can be noted.

vaginal mucosa (Fig 18.1). Therefore, the vagina should be considered as a fibromuscular connective tissue tube with mucosal lining. The support of the vagina is to the pubocervical fascia and the rectovaginal septum, not to the vaginal mucosa. Although the vaginal mucosa can be stretched to an enormous degree, the fascial connective tissue cannot. In general, if the fascia is under stress, it cannot be stretched or attenuated much; it tends to break or tear in one or more isolated areas. Once there is a break or tear in the fascial layer, the mucosal lining stretches and prolapse occurs. The support mechanism of the vagina comes from two different systems: the striated muscles of the pelvic floor, with primarily the levator ani muscle providing the active support, and the endopelvic fascia, with its peripheral attachments providing the passive support. When a woman is standing, this supporting system maintains the upper two thirds of the vagina in a nearly horizontal position resting on the levator muscle. The supporting mechanism of the pelvic floor is discussed in detail in Chapter 16. Since the surgical repair of the prolapse of the vagina greatly depends on the strength of the endopelvic fascia, we will briefly review this passive supporting system of the vagina. The support of the upper one third of the vagina comes from the uterosacral

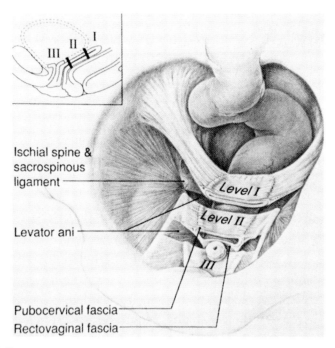

Ischial spine &
sacrospinous
ligament

Level I

Level II

Levator ani

III

Pubocervical fascia
Rectovaginal fascia

FIGURE 20.2

Level of support of the upper and mid vagina. In level 1 (suspension), the
endopelvic fascia suspend the vagina from the lateral pelvic walls. Fibers of level
1 extend both vertically and posteriorly toward the sacrum. In level 2 (attachment), the vagina is attached to the arcus tendineus fascia pelvis and the
superior fascia of the levator ani muscles. (Reproduced by permission from
DeLancey JOL. Anatomic causes of vaginal prolapse after hysterectomy. Am J
Obstet Gynecol 1992;166:1717–1728.)

and cardinal ligaments. The middle third of the vagina is held in place
by the lateral attachments of the pubocervical fascia to the arcus
tendineus fascia of the pelvis (white line) anteriorly, and the posterior
vaginal wall is supported by lateral attachment of the rectovaginal septum
to the fascia overlying the iliococcygeal muscle. In the lower third of the
vagina, the pubocervical fascia blends into the urogenital diaphragm and
the rectovaginal septum merges with the perineal body; laterally the
lower third of the vagina merges with the fascia overlying the medial
margins of the pubococcygeus (Fig 20.2).

SURGICAL CONSIDERATIONS OF VAGINAL VAULT SUSPENSION

Upper Third of the Vagina

For re-establishment of upper and middle third vaginal support, the laparoscopic approach provides the best evaluation of existing anatomic defects. There are several alternatives in repairing defects in the upper one third of vagina, as discussed below.

High McCall Vaginal Vault Suspension: High McCall vaginal vault suspension is simply re-attachment of the broken ends of the uterosacral ligaments to a reconstructed vaginal vault. Identification of the broken ends of the uterosacral ligaments can always be done laparoscopically by pushing the rectosigmoid colon cephalad toward the upper part of the abdomen. This offers the most physiologic resuspension of the vaginal vault.

Sacrospinosus Vaginal Vault Suspension: Sacrospinosus vaginal vault suspension attaches the upper and lateral margin of the rectovaginal fascia to the sacrospinosus ligament. The sacrospinosus ligament can be more easily identified laparoscopically than either abdominally or vaginally.

Sacral Colpopexy: The sacral colpopexy attaches the vaginal vault to the hollow of the sacrum with either autologous (e.g., fascia lata, rectus fascia, etc) or synthetic (e.g., Gortex strip, Mercilene or Marlex mesh) materials. The laparoscopic approach to sacral colpopexy is cumbersome and potentially risky. This procedure is discussed in more detail later in this chapter.

Middle Third of the Vagina

For repair of the middle third vaginal supporting defects, there are two structures to be considered: the pubocervical fascia and the rectovaginal septum. If the pubocervical fascia has separated from its lateral attachment to the arcus tendineus fascia, then paravaginal repair needs to be performed. If there is lateral detachment of the rectovaginal septum from the fascia overlying the iliococcygeus, then it should be reattached. The detachment of the rectovaginal septum from the pelvic side wall accounts for the majority of rectocele formations. The rectovaginal space can be opened laparoscopically and the rectum dissected away from the vagina. The rectovaginal septum and the defect can then be identified and repaired. In general, it is more difficult to reattach the rectovaginal septum to the pelvic side wall laparoscopically, especially when the location of the defect is low and close to the perineal body. The vaginal approach should be easier in this situation.

Lower Third of the Vagina

Defects in the lower third of the vagina include the detachment of the pubocervical fascia from the medial margin of the pubococcygeal muscle and the rectovaginal septum from the perineal body. The former can be repaired laparoscopically by reattaching the superior sulcus of the vagina to the medial margin of the pubococcygeal fascia with the most ventral stitches in the paravaginal repair. Defects between the rectovaginal septum and the perineal body should be done vaginally.

PREOPERATIVE EVALUATIONS

Preoperative work-up should include a detailed history and physical examination, with particular emphasis on neurologic history and current medications. Previous operative reports should be reviewed if obtainable. Pelvic examinations should include the evaluation of the motor and sensory dermatome of S_2, S_3, and S_4. All pelvic floor defects should be carefully assessed, and the presence and severity of various defects recorded on the patient's chart in detail to serve as a reminder during the intraoperative confirmation of each defect. Residual urine is obtained with a straight catheter and approximately 200 to 300 mL of warm sterile water is instilled into the bladder. Prolapses are reduced with the examiner's fingers, using special care to avoid compressing the base of the bladder. The status of the patient's stress urinary incontinence must be carefully evaluated. Urinalysis, urine culture, serum blood urea nitrogen, and creatinine should be obtained for all patients.

TECHNIQUE OF LAPAROSCOPIC VAGINAL VAULT SUSPENSION

For the following techniques of vaginal vault suspensions, the patient's position on the operating table and the trocar placement sites are the same as for laparoscopic retropubic colposuspension (Chapter 17) and paravaginal suspension (Chapter 18). For detailed description, readers should refer back to these chapters. In addition to the regular laparoscopic equipment, the rectal probe and vaginal manipulator, which is a wet 4×4 sponge on the tip of a sponge forceps (Fig 20.3), are two very important instruments used during laparoscopic vaginal vault suspensions.

Laparoscopic Sacrospinosus Ligament Suspension

Using video laparoscopy with a monitor, the operator places two fingers inside the vagina and palpates the right ischial spine and the sacrospinosus ligament (Fig 20.4). The locations of the right ischial spine and the sacrospinosus ligament are noted and marked through the laparoscope. A rectal probe is then placed into the rectum, and the

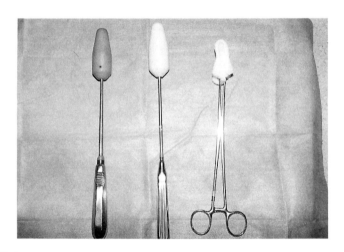

FIGURE 20.3

The rectal probe and vaginal probes (a 4×4 sponge on the tip of the sponge forceps) are two very important tools for pelvic floor reconstruction.

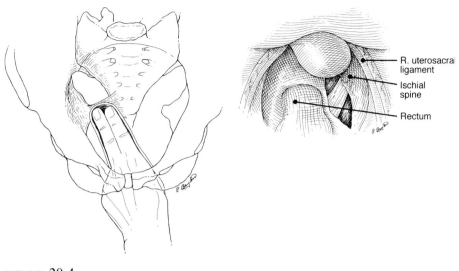

FIGURE 20.4

The operator places two fingers inside the vagina and palpates the ischial spine and sacrospinosus ligament while viewing through the laparoscope.

rectum is pushed toward the left side of pelvis. A longitudinal or transverse incision is made over the peritoneum covering the sacrospinosus ligament on the right side. The right pararectal space is entered, and the pararectal space is dissected toward sacrum. The sacrospinosus ligament can be easily identified and confirmed by placing the fingers back into the vagina and palpating the ischial spine and sacrospinosus ligament. The enterocele should be repaired and cul-de-sac obliterated prior to the vault suspension. A no. 2 Gortex suture (W.L. Gore), with a CV-2 needle is used to suture through the sacrospinosus ligament. The suture is placed at least 2 to 3 cm medially, away from the ischial spine and close to the sacrum to avoid injury to the pudendal nerve and vessels (Fig 20.5). A double bite is taken. The suture is then passed twice through the posterior wall of the vagina just below the tip of the vaginal vault, making sure the rectovaginal septum is included inside the suture while avoiding the vaginal mucosa, after which the suture is tied with the extracorporal knot-tying technique with a knot pusher. During the knot tying, the assistant places his or her fingers or a vaginal probe inside the vagina and pushes the tip of the

Laparoscopic Vaginal Vault Suspension   355

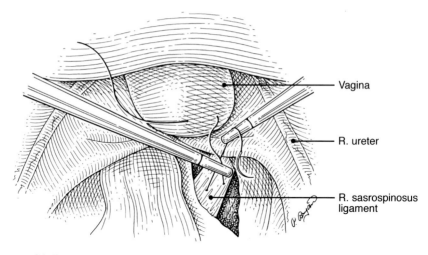

Vagina

R. ureter

R. sasrospinosus ligament

FIGURE 20.5

A permanent suture is placed through the sacrospinosus ligament away from the ischial spine. The strength of the suture should be tested by pulling on it forcefully to make sure that it is anchored deep into the sacrospinosus ligament.

vagina to the right sacrospinosus ligament. No gap should be left between the sacrospinosus ligament and the vagina (Plate 36).

Laparoscopic High McCall Vaginal Vault Suspension

During laparoscopic high McCall vaginal vault suspension the patient is placed in a 15 to 20-degree Trendelenburg's position. Both ureters must be identified and ideally dissected out from the pelvic brim all the way to the deep pelvis. The vaginal probe is inserted into the vagina, and the vagina is pushed toward the patient's head to facilitate the delineation of the enterocele, which is first repaired as described previously. The uterosacral ligaments on both sides are identified and are traced all the way to the presacral region. This can be accomplished even in an obese patient by pulling the sigmoid colon back toward the upper abdomen. With a gentle upward push of the vaginal probe toward the sacrum, the level of the presacral uterosacral ligaments to which the vaginal vault reaches is noted (Fig 20.6). The uterosacral ligament on the left side is then sutured through with no. 2 Gortex suture approximately 2 cm above the enterocele suture, and a second and third bite are taken

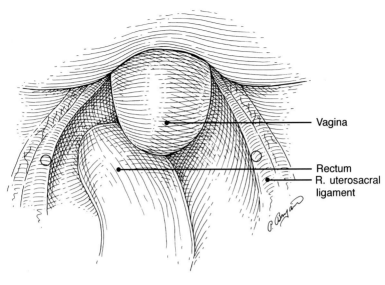

FIGURE 20.6

The vagina is pushed gently toward the sacrum. The level of the presacral uterosacral ligament to which the tip of the vaginal vault reaches is noted.

through the same structure with approximately 0.5 to 1.0 cm toward the cul-de-sac. The suture is then passed through the posterior wall of the vagina, making sure the rectovaginal septum is included but without going into the vaginal canal. With several bites on the posterior vaginal wall, the suture reaches to the right uterosacral ligament. Double or triple bites of the right uterosacral ligament are also taken. The suture is then passed through the peritoneum on both channels of the rectosigmoid colon and returned to the left uterosacral ligament, making a pursestring (Fig 20.7). The suture is then tied using the extracorporal knot-tying technique with a knot pusher. Care must be taken not to leave any peritoneal gap, which may result in a future enterocele formation. A second and third suture using the same suture material are placed in the same fashion through the uterosacral ligaments (Fig 20.8). The last suture should be placed through both sides of the uterosacral ligaments at the highest level reached by the tip of the vagina without undue tension placed on the vagina. This level frequently is right at the presacral region close to the origin of the uterosacral ligaments. The high

Laparoscopic Vaginal Vault Suspension   357

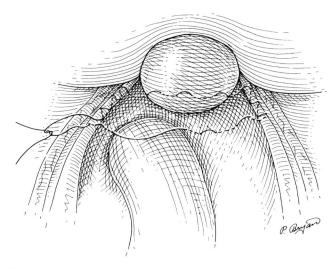

FIGURE 20.7

The first pursestring suture is placed approximately 2 to 3 cm above the enterocele suture. The suture includes both uterosacral ligaments, the rectovaginal septum, and the peritoneum of the channels on both sides of the rectosigmoid colon.

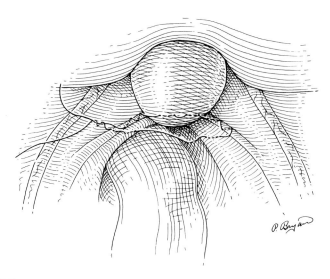

FIGURE 20.8

The second and third high McCall sutures are placed approximately 2 to 3 cm above the first suture.

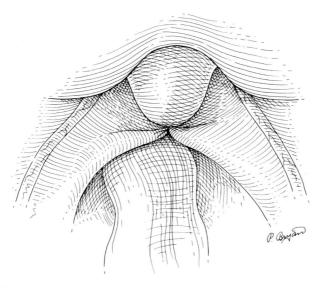

FIGURE 20.9

Laparoscopic view at the completion of high McCall vaginal vault suspension.

McCall vaginal vault suspension for complete vaginal eversion usually requires at least three or four pursestring sutures (Plate 37 and Fig 20.9). Both ureters need to be carefully monitored during the procedure. Special care also must be taken to avoid constricting the sigmoid colon with sutures.

Laparoscopic Sacral Colpopexy

Step 1. Preparation of the Vagina: The vaginal probe is placed inside the vagina and the vaginal vault lifted toward the patient's head. The peritoneum covering the vaginal tip is opened and stripped away until both the pubocervical fascia and the rectovaginal septum are identified. The bladder is dissected from the pubocervical fascia and the rectum is dissected away from the rectovaginal septum so that at least 3 to 4 cm of the vagina is exposed. If there is a gap between the pubocervical fascia and the rectovaginal septum, the pubocervical fascia and rectovaginal septum are sutured together in an anterioposterior fashion with a few interrupted sutures.

Step 2. Preparation of the Sacral Area: The sigmoid colon is pushed to the left side and the hollow of the sacrum just below the promontory is exposed. The peritoneum covering this area is opened longitudinally, curving slightly toward the right side to avoid the sigmoid colon. The incision is then extended toward the vagina. The presacral space is exposed and the longitudinal presacral ligaments are identified. The important anatomic landmarks, such as the right ureter and presacral vessels, need to be clearly identified.

Step 3. Preparation of the Graft Material: A 2.5 × 10 cm synthetic material, such as Mercilene or Gortex mesh is rolled up and introduced into the peritoneal cavity through any 10-mm trocar sleeve.

Step 4. Suturing of the Graft to the Posterior Vaginal Wall: Using permanent suture material, one end of the graft is sutured to the posterior wall of the vaginal vault. Taking adequate bites of the vaginal tissue while avoiding vaginal mucosa is important. At least three to five interrupted stitches should be placed to ensure adequate anchoring of the graft to the vagina.

Step 5. Suturing of the Graft to the Longitudinal Presacral Ligament: The vaginal probe is removed, and the grafting mesh is adjusted to hold the vagina in its horizontal position with the tip of the vagina point toward the hollow of the sacrum without undue tension. With the presacral vessels in full view, the other end of the graft is sutured to the longitudinal ligaments of the sacrum just below the promontory. Three to five sutures with permanent material are usually needed. Special care must be taken to avoid injuring the presacral vessels. Life-threatening hemorrhage can occur if these vessels are injured. A special stapling device, similar to an orthopedic thumb tag device, has been recently developed for laparoscopic use, which essentially eliminates the bleeding complication and shortens the procedure by placing the thumb tag–like staples to hold the graft to the sacrum. Unfortunately, to properly use this device, a perpendicular application of the device to the sacrum is required. Because of varying degrees of inclination of the human sacrum, it is not possible for this device to be used in every patient.

Step 6. Closure of the Peritoneum: The peritoneum is sutured over the graft from the sacrum toward the vagina. The graft should be buried under the peritoneum as much as possible to prevent dense adhesion formation.

DISCUSSION

Because patients with massive vaginal eversion usually have multiple pelvic floor defects, identification and repair of all pelvic floor defects during the initial surgery is crucial to prevent subsequent surgery, with its attendant surgical risk, pain, and expense. As stated previously, laparoscopic surgery provides unique advantages in identifying and confirming existing pelvic floor defects before the procedure begins as well as at the end of the surgery. Positive intra-abdominal pressure serves to help the surgeon to ensure that all defects have been repaired. This can be confirmed visually and by palpation.

DeLancey studied patients with posthysterectomy vaginal eversions and concluded that the upper third of the vagina is supported by vertical fibers of the paracolpium (see Suggested Readings, DeLancey, 1992). Support of the paracolpium in the midvagina is provided by attachment to the arcus tendineus of the pelvic side walls and the fascia of the levator ani muscle, and in the lower vagina by fusion to the perineal body and its muscular and fibrous attachments. Since the important support of the midportion of the vagina comes from the attachment of the vagina to the pelvic side walls, we believe that reattachment of the vagina to the pelvic side walls should be part of the repair for massive vaginal eversion. All our patients with massive eversions of the vagina also underwent paravaginal suspensions to ensure adequate support of the midvagina. Burch-type colposuspension also was performed on all our patients who exhibited stress urinary incontinence during the preoperative work-up after the prolapses were reduced. This preventive measure has reduced the incidence of postoperative stress urinary incontinence in our patients.

Laparoscopic sacropexy of the vaginal vault is technically more difficult. It involves a graft to the hollow of the sacrum below the promontory, which may result in life-threatening hemorrhage if the presacral vessels are injured when the graft is sutured to the anterior longitudinal ligaments of the bony sacral promontory. Infection and graft rejection also have been reported even years after surgery. Our preference is to perform either a high McCall type of vaginal suspension or sacrospinosus vaginal vault suspension.

The sacrospinosus ligament can be easily accessed through laparoscopy. The sacrospinosus ligament and the coccygeus muscle are basically the same structure, extending from the ischial spine on each side to the lower portion of the sacrum and coccyx, where it attaches to the sacrotuberous ligament. Laparoscopic suspension of the vaginal vault to the sacrospinosus ligament actually is one of the easiest parts of pelvic floor reconstructive surgery. Unlike vaginal sacrospinosus vault suspension, the right side rectal pillar does not have to be perforated before the sacrospinosus ligament can be identified. Laparoscopically, the right side sacrospinosus ligament can be identified easily after the covering peritoneum is opened and the subserous areola tissue is dissected. However, during suture placements, special care must be taken not to put the sutures too close to the ischial spine because of possible injury to the pudendal nerve and vessels. Using the rectal probe, the rectum must be pushed to the left side. The rectal probe should be placed inside the rectum all the time to aid in identification of the rectum during dissecting the subserous areola tissue around the sacrospinosus ligament and during the suture placement. However, patients with an anthropoid or android type of pelvis are not good candidates for sacrospinosus suspension due to the short distance between the sacrospinosus ligaments and the introitus. Sacrospinosus vaginal suspension in such patients would result in a shortened vagina. High McCall-type vaginal vault suspension is a preferable alternative for these patients. The advantages of the high McCall vaginal vault suspension include the following factors:

1. Safety. There is no danger of vessel or nerve injury with this procedure. However, constant surveillance of the ureters during the procedure and leaving at least two finger-breadth clearance

above the rectosigmoid colon to prevent constricting the colon with sutures must be done.

2. A more physiologic position of the vagina. This procedure retains the vagina in a midline and horizontal position, which is more physiologically correct compared with the sacrospinosus ligament suspension.

3. A satisfactory vaginal depth is maintained. This procedure provides the ability for the vagina to go high to the sacral region, where the uterosacral ligament originates.

CONCLUSION

Because multiple defects associated with vaginal vault eversion are the norm rather than the exception, it is important to repair of all pelvic floor defects concomitantly. Surgical goals for vaginal vault eversion include restoration of normal horizontal vaginal axis and depth, relief of symptoms of pressure, and maintenance of satisfactory sexual function. Regardless of the method of suspension used to suspend the upper vagina, reattachment of the middle vagina to the pelvic side walls should be an integral part of vaginal suspension. This will minimize the occurrence of cystoceles, a frequent sequelae of vaginal vault suspension. Study of the anatomy and physiology of the pelvic floor supporting system clearly indicates that the active and dynamic support for pelvic organs comes from the levator ani and other striated muscles of the pelvic floor. Unfortunately, we still do not have satisfactory ways to restore the levator function after they have been damaged. Current surgical practice for pelvic floor defects primarily relies on the strength of the endopelvic fascia and certain ligaments, which can only provide suspension and passive, instead of active, support of the pelvic organs. This clearly is not ideal for providing the kind of support needed to offset the dynamic nature of pelvic stress. Current advances and increased understanding of the neurophysiology, neuroanatomy and biophysics of the pelvic floor give us hope that the prevention and management of pelvic floor defects might be more rational and effective in the future.

SUGGESTED READINGS

Baden WF, Walker TA, Lindsey JH, et al. The vaginal profile. Tex Med 1968;64:56–58.

Cruikshank SH. Sacrospinous fixation—should this be performed at the time of vaginal hysterectomy? Am J Obstet Gynecol 1991;164:1072–1076.

DeLancey JOL. Anatomic causes of vaginal prolapse after hysterectomy. Am J Obstet Gynecol 1992;166:1717–1728.

DeLancey JOL, Richardson AC. Anatomy of genital support. In: Benson TJ, ed. Female pelvic floor disorders: investigation and management. New York: WW Norton, 1992:19–26.

Dunton JD, Mikuta J. Posthysterectomy vaginal vault prolapse. Postgrad Obstet Gynecol 1988;8:1–6.

Falk HC. Uterine prolapse and prolapse of the vaginal vault treated by sacropexy. Obstet Gynecol 1961;18:113–115.

Feldman GB, Birnbaum SJ. Sacral colpopexy for vaginal vault prolapse. Obstet Gynecol 1979;53:399–401.

McCall ML. Posterior culdeplasty: surgical correction of enterocele during vaginal hysterectomy; a preliminary report. Obstet Gynecol 1957;10:595–602.

McGuire EJ, Gardy M, Elkins T, DeLancey JOL. Treatment of incontinence with pelvic prolapse. Urol Clin North Am 1991;18:349–353.

Morley G, DeLancey JOL. Sacrospinous ligament fixation for eversion of the vagina. Am J Obstet Gynecol 1988;158:872–881.

Nagat I, Kato K. Sacrospinous ligament fixation of vaginal apex for repair operation of uterine prolapse—operative procedure and postoperative outcome evaluated with score system and x-ray subtration colpography. Acta Obstet Gynaecol Jpn 1986;38:29–38.

Nezhat CH, Nezhat F, Nezhat C. Laparoscopic sacral colpopexy for vaginal vault prolapse. Obstet Gynecol 1994;84:885–888.

Nichols DH. Sacrospinous fixation for massive eversion of the vagina. Am J Obstet Gynecol 1982;142:901–904.

Nichols DH. Surgery for pelvic floor disorders. Surg Clin North Am 1991;71:927–946.

Nichols DH, Milley PS, Randall CL. Significance of restoration of normal vaginal depth and axis. Obstet Gynecol 1970;36:241–246.

Nichols DH, Randall CL. Vaginal surgery. 2nd ed. Baltimore: Williams & Wilkins, 1989:284–303.

Parsons L, Ulfelder H. An atlas of pelvic operations. 2nd ed. Philadelphia: WB Saunders, 1968:280–283.

Richter K, Albrich W. Long term results following fixation of the vagina on the sacrospinal ligament by the vaginal route (vaginaefixatio sacrospinalis vaginalis). Am J Obstet Gynecol 1981;141:811–816.

Shull BL. Clinical evaluation of women with pelvic support defects. Clin Obstet Gynecol 1993;36:939–951.

Shull BL, Capen CV, Riggs MW, Kuehl TJ. Preoperative and postoperative analysis of site-specific pelvic support defects in 81 women treated with sacrospinous ligament suspension and pelvic reconstruction. Am J Obstet Gynecol 1992;166:1764–1771.

Shull BL, Capen CV, Riggs MW, Kuehl TJ. Bilateral attachment of the vaginal cuff to iliococcygeus fascia: an effective method of cuff suspension. Am J Obstet Gynecol 1993;168:1669–1674.

Smith ARB, Hosker GL, Warrell DW. The role of partial denervation of the pelvic floor in the etiology of genitourinary prolapse and stress incontinence of urine: a neurophysiological study. Br J Obstet Gynecol 1989; 96:24–28.

Symmond RE, Pratt JH. Vaginal prolapse following hysterectomy. Am J Obstet Gynecol 1960;79:899–909.

Symmonds RE, Williams TJ, Lee RA, Webb MJ. Posthysterectomy enterocele and vaginal vault prolapse. Am J Obstet Gynecol 1981;140:852–859.

Timmons MC, Addison WA, Addison SB, Cavenar MG. Abdominal sacral colpopexy in 163 women with posthysterectomy vaginal vault prolapse and enterocele. J Reprod Med 1992;37:323–327.

Vancaillie TG, Butler DJ. Laparoscopic enterocele repair—description of a new technique. Gynecol Endoscopy 1993;2:211–216.

Wiskind AK, Creighton SM, Stanton SL. The incidence of genital prolapse after the Burch colposuspension. Am J Obstet Gynecol 1992;167:399–405.

Index

Bladder (*cont.*)
laparoscopic injuries to, 190, 281–282
management of, 283–284
prevention of, 282–283
mobilization of, 245
medial, 335
off cervix, 234
overdistention of, 100
reflection of, 176–179
retraining of, 323
retropubic coloposuspension injury of, 322
support for, 330–331
surgical penetration of, 334
Bladder flap, 243–245
Bladder neck support, loss of, 299–300
Bladder pillar, 178f
Blend waveforms, 53–55
Blood
loss in supracervical hysterectomy *vs.* LAVH, 250–251
volume, 90–91
Blood vessel(s). *See also specific vessels*
laparoscopic injury of, 278–281
pelvic, 15–16
perforation of, 162
Bovie, William T., 48
Bowel. *See also* Colon; Small intestine
disorders of, 86
laparoscopic injuries to, 190–191, 287–291
perforation of, 162
postoperative function of, 98
preoperative preparation of, 95–96
surgery, for endometriosis, 201–202
Breast cancer, 263
Broad ligament, 15, 129
incision of, 156, 158
opening in, 247f
Burch procedure, 316–327

Burch stitch, 336
Burn
alternate site, 60
with electrode insulation failure, 62–63
with electrosurgical current, 60

Camera
equipment, 37–42
resolution of, 40
Cancer
breast, 263
cervical, 240
screening tests for, 86
Capacitive coupling, 63–64
Carbon dioxide, 83–84
Carboperitoneum, 205
Carcinoma
cervical, 257
endometrial, 257
FIGO staging of, 262
laparoscopic management of, 258f, 259f
ovarian, 257
laparoscopy for, 264–265
uterine, 256–257
Cardinal ligament, 303f
suturing of, 182f
Cardinouterosacral ligaments, 303
Cardiopulmonary disease, 85
Cardiovascular collapse, postoperative, 101
Cardiovascular disorders, postoperative, 100–101
Catheterization
unexplained hematuria during, 282
ureteral perforation with, 284–285
Cervical fibroid, 135
Cervix, 15
cancer of, 240
carcinoma of, 257

Intra-abdominal pressure, increased, 302
  during laparoscopy, 326
Irrigation/suction control system, 153

Kalk, H., 107
Kelly, Howard, 313
Kleppinger-type forceps, 34
Knot pusher, 38f
  for LAVH, 153
Knot tying
  extracorporal, 321
  instruments for, 37

Laboratory assessment, preoperative, 90–92
Laparoscopic dissection, lateral pelvic spaces, 22–27
Laparoscopic en bloc resection, 211–213
Laparoscopic hysterectomy. *See also* Vaginal hysterectomy, laparoscopic-assisted
  benefit of, 80
  classification of, 170–171
  complications of, 4, 80, 277–295
    rates of, 277–278
  consumer interest in, 4
  contraindications for, 171
  cost of, 7–8, 191
  definition of, 170
  economics of, 42–44
  efforts to discredit, 6
  for extensive endometriosis 194–223
  first in U.S., 277
  first presentation of, 3
  future of, 8–9
  goal of, 227
  in gynecological surgery, 3–9

instruments for, 172
for large myomatous uterus, 227–237
laser applications for, 76–79
morbidity of, 82
operating equipment for, 32–37
operating room setup for, 28–31
operative environment for, 5
pathologies in, 187t
postoperative care in, 80, 96–101
preoperative care in, 80, 81–96
procedures concomitant with, 188t
randomized control trials for, 6–7
reducing risk in, 4–5
supracervical, 149, 238–253
techniques of, 8
times for, 222–223
ureteral protection in, 5
versus vaginal hysterectomy, 5–6
video and camera equipment for, 37–42
Laparoscopic landmarks, retroperitoneal, 24
Laparoscopic techniques
  in difficult cases, 115–122
  history of, 106–107
  in ureteral dissection, 133–140
Laparoscopy
  early textbook on, 107
  electrical energy in, 61–66
  electrosurgical energy in, 47–48
  initiation in endometriosis surgery, 204–205
  open, 114, 117
  in patient with previous surgery, 117–118
  as risk factor, 83–84
  tumor dissemination during, 265–266
Laparotomy, costs of, 7
Large intestine. *See* Colon

378   Index